Soluble Factors Mediating Innate Immune Responses to HIV Infection

Edited by

Massimo Alfano
AIDS Immunopathogenesis Unit,
Department of Immunology,
Transplantation and Infectious
Diseases,
San Raffaele Scientific Institute,
20132 Milan,
Italy

Soluble Factors Mediating Innate
Immune Responses to HIV Infection

Editor: Massimo Alfano

eISBN: 978-1-60805-006-2

ISBN: 978-1-60805-580-7

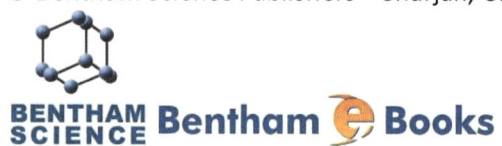

BENTHAM SCIENCE Bentham e Books

CONTENTS

FOREWORD

Human Immunodeficiency Virus (HIV) and AIDS pathogenesis have been under investigation for almost three decades. Substantial scientific and medical data have been collected on the structure of the virus and its replication cycle in infected cells. In addition, our understanding of the pathogenesis of HIV infection has greatly improved: It depends on virus-induced immune suppression as well as the formation of cellular virion reservoirs. The role of non-viral factors in AIDS pathogenesis was first identified 20 years ago with the description of soluble factors, the cytokines, which modulate HIV-1 replication in infected cells. Since then, more soluble factors have been discovered, capable of either stimulating or inhibiting HIV replication. Two critical anti-viral arms of HIV-specific CD8+ T cells (cytolytic and non-cytolytic) were shown to play a significant role in HIV prevention, and were associated with asymptomatic survival and slower disease progression. The activity of cytokines and their role in modulating HIV infection have been investigated *in vitro* and *in vivo*, both in animal models and human tissues such as gut and lymphoid tissue. Moreover, modalities of using cytokines as immunotherapy, either alone or in combination with anti-retrovirals, have been described. Leukocytes and epithelial cells produce defensins, which are innate effectors and immunomodulators during HIV infection, taking a variety of actions against microorganisms. They also act as immunomodulators involved in inflammation, tissue repair, and angiogenesis. Other soluble factors, such as the high mobility group box 1 (HMGB1) protein and urokinase plasminogen activator and its receptor (uPA/uPAR system), have a critical task between innate and adaptative immunity, and may possibly interfere with HIV-1 infection. Alpha 1-antitrypsin levels, which are deficient in HIV-1 disease, and rate-limiting for CD4+ T lymphocytes, could be a therapeutic target. Research for a better understanding of the role of vitamin D during HIV infection and disease progression to AIDS is ongoing. The complement system, a prominent component of the innate immunity, is likely to aid in the control of HIV replication, although the virus has developed escape mechanisms to avoid complement-mediated destruction.

Among the cells of the innate immune system, macrophages, NK cells, and dendritic cells (DC) have been shown to be actively involved in the defence against HIV infection. Many cellular and environmental factors influence viral replication in cells of the innate immune system. These factors include: status of cellular activation, macrophage or DC/T cell interaction, cytokines and chemokines, immune complexes, and opportunistic pathogens. The effects of soluble factors and the innate immune cells on HIV pathogenesis also depend on the localization of the immune cells. Regarding viral replication, cellular activation status, and expression of chemokine receptors on the cell surface, macrophages do not behave in the same manner as viral reservoirs in lymph nodes, intestinal tissue, lung, and central nervous system. Therefore, in addition to the adaptative immune system, a complex network of soluble factors and innate immune cells appears to be a critical component in disease development. A better understanding of the pivotal role played by soluble factors in mediating innate immune responses to HIV infection should ultimately enable the development of new antiretroviral treatments. These treatments would make it possible to target not only the virus but also to modify its cellular environment, leading to a more complete control of HIV replication.

The present book strategically places the soluble factors and innate immune cells at the forefront of AIDS pathogenesis. Reading this book is essential to the understanding of the future development of therapeutic approaches for HIV infection.

Georges Herbein,
University of Franche-Comté
Besançon
France

PREFACE

The Human Immunodeficiency Virus (HIV) infection represents one of the biggest challenges faced by the scientific community in recent years. HIV was discovered in the early '80s and has caused one of the most dramatic epidemics (known as the Acquired ImmunoDeficiency Syndrome, AIDS) of the last (and current) century. Very extensive knowledge has been accumulated on the virus as well as on the deleterious effect of viral proteins for the host, leading to efficient therapies controlling viral replication. However, in the face of the great advances in antiretroviral therapy scientists and physicians still do not have effective countermeasures for preventing infection with microbicides or vaccines and for eradicating the infection in those who have already acquired HIV, while the selection of drug-resistant strains, as well as side-effects, represent frequent problems for those under antiretroviral regimens.

The earliest defense against microbial infections is represented by the responses of the innate immune system that is finely tuned by different cellular types and several soluble factors. Related to HIV infection, soluble molecules of the innate immune system target multiple steps in the virus life cycle, sometimes in favor of the host and sometimes of the virus, for example for cytokines and the complement system. On the other hand, it has been clearly demonstrated that the potency of early immune responses profoundly regulates the levels of HIV replication and spreading and, overall, the speed of disease progression towards AIDS. Findings obtained with clinical trials based on α_1-antitrypsin or IL-2 therapy in HIV individuals have clearly shown that strategies aimed at the manipulation of the immune system responses are feasible ways to enhance the control of virus replication, for example by boosting the ability of CD8+ T cells to release soluble, non-lytic anti-viral factors (CAF). Therefore, better characterization of the interactions between soluble factors mediating innate immune system responses and HIV might lead to the design of immunological compounds boosting the innate immune system against HIV. Most of these soluble mediators owing to anti-viral activity are independent of co-receptor usage, drug-resistance mutations, thus widening their therapeutic window in all stages of disease. In addition, a better comprehension of anti-viral activities delivered by innate immune response might turn fundamental for the design of anti-HIV vaccines.

Common denominator of all chapters described in this e-book is the mutual interaction between innate immunity and HIV infection, a topic that has been investigated from the late '80s. Different authors describe different soluble factors responsible for the regulation of HIV infection and replication in various cell types and model systems of infection.

Therefore, this e-book provides a very detailed description about the role of innate immune responses regulating HIV replication according to the studies of several international experts. I do hope that this book will be a key reference text for a wide range of scientists, such as graduate students, for which it represents a good starting point, as well as for investigators in general, for whom it may represent a collection of the state of the art of 20 years of HIV research.

Massimo Alfano
AIDS Immunopathogenesis Unit
Department of Immunology
Transplantation and Infectious Diseases
San Raffaele Scientific Institute
20132 Milan
Italy

CONTRIBUTORS

Massimo Alfano, Ph.D.
AIDS Immunopathogenesis Unit, Department of Immunology, Transplantation and Infectious Diseases, San Raffaele Scientific Institute, 20132 Milan, Italy.

Zoltàn Banki, Ph.D.
Department of Hygiene and Medical Microbiology, Innsbruck Medical University, A-6020 Innsbruck, Austria.

Chloe Borde, Ph.D.
Centre de Recherche des Cordeliers, Universitè Pierre et Marie Curie, Paris, F-75006 France; Université Paris Descartes, Paris, F-75006 France ; INSERM Paris, F-75006 France.

Cynthia L. Bristow, Ph.D.
Institute for Human Genetics and Biochemistry, Laboratory for AIDS Virus Research, Department of Medicine, Weill Medical College of Cornell University, New York, NY 10065, USA.

Antonio Caruz, Ph.D.
Immunogenetics Unit, Faculty of Sciences, Universidad de Jaén, Pasaje Las Lagunillas s/n 23071-Jaén, Spain.

Theresa L. Chang, Ph.D.
Department of Medicine, Division of Infectious Diseases, Mount Sinai School of Medicine, Box 1090, One Gustave L. Levy Place, New York, NY, 10029, USA.

Jose Cortes, M.D.
Beth Israel Medical Center, New York, NY 10003, USA.

Jesper Eugen-Olsen, Ph.D.
Clinical Research Centre 136, Copenhagen University Hospital Hvidovre Hospital, 2650 Hvidovre Denmark.

Joan Fibla, Ph.D.
Human Genetics Unit, Departament de Ciències Mèdiques Bàsiques, Universitat de Lleida and Institut de Recerca Biomèdica de Lleida, 25199 LLEIDA, Catalunya, Spain.

Aaron Franklin, B.S.
University of Toledo College of Medicine, Toledo, OH 43614, USA.

Joel Gozlan, M.D., Ph.D,
Laboratoire de Virologie, Hôpital Saint-Antoine, Paris, F-75012 France; Centre de Recherche des Cordeliers, Université Pierre et Marie Curie, Paris, F-75006 France; Universitè Paris Descartes, Paris, F-75006 France; INSERM Paris, F-75006 France.

Eva Haastrup, M.D.
Department of Clinical Immunology, Copenhagen University Hospital, Rigshospitalet, Copenhagen, Denmark.

Mary E. Klotman, Ph.D.
Department of Medicine, Division of Infectious Diseases, Mount Sinai School of Medicine, Box 1090, One Gustave L. Levy Place, New York, NY, 10029, USA.

Anne Langkilde, M.Sc.
Clinical Research Centre 136, Copenhagen University Hospital Hvidovre Hospital, 2650 Hvidovre, Denmark.

Katherine Lau, Ph.D.
Retroviral Genetics Division Center for Virus Research, Westmead Millennium Institute, Westmead Hospital, Westmead NSW 2145, Sydney, Australia.

Vincent Marechal, Ph.D.
Centre de Recherche des Cordeliers, Universitè Pierre et Marie Curie, Paris, F-75006 France; Université Paris Descartes, Paris, F-75006 France; INSERM Paris, F-75006 France.

Roya Mukhtarzad, M.D.
Kingsbrook Jewish Medical Center, Brooklyn, New York, NY 11203, USA.

Sisse Rye Ostrowski, M.D., Ph.D.
Department of Clinical Immunology, Copenhagen University Hospital, Rigshospitalet, Copenhagen, Denmark.

Guido Poli, M.D.
Vita-Salute San Raffaele University School of Medicine, San Raffaele Scientific Institute, 20132 Milan, Italy; AIDS Immunopathogenesis Unit, Department of Immunology, Transplantation and Infectious Diseases San Raffaele Scientific Institute, 20132 Milan, Italy.

Val Romberg, Ph.D.
CSL Behring, Bern, CH3000, Switzerland.

Nitin K. Saksena, Ph.D.
Retroviral Genetics Division Center for Virus Research, Westmead Millennium Institute, Westmead Hospital, Westmead NSW 2145, Sydney, Australia.

Maly Soedjono, Ph.D.
Retroviral Genetics Division Center for Virus Research, Westmead Millennium Institute, Westmead Hospital, Westmead NSW 2145, Sydney, Australia.

Heribert Stoiber, Ph.D.
Department of Hygiene and Medical Microbiology, Innsbruck Medical University, A-6020 Innsbruck, Austria.

Maylis Trucy, Ph.D.
Institute for Human Genetics and Biochemistry, Laboratory for AIDS Virus Research, Department of Medicine, Weill Medical College of Cornell University, New York, NY 10065, USA.

Henrik Ullum, M.D., Ph.D.
Department of Clinical Immunology, Copenhagen University Hospital, Rigshospitalet, Copenhagen, Denmark.

Bin Wang, Ph.D.
Retroviral Genetics Division Center for Virus Research, Westmead Millennium Institute, Westmead Hospital, Westmead NSW 2145, Sydney, Australia.

Doris Wilflingseder, Ph.D.
Department of Hygiene and Medical Microbiology, Innsbruck Medical University, A-6020 Innsbruck, Austria.

Ronald Winston, B.S.
Institute for Human Genetics and Biochemistry, Laboratory for AIDS Virus Research, Department of Medicine, Weill Medical College of Cornell University, New York, NY 10065, USA.

Jing Qin Wu, Ph.D.
Retroviral Genetics Division Center for Virus Research, Westmead Millennium Institute, Westmead Hospital, Westmead NSW 2145, Sydney, Australia.

Li Zou, Ph.D.
Retroviral Genetics Division Center for Virus Research, Westmead Millennium Institute, Westmead Hospital, Westmead NSW 2145, Sydney, Australia.

CHAPTER 1

CD8 Antiviral Soluble Factors and Human Immunodeficiency Virus (HIV) Control

Nitin K. Saksena*, Jing Qin Wu, Katherine Lau, Li Zhou, Maly Soedjono and Bin Wang

Retroviral Genetics Division, Center for Virus Research, Westmead Millennium Institute, The University of Sydney, Westmead NSW 2145.

Abstract: CD8 antiviral activity is a subject of intense studies. Two very critical anti-viral arms of HIV-specific CD8+ T cells (cytolytic and non-cytolytic) have been shown to play a significant role in protection against HIV and appear to associate with asymptomatic survival and slower disease progression. The cytotoxic CD8+ T cells (CTL) recognize and eliminate HIV-infected cells displaying MHC class-I proteins. Along with recognition and elimination of HIV-infected cells, CD8+ T cells potentially influence various stages in HIV life cycle. For instance the chemokines produced by CD8+ T cells block the entry of the virus into T cells and macrophages. The activated CD8+ T cells also produce soluble factors that act at the transcriptional level. In contrast, the non-cytolytic CD8+T cells from HIV+ individuals suppress virus replication in CD4+ T cells *in vitro*, involving interplay of soluble factors such as chemokines and other antiviral factors such as unidentified soluble CD8 Antiviral Factor (CAF), urokinase-type plasminogen activator (uPA) and antiviral membrane-bound factor. In light of these factors, it is clear that the cell-mediated immune responses are critical in controlling HIV replication *in vivo*. Although the constituents of antiviral activity of CD8+ T cells remain largely elusive, the restoration of this activity during Highly Active Antiretroviral Therapy (HAART) and IL-2 treatment confers significant improvement in antiviral activity. The aim of this chapter is to provide a comprehensive and unbiased snapshot of antiviral potential of these cells and mechanisms involved in conferring this protective activity in HIV+ individuals and its overall relevance in HIV disease.

INTRODUCTION

The CD8 T-cells act against HIV strains in two principal ways during primary infection by: 1. killing HIV-infected cells and 2. secreting soluble factors, such as chemokines and other unknown factors, which suppress viral replication. HIV-specific CD8 T-cells have the ability to recognize specific HIV sequences, which is copied and primes the CD8+ T cells to save the host against future encounters with similar strains. Although soluble non-cytolytic activity mediated by soluble factors is potent in inhibiting HIV without MHC restriction, it also described that this function can be carried out by the CTLs as well, which upon CD3 stimulation can produce soluble factors that impinge on viral replication in MHC-mismatched target infected cells. The cell supernatant from activated CTLs is also highly effective in viral suppression *in vitro*. In general the inhibition with active supernatant is less efficient than the cell-to-cell-contact between CTL and the target cell. Thus, overall it appears that the release of soluble factor is incumbent upon cellular activation. Even though the soluble factor release by CTLs is highly antigen-specific and MHC-restricted, the soluble factors can achieve this without MHC-restriction.

The significance of CD8+ T cells and the antiviral and/or soluble factors secreted by HIV-specific CD8+ T cells in HIV immunobiology is indisputable. HIV-infected individuals mount a powerful cytotoxic T-cell-mediated immune response against specific HIV epitopes, which confers protection to the host against disease progression. As the CD4+ T cells are the target cells for HIV, greater attention has been paid to the role of CD4+ T lymphocytes in HIV pathogenesis. Even though HIV is capable of infecting diverse blood leukocytes, yet the importance of CD8+ T cells, particularly in relation to HIV infection remains underestimated. Their sheer numbers and high level of activation during HIV infection provides the strongest support in favor of their key role in progressive and non-progressive HIV disease, reviewed in [1].

*Address Correspondence to this author Dr. Nitin K. Saksena at: Retroviral Genetics Division, Center for Virus Research, Westmead Millennium Institute, Westmead Hospital, Darcy Road, Westmead NSW 2145. Sydney. Australia. Phone: (+612) 9845 9119. Fax: (+612) 9845 9103. E-mail: nitin_saksena@wmi.usyd.edu.au.

The CD8+ T lymphocytes from HIV-1-seropositive individuals are also known to inhibit HIV-1 replication in CD4+ T lymphocytes *in vitro*. These CD8+ T lymphocytes from HIV+ individuals are 'primed' against HIV-1 antigens, conferring partial HIV-specific resistance during infection through the secretion of HIV-specific soluble factors. Previously, in support of this [2, 3] it has been shown that the stripping of CD8+ lymphocytes derived from the whole PBMC fraction obtained from HIV-1-seronegative individuals can also result in a significant increase of HIV-1 replication in the remaining fraction, supporting their significant and definitive role in the immunologic defense against HIV. The CD8+ lymphocytes control viral replication either by direct antigen-specific cytolysis or through the secretion of soluble antiviral factors, which are highly HIV-specific or in other cases specific to the infectious agent. Thus, the cytotoxic and non-cytotoxic arms of the CD8+ T cells play a significant role in controlling HIV. Although the CD8 antiviral activity has been very well characterized and remains an intense subject of study in the field of innate and adaptive immunity, yet the biochemical components of this potent antiviral activity remain undefined, to date. As a consequence, the identity of CAF has remained elusive. The antiviral or non-cytolytic activity of CD8+T cells has been referred to with different terminologies, such as CNAR (CD8+ cell non-cytotoxic anti-HIV response) or CASA (CD8+ anti-HIV suppressor activity) (CASA is synonymous to CNAR), with CAF (CD8+ antiviral Factor) being the most commonly used terminology for this unidentified group of anti-HIV soluble factor(s). CAF secreted by CD8+ T cells in culture supernatants confers a potent anti-HIV activity against primary CD4+ T cells infected with a variety of beta chemokine insensitive HIV-1 strains *in vitro*.

In contrast, the antigen-specific cytotoxic T-lymphocytes (CTL) mediate direct killing of virus-infected cells through a cytolytic mechanism.

This review, in the subsequent sections, makes an attempt to discuss several mechanisms and hypotheses in regards to CD8 antiviral factors at various stages of HIV disease, and provide comprehensive discussion highlighting the relevance of interactions between CD8+T cells and in innate and adaptive immunity.

HIV INFECTION OF THE CD8+ T CELLS: CONTROVERSY AND CLARIFICATION

HIV is able to infect diverse blood leukocytes, but controversy has persisted regarding the infection of CD8+ T cells for quite sometime. Recent work has shown that HIV is capable of productively infecting CD8+ T cells. All initial descriptions of CD8[+] T cells came from *in vitro* experiments [4-7], which were followed by evidence that CD8[+] T cells can harbour and express HIV-1 *in vivo* [8, 9], and may also express small amounts of CD4 RNA [10]. It has since been confirmed that CD8[+] T cells harbor considerable amounts of HIV provirus [8, 11], suggesting their susceptibility to HIV.

So far, the HIV infection of CD8[+] T cells has mainly focused on the mechanism of viral entry, and the origins of CD8[+] cell infection [1]. It is believed that the CD8[+] T cells become infected through a conventional CD4-dependent mechanism during their maturation in the thymus. The most plausible explanation could be the infection at the double-positive (DP) stage, where CD4 is co-expressed on the CD8 cell surface. Implants of human thymic tissue containing infected DP thymocytes in SCID mice have been shown to produce infected single positive (SP) CD8[+] T lymphocytes in the peripheral circulation [12, 13]. HIV-1 proviral DNA is also preferentially distributed in the naïve (CD45RA[+]) subset of CD8[+] T cells, further supporting the thymus as a source of CD8[+] T cell infection [14].

In addition to possible intrathymic mechanisms, stimulation of highly purified CD8[+] T cells with mitogens, allogeneic dendritic cells or anti-CD3 and anti-CD28 antibodies *in vitro* leads to *de novo* synthesis of CD4 and susceptibility to HIV-1 infection [14, 15]. Activated subsets of circulating CD8[+] T lymphocytes express high frequencies of CD4 *in vivo*, rendering these cells vulnerable to virus-mediated destruction [9, 16-18]. Reports of CD8[+] T cell-mediated, CD4 independent entry into CD8[+] T cells have also been provided by Saha and colleagues, who showed specifically the role of CXCR4 in CD8+ T cell infection by a peculiar CD8-tropic HIV isolate. Multiple CD8[+] clones generated from patients with AIDS were characterized and it was found that several singly positive CD8 were endogenously infected by HIV [19]. Subsequent biological characterization of these isolates demonstrated CD8-mediated cell entry without the requirement for any known chemokine co-receptor [19]. Recent work by this group has led to the further characterization of CD4-

independent entry of HIV-1 in CD8+ T cells [20].

In addition to clarification of CD8$^+$ T cell entry mechanisms, several studies have focused on quantitative aspects of CD8$^+$ T cell infection by HIV. Several reports have sought to compare the abundance of HIV provirus in CD8$^+$ T cells with those of other leukocytes. These reports have concluded that CD8$^+$ T cells harbor substantial amounts of provirus. Livingstone and colleagues found that in late stage disease, infection in CD8$^+$ T cells accounted for between 66% and 97% of total proviral DNA, and observed a strong inverse relationship between CD8$^+$ T cell count and the frequency of CD8$^+$ T cell infection [8]. Similarly, more recent reports have further confirmed that CD8$^+$ T cells do contain significant amounts of provirus [21]. Additional studies have also attempted to clarify the distribution of proviral DNA in specific CD8$^+$ T cell subsets. One report demonstrated a preferential distribution of HIV in the naive (CD45RA$^+$) subset of CD8$^+$ T cells compared to the memory/effector (CD45RO$^+$) population. In contrast to all previous findings, it has been suggested that naïve and memory CD8$^+$ T cells are rarely infected by HIV [22].

There is debate over whether the infection of CD8$^+$ T cells contributes significantly to the immunodeficiency observed in AIDS. This stems from the existence of a number of other possible mechanisms that could account for the numerical decline and functional impairment of CD8$^+$ T cells observed on disease progression. These include increased susceptibility to apoptosis from alterations in the cytokine milieu in lymphoid tissue, bystander effects from neighbouring productively infected CD4$^+$ T cells, or toxicity from the release of HIV derived proteins such as gp120 or Tat [23, 24]. Loss of CD4$^+$ T cell helper function leading to impaired clonal expansion and function of CD8$^+$ T lymphocytes on antigenic pressure also contributes [25]. Thymic destruction of precursor CD8+ T cells has been proposed as an explanation for the eventual failure of CD8+ T cell homeostasis, the decline in circulating numbers of first naïve and then memory CD8$^+$ T cells upon disease progression [26], and the recovery in naïve CD8$^+$ T cell numbers on commencement of antiretroviral therapy [27].

Viral Evolutionary Processes in HIV-Infected CD8+ T cells

Previous analyses have shown the compartmentalization of HIV in CD4$^+$ T cells, CD8$^+$ T cells and monocytes in patients receiving HAART [28-30]. To investigate whether this compartmentalization impacts significantly at the functional level during therapy, Potter *et al.* [28], conducted a detailed phylogenetic and evolutionary analysis of viral populations derived from multiple blood leukocytes. Mutations in the protease (PR) and reverse transcriptase (RT) genes from the virus in each compartment were analyzed to identify cellular reservoirs of HIV-1 drug resistance, and to clarify the trafficking of viral strains between cell-free and cell-associated compartments. Their analyses revealed that HIV populations from individual blood cell compartments were in many cases genetically distinct. This was evident in most patients, particularly those who displayed cellular compartmentalization of drug resistance mutations. Most notably, virus isolated from CD8$^+$ T cells was phylogenetically distinct in a number of subjects, and branched separately from other blood cell types. In addition, they also demonstrated reduction in HIV drug resistant HIV strains uniquely in CD8 compartment. Interestingly, in some patients, the PCR amplification of virus from CD8$^+$ T cells and monocytes was unsuccessful despite repeated attempts. This phenomenon was unique to patients who showed low to undetectable plasma viremia with moderate to high CD4$^+$ and CD8$^+$ T cell counts. This suggests that the infection of CD8$^+$ T cells and monocytes may be less prominent during low plasma viremia phase and elevated T cell counts. There appears to be some correlation between compartmentalization of HIV variants with lower levels of drug resistance in CD8$^+$ T cells and the contribution of this compartment to plasma virus. It was also interesting to note that in patients with extremely low CD4$^+$ T cell counts, CD8$^+$ T cells and monocytes were more closely related to the plasma population than HIV clones from CD4$^+$ T cells. This suggested that additional leukocyte reservoirs might play a more significant role in the absence of viable numbers of CD4$^+$ T cells. Overall, the data of Potter *et al.* [29, 30] has demonstrated that in most cases HIV variants isolated from CD8$^+$ T cells and monocytes are often genetically distinct from those found in CD4$^+$ T cells and other cellular compartments.

At present, there is no clear explanation for the notable absence of drug resistance mutations in virus derived from CD8$^+$ T cells observed in some HIV patients receiving HAART. One possibility is that antiretroviral drugs were less efficient in targeting CD8$^+$ T cell compartment in some individuals leading to a decrease in the selective pressure for the development of drug resistant variants. However, if this were the case, it would also be likely that drug resistant viral strains could arise due to replication in suboptimal drug concentrations. An alternative explanation could be that drug resistant strains were not tropic for CD8$^+$ T cell entry. It is also conceivable that these strains represent 'archival species' established in memory CD8$^+$ T cell subsets soon after primary seroconversion. Several studies have demonstrated that latently infected memory CD4$^+$ T cell reservoirs are established soon after infection [31] and can be activated by pro-inflammatory cytokines *in vitro* and potentially *in vivo* [32]. Viral strains derived from latent memory CD4$^+$ T cells have been shown to contain few antiretroviral drug resistance mutations compared to the predominant viral population suggesting the absence of ongoing replication [33, 34]. The marked absence of drug resistance mutations in the CD8$^+$ T cell viral population of a number subjects was also indicative of reduced HIV turnover and evolution. This raises the possibility that wild type HIV variants isolated from the CD8$^+$ compartment of these patients may derive from memory CD8$^+$ T cell subsets. However, this was not confirmed in the study by [28], as the individual contribution of the memory CD8$^+$ T cell subset was not assessed. Other factors that are likely to contribute to the lack of HIV drug resistance in CD8$^+$ T cells include tissue distribution, persistence and/or slower HIV replication. CD8$^+$ T cell infection appeared to be productive in a number of other patients further complicating this issue. Nonetheless, these findings on the infection of total CD8$^+$ T cell populations are of significant biological relevance to the clinical management of HIV patients. The protection of CD8$^+$ T cells from HIV-1 infection during HAART should lead to better T-cell responses and is crucial for long lasting CD8-mediated antiviral activity and natural immunity in infected patients.

Role of CD8+ T Cells in Acute HIV/SIV Infection

Vigorous immune responses accompanied by the proliferation of selected T cell receptor V beta (BV)-expressing CD8+ T cells characterize acute HIV infection. Such 'expansions' can persist during chronic HIV infection and are likely to result in the dominance of some selected clones. The oligoclonal expansion of CD8+ T cells *in vivo* is HIV specific during chronic HIV infection and the clonal population is usually consistent with antigen-driven expansions of CD8+ T cells [35].

In greater number of HIV-infected individuals the acute HIV infection is usually presented as a transient symptomatic illness, together with elevated levels of HIV-1 replication and an expansive HIV-specific immune responses. Understanding the true role of CD+8 T cells *in vivo* is vital for understanding HIV pathogenesis and for the designing of future vaccine candidates for HIV control. A plethora of clinical evidence suggests the potential role of cellular immune responses in the control of HIV replication in infected individuals. Recently, evidence attesting the role of CD8+ T cells in controlling SIV replication in macaques was shown [36, 37]. Here, the CD8+ T lymphocytes were depleted in rhesus macaques infected with SIV-mac251 and the effect of CD8+ T cell depletion was assessed on plasma viral load and p24 antigenemia. The animals that were depleted of CD8+ lymphocytes for more than 4 weeks failed to control viral RNA and p24 antigenemia and developed disease. These data imply that acute viremia is a consequence of response from SIV-specific CD8+ T cells and not a consequence of waning CD4+ T cell numbers. Incomplete CD8+ T cell depletion *in vivo*, due to variability in plasma viremia, has hampered interpretation of the exact role of CD8+ T cells in acute SIV infection [38]. In contrast, Matano *et al.* [39] depleted CD8+ T cells from a SIV-infected animal during early infection and showed a role for CD8+ T cells in plasma viremia clearance.

A number of factors, such viral fitness, host genetics, and host immune responses are some factors that modulate acute infection and are known to influence viral replication and defining the viral set point during acute infection. Although the induction of HIV-1-specific CD8(+) T cells during acute infection is associated with a decline in viremia, the role CD8+ T effectors in subsequently establishing the viral set point remains unknown. Cao *et al.* [40] analyzed two acutely infected HIV patients with the same initial Tat-specific CD8+ T cell response. They analyzed their CD8+ T cell responses over time in relation to viral load and sequence evolution. In one patient following the initiation of treatment during acute infection, the frequencies of Tat-specific CD8+ T cells gradually diminished but persisted, and the Tat epitope sequence was largely unaltered. Interestingly, in the second patient, who declined treatment, Tat-specific CD8+ T cells also declined to below detection levels, in tandem with Gag-specific CD4+ T cell loss, as plasma viremia reached a set point. This *in vivo* event temporally coincided with the emergence of an escape variant within the Tat epitope with an additional Vpr epitope. As a consequence, new CD8+ T cell responses emerged with no further decline in plasma viremia. These data suggest that, in the absence of treatment, the initial CD8+ T cell responses have the greatest impact on reducing viremia, and that later, continuously evolving responses are less efficient in further reducing viral load. These results also imply that T cell help is one of the principal contributors to the antiviral efficiency of the acute CD8+ T cell response.

Further, there is supporting evidence showing a massive, oligoclonal expansion of CD8+ T cells during the acute phase of infection [41], which coincides with the appearance of HIV-1-specific CD8+ T and the initial decline in plasma viremia [42]. These HIV-specific CD8+ T cells can potentially eliminate HIV-1-infected cells directly by MHC class I-restricted cytolysis or by a non-cytotoxic mechanism through the secretion of soluble factors [43]. Thus, the biological relevance of CD8+T cell immune responses is evident from both human and non-human primate studies in acute HIV/SIV infection.

CD8+ T cell Responses and their Significance in Chronic HIV/SIV Infection

HIV-infected, therapy naïve, long-term non-progressors (LTNP) usually display strong CD4+ T-cell lymphoproliferative responses to HIV-1 gag antigens [7, 44, 45]. In addition, these patients also maintain a strong lymphoproliferative capacity of HIV-specific CD8+ T-cells [46]. This is known to enhance the function of effector CTL [47]. Disappointingly, the large majority of HIV patients with chronic HIV-1 infection show signs of functional impairments in both CD4+ and CD8+ HIV-reactive T-cells, which is attributed to the continued low-level viral replication and possibly a simultaneous slow decline in the number of CD4+ T cells. Animal model studies have also demonstrated that although HIV-specific CD8+ T cell numbers are maintained by sustained viral replication, the maturation of CTL becomes skewed [48]. At present the functional aspects of HIV-specific CTL *in vivo* are poorly understood. Considerable evidence exists to show that HIV-1, through mutation of viral sequences recognized by CTL epitopes, can evade host immune responses [49], and these molecular changes provide HIV with an arsenal to counteract the host immune system at various stages of HIV disease and therapy. Both CD4 and CD8+ T cell responses are crucial to the success of HAART, but as the HIV-specific CD4+ T cell responses seem to improve with HAART over time, the CD8+ T cell responses show a decline due to decreasing antigenemia and possibly due to the deleterious effects of some drugs on CNAR activity. As a consequence the defenses of these cells weaken and are not sufficient and potent enough to prevent surges in viral replication in the absence of HAART [50].

MECHANISM OF NON-CYTOLYTIC INHIBITION OF HIV BY CD8+T CELLS: EVIDENCE SUPPORTING THE ROLE OF SOLUBLE CD8 ANTIVIRAL FACTORS

Inhibition Through HIV Transcription

The inability to recover virus from asymptomatic HIV-infected individuals unless CD8+ T lymphocytes are first removed, led to the discovery of CD8-mediated suppressor responses [2]. When CD8+ effector cells were added back to the assay virus replication was again suppressed in a dose dependant manner. Subsequently, it has been shown [51, 52] that CD8+ T cells from HIV-infected individuals are able to suppress HIV replication in cultured CD4+ cells by a non-cytolytic mechanism that involves a secreted CAF. These studies demonstrated an arrest of HIV replication at the level of viral transcription. This was shown by culturing naturally-infected CD4+ T cells that were actively producing HIV with either autologous CD8+T cells or a 50% dilution of culture fluids derived from these cells, resulting in a greater than 80% reduction in the number of cells expressing HIV antigens and RNA. This effect was observed within 2 days of exposure to CD8+ T cells, but required 6 days in the presence of CAF-containing culture fluids to attain similar level of HIV suppression. Northern blot analysis of CD4+ T cell extracts showed that all viral RNA species (unspliced/ single and double spliced) were reduced in quantity accordingly. CAF-containing culture fluids showed a direct inhibitory effect on HIV long terminal repeat (LTR)-driven transcription in HIV-infected 1G5 cells. These experiments suggest non-cytolytic inhibition of HIV by CD8+ cell antiviral activity through the suppression of HIV transcription. More recently, it has been shown [53] that the non-cytotoxic anti-HIV response of CD8+ T cells, demonstrable *in vitro*, does not affect any of the virus replication steps leading to the integration of HIV provirus, but specifically interrupts the expression of viral RNA.

HIV Suppression Through STAT1 Activation

Chang TL *et al.* [54] showed the CD8 soluble factor-mediated suppression of HIV to occur via STAT1 activation. Their results reveal that CAF-induced expression of interferon regulatory factor 1 (IRF-1), and that the IRF-1 gene induction was STAT1 dependent. Taken together, the results of Chang *et al.* suggest that CAF activates STAT1, leading to IRF-1 gene induction and inhibition of gene expression regulated by the HIV-1 LTR.

Evidence for the Existence of an Antiviral Membrane-Bound Factor for Non-Cytolytic CD8+T Cell Activity

Recently, Chang and colleagues [55] have shown an elegant demonstration of non-cytotoxic suppression of HIV-1 transcription being achieved by exosomes secreted from CD8+ T cells. Despite evidence indicating the dependence of the activity with cell-to-cell contact, the possibility of a membrane-mediated activity repressing transcription from the viral promoter remains unexplored. They, therefore, investigated whether this inhibition of HIV-1 transcition was elicited by a membrane-bound determinant. Using a CD8+ T cell line displaying potent non-cytotoxic HIV-1 suppression activity, they have identified a membrane-localized HIV-1 suppressing activity that is concomitantly secreted as 30-100 nm sized endosome-derived tetraspanin-rich vesicles known as exosomes. Purified exosomes from CD8+ T cell culture supernatant non-cytotoxically suppressed CCR5-tropic (R5) and CXCR4-tropic (X4) replication of HIV-1 *in vitro* through a protein moiety. Similar antiviral activity was also found in exosomes isolated from two HIV-1 infected subjects. The antiviral exosomes specifically inhibited HIV-1 transcription in both acute and chronic models of infection. This is the first powerful demonstration showing the existence of an antiviral membrane-bound factor consistent with the hallmarks defining non-cytotoxic CD8+ T cell suppression of HIV-1.

Other Side of the Coin for CD8 Antiviral Factors in HIV Disease: Novel CD8 Antiviral Mechanisms

Elevated levels of soluble urokinase-type plasminogen activator (uPA) receptor, CD87/u-PAR, can predict survival of HIV+ individuals. Recently, Wada *et al.* [56] purified an HIV-1 suppressing activity from the culture supernatant of an immortalized CD8+ T cell clone, derived from an HIV-1 infected long-term nonprogressor, and identified this activity as the amino-terminal fragment (ATF) of urokinase-type plasminogen activator (uPA). ATF is catalytically inactive, but can suppress the release of viral particles from the HIV-1 infected cell lines via binding to its receptor CD87. In contrast, cell proliferation and the secretion of an HIV-1 LTR driven reporter gene product were not affected by ATF. These findings suggest that ATF may inhibit the assembly and budding of HIV-1. Supporting this It has also been confirmed by several studies that a serine protease (uPA) possesses anti-HIV activity, which functions by blocking the release/budding of virions [56, 57]. This anti-HIV activity of uPA is due to an intracellular signaling mediated by its receptor uPAR, but not by its enzymatic activity. At this stage, it is difficult to explain the functional link between findings described in the paper by Mackewicz *et al.* [58], and recent findings reported previously by Tumne *et al.* [55], Wada *et al.* [56], Alfano *et al.* [57, 59]. But these disparate antiviral activities will be discussed and clarified in detail in the subsequent chapters.

Clarifications on the Possible Nature of Soluble Factor-Mediated Antiviral Activity of CD8+ T Cells

Recent studies [60] have shown that CAF activity is different from other antiviral factors (defensins) reported from CD8+ T cells. The alpha-defensin-1 inhibits HIV-1 infection following viral entry but alpha-defensins 1 to 3 are not responsible for the HIV-1 transcriptional inhibition imparted by CAF. A recent report by [61] also demonstrate that alpha-defensins specifically block the initial phase of the HIV infectious cycle and modulate the expression of CD4, a critical receptor in the physiology of T-cell activation.

Further, it has also been shown that the alpha-defensins exhibit anti-HIV activity on at least two levels: directly inactivating virus particles; and affecting the ability of target CD4 cells to replicate the virus. While they could demonstrate alpha-defensins in neutrophils and monocytes, no evidence was seen for the production of these peptides by CD8+ T cells. Further, no messenger RNA encoding these proteins was detected in purified CD8 T cells, nor did these cells produced intracellular or extracellular alpha-defensin peptides. Furthermore, antibodies specific for human alpha-defensins 1, 2, and 3 did not block the antiviral activity of CAF-active CD8 cell culture fluids. These data suggest that alpha-defensins are not produced by CD8 cells and are not the components of the elusive CAF, but they possess potent anti-HIV activity and are a vital part of soluble anti-HIV arsenal of neutrophils and monocytes [58].

CAF Antiviral Activity is Mediated by Protein

In the context of HIV, cell culture studies have shown that three beta chemokines RANTES, MIP-1beta and MIP-1 alpha are known to be important anti-HIV factors produced by CD8+ T cells, which do not kill the infected cells. These beta chemokines can act individually in blocking HIV replication, but the presence of all three in excess of 500 pg to 500 ng is more effective in blocking HIV replication, which works at the level of cell surface inhibition of CCR5 binding to the envelope glycoprotein [62]. Thus, in summary all the cytokines known in the context of HIV disease (IL-1-IL-13, IL15, IL-16, TNF alpha and beta, INF-alpha, beta and gamma, TGF-beta, GM-CSF, G-CSF, RANTES< MIP-1alpha and beta, MCP-1, 2, 3, GRO-alpha and beta, LIF, IP-10 and lymphotactin) lack identity to the elusive CAF factor produced by CD8+ T cells.

Recently, it has been shown that the HIV replication by EBV-specific CD8(+) T lymphocytes corresponded to a CAF-like activity, suggesting that CAF production may not be restricted to CTL induced during HIV disease [63, 64]. Moreover, CAF may act after reverse transcription, at least for X4 isolate replication inhibition. Geiben-Lynn R [65] performed detailed analysis of CTL as well as bulk CD8+ T lymphocytes from six HIV-1-infected individuals and from six HIV-1-seronegative individuals. Their kinetic studies showed that secreted suppressive activities of HIV-1-specific CTL and bulk CD8+ T lymphocytes from all HIV-1-infected persons were significantly higher than that of supernatants from seronegative controls. This suppressive activity was blocked by monensin and brefeldin A, was heat labile, and appeared distinct in pattern from that of chemokines (MDC, I-309, MIP-1alpha, MIP-1beta, and RANTES), cytokines (gamma interferon, tumor necrosis factor alpha, and granulocyte-macrophage colony-stimulating factor), and interleukins (interleukin-13 and interleukin-16). The suppressive activity was predominant in supernatants in which molecules were size restricted to greater than 50 kDa. Their data provides a functional link between CD8(+) cells and CTL in the non-cytolytic inhibition of HIV-1 and demonstrates that suppression of X4 virus is mediated through protein(s). To date, these are the only mechanisms known for the non-cytolytic inhibition of HIV by CD8+ T cells and the actual identity of protein(s) conferring this activity remains unknown.

Does Non-Cytotoxic Activity Mediated by CD8+T Cells Require Interaction with other Cell Types? Possible Role of DCs in the Enhancement of Non-Cytotoxic anti-HIV Responses

Dendritic cells (DCs) have a number of roles in HIV pathogenesis, including initial HIV uptake and transport to lymphoid tissue, stimulating HIV replication in T cells and priming CD4+ and CD8+ T lymphocyte mediated immunity. As a result of HIV-1 infection, DCs are able to infect and subsequently induce anergy or apoptosis of naïve T cells, which contributes to the early loss of HIV-specific CD4+ and CD8+ T cells [66].

Recently, Castelli *et al.* [67] have shown a powerful demonstration suggesting that mature dendritic cells can enhance CD8 cell non-cytotoxic anti-HIV responses, which implies the role of IL-15. It is already known that The CD8 cell non-cytotoxic anti-HIV response (CNAR) is associated with a long-term healthy clinical state in HIV-infected individuals.

With time, the CNAR is reduced in concomitance with HIV disease progression. CD8+T cells from healthy HIV-infected individuals display potent ability to suppress viral replication without killing the infected cells. HIV-infected individuals who progress to HIV disease display diminishing CD8+T cell non-cytotoxic antiviral response (CNAR). The underlying reasons for this profound loss of this vital antiviral activity are not known. One reason for the loss of CNAR could be attributed the decrease in a T helper 1 (TH-1) cell cytokine profile, which is seen to persist over time in HIV+ individuals and this switches to TH-2 type of immune response This response is characterized by the production of interleukin-4 (IL-4), IL-5, and IL-10. TH-1 cell cytokines, in particular IL-2, are vital in sustained maintenance of CNAR, whereas theTH-2 cytokines inhibit its activity. Since IL-2 production by lymphocytes is a consequence of their interaction with dendritic cells (DCs), it is likely that this compromise in the functional aspect of DC could result in the loss of CNAR over time. Supporting this, it already documented that the there is significant decrease in DC numbers accompanied by functional impairment following HIV infection [67].

Low CD4+ T cell counts can also contribute to profound loss in CD8+ T cell activity and it is known that the ratio between CD4+ and CD8+ T cells is of vital importance in maintaining both CD8 and CNAR activity. Therefore, it appears that the CD40 ligand (CD40L), a surface protein expressed on CD4+ T cells following activation, is present in low levels, which fails to force maturation of DCs via CD40 in order to induce CD8+ cell immune responses, in particular, CNAR. Dendritic cells mature and secrete IL-15 and IL-12 upon activation by CD40L. IL-15 regulates differentiation and expansion, particularly the memory subsets of CD8+ T cells, whereas IL-12 can cause the differentiation of T cells into TH-1 type cells, which are vital for the secretion of large amounts of interferon. This secretion of interferon, in turn, plays a significant role in enhancing CD8+ T cell responses and CNAR. Thus, it is apparent from the data of Castelli *et al.*, that improving DC/T-cell interactions can possibly lead to a better restoration and enhancement of CNAR in HIV-infected individuals.

CLINICAL SIGNIFICANCE OF CD8+ T CELLS AND SOLUBLE ANTIVIRAL FACTORS.

Influence of Highly Active Antiretroviral Therapy (HAART) on CAF-Mediated Antiviral Activity and its Implications in Anti-HIV Treatment.

It has been shown that [68] the suppressor activity of CAF during antiretroviral therapy was associated with the loss of viremia. This analysis consisted of 32 patients receiving mono-and dual-therapy for a period of 52 weeks, in addition to another 52 weeks with HAART. Prior to therapy, CAF (or CASA as referred to by the authors) correlated inversely with HIV RNA. Dual therapy yielded greater and more sustained changes in CASA, but HAART decreased CASA to levels seen in uninfected individuals. The magnitude of HIV RNA suppression correlated significantly with a decrease in activated CD8+ T lymphocytes (CD38+HLADR+), an increase in CD4+ T lymphocytes (CD45RA+62L+), and an increase in the delayed hypersensitivity score. Overall, the numbers of T lymphocytes did not correlate with changes in CASA activity but CASA augmented with the improvement in immune system and was dependent on ongoing HIV replication *in vivo* or antigenic stimulation. Further, Wilkinson *et al.* [69] constructed a panel of 22 CD8+ T cell lines, with a broad range of CD8+ anti-HIV-1 suppressor activity (CASA), which were generated from a single patient with HIV infection. It was shown that the strong CASA activity was mainly associated with rapidly replicating CD8+ T cells of the phenotype CD8+CD28+Ki67+ that expressed greater levels of IL-2 and the ligands RANTES and I309.

Previously, Gray CM *et al.* [70] have also shown a strong correlation between reduced viral load and loss of activated CD8+CD38+HLA-DR+ cell numbers in the absence of protease inhibitors. Only dual therapy was used in the study of ten HIV-infected asymptomatic patients. These studies are further supported by data from Stanford SA *et al.* [71], which showed the impact of HAART on the plasma HIV-1 RNA levels, CD4+ and CD8+ T lymphocyte counts, and the CD8+ T cell anti-HIV response. Individuals treated with HAART within 6 months of infection showed rapid reductions in HIV-1 RNA levels along with modest increases in CD4+ T cell number and decreases in CD8+ T cell numbers. A significant reduction in the level of CD8+ T cell-mediated non-cytotoxic suppression of HIV replication was observed over time in most participants receiving HAART. Importantly, those individuals who did not receive therapy showed low but detectable HIV-1 RNA levels with no reduction in their CD8+ T cell antiviral response. Taken together, it appears from these that either continued antigenic challenge is required for a sustained CD8+ cell-mediated anti-HIV activity, or that HAART or certain drug regimen in HAART have some direct or indirect bearing on CD8-mediated antiviral inhibition. In addition, associated with improving immune function in the absence of viremia, Ogg and co-workers found a significant inverse correlation between HIV-specific CTL frequency and plasma RNA [72].

Recently, Torres KJ [73] investigated whether HAART has different effects on CNAR in patients at the intermediate and late stages of HIV infection. They studied untreated healthy HIV-infected subjects at baseline and regular intervals for at least 48 weeks following initiation of HAART. Baseline CNAR activity in all subjects correlated inversely with viral load and directly with CD4 T+ cell counts. The level of CNAR in the late stage group was significantly lower than in the intermediate-stage and the healthy reference group (p < 0.01). Following initiation of HAART, CNAR activity was increased significantly during HAART, but only in the late-stage group (p < 0.01). This increase in CD8+ T cell function was seen within 4 weeks of treatment initiation and resulted in levels of CNAR activity almost equal to those observed in the healthy reference subjects. Their findings suggest a beneficial effect on CNAR in those individuals with reduced activity, especially in late-stage infection. But they do not clarify, if HAART may also have some adverse effect on CD8-mediated antiviral inhibition in patients who are doing well.

How Protease Inhibitors Affect Soluble Factor-Mediated Antiviral Activity of CD8+ T Cells?

As discussed above that HAART therapy may have some bearing on CD8+ T cell antiviral activity, recent studies by Stanford *et al.* [71] and Wilkinson *et al.* [68], have shown that HAART has an effect on CD8+ T cell non-cytotoxic antiviral activity, but it is unclear whether some anti-HIV drugs have a deleterious effect on this antiviral activity. One of the protease inhibitors leupeptin, which is not a prescribed drug in the HAART regimen for treatment, was shown to block CNAR activity by up to 95%, *in vitro*. The effect was shown to be dose-dependent and was observed in up to 70% of the CAF and CNAR assays by using fluids and cells from several different subjects. Pretreatment of CD8+ T cells with leupeptin reduced CNAR, further supporting an inhibitory effect on a CD8+ T cell product. Leupeptin did not affect cell growth, expression of activation antigens, or viability of cells (both CD4+ and CD8+ T lymphocytes). Thus it appears that a part of the CD8+ T cell non-cytotoxic response may involve the activity of a protease or a protein that is capable of interacting with certain protease inhibitors, in particular leupeptin [58]. In light of these data, an assessment of the effect(s) of each of the protease inhibitors and combination drugs on CNAR activity needs to be evaluated, as it may provide strategies to maintain this activity and lead to better immune restoration during HAART therapy. In turn, this may also provide better long-term clinical management of HIV patients and may possibly provide better drug choices.

Relationship Between CD4+ T Cell Depletion and Failure of CD8+ T Cell to Combat HIV

During primary infection, HIV-1 infects CD4+T cells, as well as cells of monocyte/macrophage lineage through the mucosal tracts. In this period, neutralized infecting virions as well as the selection of resistant variants and latently infected pool of CD4+ T cells are established [32]. By the time of the chronic phase, the memory CD4+ T cell pool is already shrunk. The escaped HIV-1 variants may initiate another round of antigen stimulation, immune cell activation, neutralization and escape. While the activation process keeps on repeating, CD4+ T cells are under a continuous and large-scale destruction [74]. However, the high death rate of CD4+ T cells due to the chronic immune activation alone cannot explain the depletion of CD4+ T cells. It is the impaired production of new cells combined with continuous destruction of mature cells that leads to the progressive depletion of CD4+ T cells. It has been observed that HIV infection does lead to the impaired production of new T cells by disrupting the bone marrow, thymus [75] and peripheral organs [76].

The thymus is one of the sites for T cell production in the adult life. When HIV-1 is established within the thymic epithelium and the remainder of the thymic stroma, the specific cell populations affected may interfere with the selection process during the development of T cells, leading to immune suppression/tolerance caused by clonal deletion, clonal anergy and/or clonal suppression [77]. Thus, the impaired production in the thymus leads to the progressive shrinking of memory CD4+ T cell pool.

CD4+ T cell help is essential for both the full function and the maintenance of CD8+ T cell responses. This help is essential for the naïve CD8+ precursor CTL to differentiate into mature CTL [78]. This help may depend on cytokine secretion to some extent [79]. In addition, it has been shown that activated CD4+ T cells specifically interact with DC through CD40L-CD40 binding, hence activating DC into a potent inducer of the CTL response [80, 81]. It has been observed that the absence of CD4+ T cells is associated with a lower level of IFN-γ production by HIV-specific CTL [82], impaired CTL function and the wane of CTL activity in the late stages. Vigorous CTL responses are associated with high levels of CD4+ T cells [83]. In CD4+ T-cell depleted mice, although antiviral CD8+ T cells persist, their function is impaired [84, 85], have shown that CD8+ T cells primed without CD4+ T cells are less capable of secondary expansion upon *in vitro* re-stimulation. The study by Janssen *et al.* [86] has demonstrated that CD8+ memory T cells primed in CD4+ T-cell-depleted mice have a defective recall response leading to reduced protective immunity, even when transferred into normal hosts, whereas CD8+ memory T cells primed in normal mice can mount a recall response when transferred into a CD4+ T cell deficient host.

It has been noted that HIV-1-specific CD8+ T cells lose the ability of proliferation with ongoing viral replication after acute infection. Lichterfeld [87] has shown that this functional defect can be induced *in vitro* by depletion of CD4+ T cells. Further, it can be corrected during chronic infection *in vitro* by addition of autologous CD4+ T cells isolated during acute infection and *in vivo* by vaccine-mediated induction of HIV-1-specific CD4+ T helper cell responses. These data demonstrate that HIV-1-specific proliferation of CD8+ T cells critically depends on the presence of antigen-specific CD4+ T cells.

Clinical Correlation of CD8+ T Cells with Plasma Viremia and Proviral DNA in HIV Patients

Acute HIV-1 infection leads to rapid expansion of HIV-1-specific CD8+ T cells [88], which is followed by a rapid and dramatic decline of the viremia [42, 89]. In chronic infection, stronger and broadly diversified HIV-1-specific CD8+ T cell responses have been detected, yet the viremia remains high [46, 90, 91]. Hazenberg *et al.* [92] have carried out a longitudinal analysis in patients before and during HARRT to investigate the proliferation in peripheral blood CD4+ and CD8+ T cells by detecting the Ki-67 nuclear antigen expression [92]. In untreated HIV-1 infection, the percentage and number of Ki-67+CD8+ T cells were significantly increased compared with values from healthy individuals. Immediately on reduction of plasma HIV-RNA load by HAART, the percentage and the total number of Ki-67+CD8+ T cells declined [27]. Lieberman's study [93] has shown that high proportions of CD38+DR+CD8+ T cells are correlated with high levels of plasma HIV RNA, whereas the expression of CD57+ and CD62L-CD45RA+CD8+ T cells are correlated with low viral loads. Besides these activation markers, granzyme can be detected as a marker of CTL activation. Naïve CD8+ T cells do not express granzyme required for target cell lysis, which is expressed within a few days of activation. Compared with healthy donors, peripheral CD8+ T cells in HIV-1-infected subjects have an unusually high percentage of CD8+ cells containing cytolytic granules as measured by staining for the granzyme A, the most abundant granule protease among the granzyme [94]. The overwhelming majority of HIV-1-specific CD8+ T cells express granzyme A [95, 96]. Although the percentage of CD8+ T cells staining for granzyme A did not correlate with plasma viral RNA, it did correlate negatively with CD4+ T cell counts [93].

Further, an elegant study by Salerno-Goncalves *et al.* [97] has measured CD8 antiviral activity in 22 asymptomatic human immunodeficiency virus type 1-infected patients (10 rapid progressors and 12 slow progressors) and its effect on the proviral load of CD4+ T cells homogeneously superinfected by the same dose of a non-syncytium-inducing virus in the presence or in the absence of autologous CD8+ T cells. They demonstrated that the antiviral activity of CD8+ T cells was highly predictive of the rate of peripheral CD4+ T-cell decline and reducing proviral DNA integration in autologous CD4+ T cells. These findings show a strong correlation between the antiviral activity of CD8+ T cells of HIV-infected patients (as measured by the CD4+ T-cell proviral DNA decrease) and the rate of peripheral CD4+ T-cell count decline in the next 3 years. This proviral DNA in rapid and slow progressors correlated clinically with plasma viremia levels. They also imply that such an activity could be the sum of various HIV-specific CD8+ T-cell activities, but they failed to find any correlation with the Gag-specific CTL activity.

Secretion of CD8 Soluble Antiviral Factor and HIV Disease Staging and Balance Between CD4+ and CD8+ T Cell Counts

CD4/CD8 T cell ratio is a more sensitive predictor of HIV infection than the CD4 T cell count alone Thus CD4/CD8 T cell ratios may prove to be vital in predicting the CD8 antiviral activity in HIV patients and SIV-infected macaques. Recently, it has been shown through a cross-sectional study that the capacity of CD8+ cells from HIV-infected patients and SIVmac-infected macaques to suppress the replication *in vitro* depends on the clinical stage of disease [98]. Little is known about changes in this antiviral activity over time in individual HIV-infected patients or SIV-infected macaques. Dioszeghy assessed changes in the soluble factor-mediated non-cytolytic antiviral activity of CD8+ cells over time in eight cynomologus macaques infected with SIVmac251 to determine the pathophysiological role of this activity. They found that CD8+ cell-associated antiviral activity increased rapidly in the first week after viral inoculation and remained detectable during the early phase of infection. This net increase in antiviral activity of CD8+ cells correlated with plasma viral load throughout the 15 months of follow-up. CD8+ cells gradually lost their antiviral activity over time and acquired virus replication-enhancing capacity. Levels of antiviral activity also correlated with the total CD4+ T-cell counts after viral set point. Further, the beta-chemokines and interleukin-16 and alpha defensins in CD8+ cell supernatants did not correlate with CD8 antiviral activity. More importantly, the soluble factor-mediated antiviral activity of CD8+ cells was neither cytolytic nor restricted to major histocompatibility complex. This is the first longitudinal study to demonstrate that the increase in non-cytolytic antiviral activity from baseline and the maintenance of this increase over time in cynomolgus macaques depend on both viral replication and CD4+ T cell count, implying the significance of balance in ratio of CD4+ and CD8+ T cells in SIV-infected monkeys and HIV-infected humans.

GENOMIC BASIS OF CD8-MEDIATED PROTECTION: CLUES FROM THE WHOLE HUMAN GENOME MICROARRAY STUDIES

It is already known that the functional impairment and numerical decline of CD8+ T cells during HIV infection has a profound effect on disease progression, but to date, only limited microarray studies have used cellular transcriptome of CD8+ T cells in order to understand the interactions of HIV and host CD8+ T cells at different disease status. Previous microarray studies in relation to HIV disease have used whole PBMC or cell lines, monocytes, macrophages, CD4+ T cells, lymphoid and gut tissue, etc [99, 100], but only a few studies have used CD8+ T cells to understand gene regulation during HIV infection. These include studies using CD8+ T cell gene expression profiling to detect genes responsible for non-cytotoxic activity of CD8+ T cells [101, 102]; the study by Martinez-Marino *et al.* identified 52 differentially expressed genes between infected subjects with high CD8+ cell non-cytotoxic anti-HIV responses and uninfected controls that lack this activity. Recently, the transcriptional profiling of CD4+ and CD8+ T cells from early infection, chronic infection and LTNP patients has been studied and interferon responses were characterized as a transcriptional signature of T cells from early and chronic HIV infected individuals [103]. It has also been shown that CD8+ T cells contain more differential genes than CD4+ T cells, which is consistent with our recent antibody microarray study illustrating that CD8+ T cells have more cell surface molecules differentiating disease status then CD4+ T cells [104].

Our recent studies [105] assessed all 48,000 human genome transcripts (encompassing all 25,000 human genes) in primary CD8+ T cells from HIV+ therapy naïve non-progressors and therapy-experienced progressors. Sixty-eight differentially expressed genes were identified and divided into eight categories according to their biological functions and relevance in HIV pathogenesis: (1) genes previously reported to be involved in HIV infection and disease (6/68); (2) Interferon induced, apoptosis and actin-related genes (11/68); (3) cell cycle, proliferation and activation genes (5/68); (4) adhesion and cell surface molecules (6/68); (5) endosome, lysosome and cytotoxicity (6/68); (6) mitochondria, lipid and carbohydrate metabolism associated genes (8/68); (7) genes lacking relevance to HIV pathogenesis (13/68) and (8) less characterized genes (13/68). Further, by geneset enrichment analysis (GSEA), the coordinated up-regulation of oxidative phosphorylation genes encoding for enzymes and genes involved in interferon responses were detected as fingerprints in HIV progressors on HAART, whereas LTNPs displayed a transcriptional signature of coordinated up-regulation of components of MAPK pathway.

CONCLUSIONS AND FUTURE PERSPECTIVES

A soluble factor produced by CD8+ T cells in HIV-infected patients is involved in part in CD8+ cell anti-HIV activity. This implies their significant participation in progressive and non-progressive HIV disease. The non-cytotoxic activity of CD8+ T cells suppresses transcription of human immunodeficiency virus type 1 (HIV-1) in an antigen-independent and MHC-unrestricted manner. But, the precise cellular and molecular factors or the biochemical constituents mediating this CD8+ T cell effector function remain obscure. While the CTL activity mediated by CD8+ T cells is protective against HIV infection, it is highly variable between different groups of HIV patients. In contrast, the antiviral arm of the CD8+ T cells is more stable and a strong predictor of HIV disease stages. This activity comprises of potent antiviral soluble factors, the actual biochemical definition of which remains poorly understood. Once characterized, these soluble factors can be used as potential markers to predict the progression and non-progression of HIV disease. In addition, these soluble factors could be important candidates, which can be used in predicting the success and failure of HAART therapy in HIV patients. Further, it is likely that a subset of CD8+ T cells mediate these antiviral soluble factors and a detailed analysis of various subsets of CD8+ T cells *in vivo* and their modulation during HIV infection will yield valuable insights to mechanisms governing the infectious process in the host. With the advent of whole human genome microarray technologies, gene expression analysis of transcriptomes of various CD8+ T cell subsets may shed greater light on how HIV subverts and manipulates the host gene machinery at the level of genes encoding these soluble antiviral factors in minor, yet physiologically and biologically important CD8+ T cell subsets.

REFERENCES

[1]   Saksena NK, Wu JQ, Potter SJ, Wilkinson J, Wang B. Human immunodeficiency virus interactions with CD8+ T lymphocytes. Curr HIV Res. 2008;6(1):1-9.

[2]   Walker CM, Moody DJ, Stites DP, Levy JA. CD8+ lymphocytes can control HIV infection in vitro by suppressing virus replication. Science. 1986;234(4783):1563-1566.

[3]   Bagasra O, Pomerantz RJ. The role of CD8-positive lymphocytes in the control of HIV-1 infection of peripheral blood mononuclear cells. Immunol Lett. 1993;35(2):83-92.

[4]   De Maria A, Pantaleo G, Schnittman SM, Greenhouse JJ, Baseler M, Orenstein JM, *et al.* Infection of CD8+ T lymphocytes with HIV. Requirement for interaction with infected CD4+ cells and induction of infectious virus from chronically infected CD8+ cells. J Immunol. 1991;146(7):2220-2226.

[5]   De Rossi A, Franchini G, Aldovini A, Del Mistro A, Chieco-Bianchi L, Gallo RC, *et al.* Differential response to the cytopathic effects of human T-cell lymphotropic virus type III (HTLV-III) superinfection in T4+ (helper) and T8+ (suppressor) T-cell clones transformed by HTLV-I. Proc Natl Acad Sci USA. 1986;83(12):4297-4301.

[6]   Mercure L, Phaneuf D, Wainberg MA. Detection of unintegrated human immunodeficiency virus type 1 DNA in persistently infected CD8+ cells. J Gen Virol. 1993;74 (Pt 10):2077-2083.

[7]   Wang B, Dyer WB, Zaunders JJ, Mikhail M, Sullivan JS, Williams L, *et al.* Comprehensive analyses of a unique HIV-1-infected nonprogressor reveal a complex association of immunobiological mechanisms in the context of replication-incompetent infection. Virology. 2002;304(2):246-264.

[8]   Livingstone WJ, Moore M, Innes D, Bell JE, Simmonds P. Frequent infection of peripheral blood CD8-positive T-lymphocytes with HIV-1. Edinburgh Heterosexual Transmission Study Group. Lancet. 1996;348(9028):649-654.

[9]   Imlach S, McBreen S, Shirafuji T, Leen C, Bell JE, Simmonds P. Activated peripheral CD8 lymphocytes express CD4 in vivo and are targets for infection by human immunodeficiency virus type 1. J Virol. 2001;75(23):11555-11564.

[10]   Semenzato G, Agostini C, Ometto L, Zambello R, Trentin L, Chieco-Bianchi L, *et al.* CD8+ T lymphocytes in the lung of acquired immunodeficiency syndrome patients harbor human immunodeficiency virus type 1. Blood. 1995;85(9):2308-2314.

[11]   McBreen S, Imlach S, Shirafuji T, Scott GR, Leen C, Bell JE, *et al.* Infection of the CD45RA+ (naive) subset of peripheral CD8+ lymphocytes by human immunodeficiency virus type 1 in vivo. J Virol. 2001;75(9):4091-4102.

[12]   Brooks DG, Kitchen SG, Kitchen CM, Scripture-Adams DD, Zack JA. Generation of HIV latency during thymopoiesis. Nat Med. 2001;7(4):459-464.

[13]   Lee S, Goldstein H, Baseler M, Adelsberger J, Golding H. Human immunodeficiency virus type 1 infection of mature CD3hiCD8+ thymocytes. J Virol. 1997;71(9):6671-6676.

[14]   Flamand L, Crowley RW, Lusso P, Colombini-Hatch S, Margolis DM, Gallo RC. Activation of CD8+ T lymphocytes through the T cell receptor turns on CD4 gene expression: implications for HIV pathogenesis. Proc Natl Acad Sci USA. 1998;95(6):3111-3116.

[15]   Yang LP, Riley JL, Carroll RG, June CH, Hoxie J, Patterson BK, *et al.* Productive infection of neonatal CD8+ T lymphocytes by HIV-1. J Exp Med. 1998;187(7):1139-1144.

[16]   Kitchen SG, LaForge S, Patel VP, Kitchen CM, Miceli MC, Zack JA. Activation of CD8 T cells induces expression of CD4, which functions as a chemotactic receptor. Blood. 2002;99(1):207-212.

[17]   Kitchen SG, Jones NR, LaForge S, Whitmire JK, Vu BA, Galic Z, *et al.* CD4 on CD8(+) T cells directly enhances effector function and is a target for HIV infection. Proc Natl Acad Sci USA. 2004;101(23):8727-8732.

[18]   Zloza A, Sullivan YB, Connick E, Landay AL, Al-Harthi L. CD8+ T cells that express CD4 on their surface (CD4dimCD8bright T cells) recognize an antigen-specific target, are detected in vivo, and can be productively infected by T-tropic HIV. Blood. 2003;102(6):2156-2164.

[19]   Saha K, Zhang J, Zerhouni B. Evidence of productively infected CD8+ T cells in patients with AIDS: implications for HIV-1 pathogenesis. J Acquir Immune Defic Syndr. 2001;26(3):199-207.

[20] Zerhouni B, Nelson JA, Saha K. CXCR4-dependent infection of CD8+, but not CD4+, lymphocytes by a primary human immunodeficiency virus type 1 isolate. J Virol. 2004;78(22):12288-12296.

[21] Semenzato G, Agostini C, Chieco-Bianchi L, De Rossi A. HIV load in highly purified CD8+ T cells retrieved from pulmonary and blood compartments. J Leukoc Biol. 1998;64(3):298-301.

[22] Brenchley JM, Hill BJ, Ambrozak DR, Price DA, Guenaga FJ, Casazza JP, *et al*. T-cell subsets that harbor human immunodeficiency virus (HIV) in vivo: implications for HIV pathogenesis. J Virol. 2004;78(3):1160-1168.

[23] Herbein G, Mahlknecht U, Batliwalla F, Gregersen P, Pappas T, Butler J, *et al*. Apoptosis of CD8+ T cells is mediated by macrophages through interaction of HIV gp120 with chemokine receptor CXCR4. Nature. 1998;395(6698):189-194.

[24] Lewis DE, Tang DS, Adu-Oppong A, Schober W, Rodgers JR. Anergy and apoptosis in CD8+ T cells from HIV-infected persons. J Immunol. 1994;153(1):412-420.

[25] Kalams SA, Walker BD. The critical need for CD4 help in maintaining effective cytotoxic T lymphocyte responses. J Exp Med. 1998;188(12):2199-2204.

[26] Roederer M. T-cell dynamics of immunodeficiency. Nat Med. 1995;1(7):621-622.

[27] Bohler T, Walcher J, Holzl-Wenig G, Geiss M, Buchholz B, Linde R, *et al*. Early effects of antiretroviral combination therapy on activation, apoptosis and regeneration of T cells in HIV-1-infected children and adolescents. AIDS. 1999;13(7):779-789.

[28] Potter SJ, Dwyer DE, Saksena NK. Differential cellular distribution of HIV-1 drug resistance in vivo: evidence for infection of CD8+ T cells during HAART. Virology. 2003;305(2):339-352.

[29] Potter SJ, Lemey P, Achaz G, Chew CB, Vandamme AM, Dwyer DE, *et al*. HIV-1 compartmentalization in diverse leukocyte populations during antiretroviral therapy. J Leukoc Biol. 2004;76(3):562-570.

[30] Potter SJ, Lemey P, Dyer WB, Sullivan JS, Chew CB, Vandamme AM, *et al*. Genetic analyses reveal structured HIV-1 populations in serially sampled T lymphocytes of patients receiving HAART. Virology. 2006;348(1):35-46.

[31] Chun TW, Engel D, Berrey MM, Shea T, Corey L, Fauci AS. Early establishment of a pool of latently infected, resting CD4(+) T cells during primary HIV-1 infection. Proc Natl Acad Sci USA. 1998;95(15):8869-8873.

[32] Chun TW, Engel D, Mizell SB, Ehler LA, Fauci AS. Induction of HIV-1 replication in latently infected CD4+ T cells using a combination of cytokines. J Exp Med. 1998;188(1):83-91.

[33] Wong JK, Hezareh M, Gunthard HF, Havlir DV, Ignacio CC, Spina CA, *et al*. Recovery of replication-competent HIV despite prolonged suppression of plasma viremia. Science. 1997;278(5341):1291-1295.

[34] Furtado MR, Callaway DS, Phair JP, Kunstman KJ, Stanton JL, Macken CA, *et al*. Persistence of HIV-1 transcription in peripheral-blood mononuclear cells in patients receiving potent antiretroviral therapy. N Engl J Med. 1999;340(21):1614-1622.

[35] Wilson JD, Ogg GS, Allen RL, Goulder PJ, Kelleher A, Sewell AK, *et al*. Oligoclonal expansions of CD8(+) T cells in chronic HIV infection are antigen specific. J Exp Med. 1998;188(4):785-790.

[36] Schmitz JE, Kuroda MJ, Santra S, Sasseville VG, Simon MA, Lifton MA, *et al*. Control of viremia in simian immunodeficiency virus infection by CD8+ lymphocytes. Science. 1999;283(5403):857-860.

[37] Jin X, Bauer DE, Tuttleton SE, Lewin S, Gettie A, Blanchard J, *et al*. Dramatic rise in plasma viremia after CD8(+) T cell depletion in simian immunodeficiency virus-infected macaques. J Exp Med. 1999;189(6):991-998.

[38] Stebbings R, Stott J, Almond N, Hull R, Lines J, Silvera P, *et al*. Mechanisms of protection induced by attenuated simian immunodeficiency virus. II. Lymphocyte depletion does not abrogate protection. AIDS Res Hum Retroviruses. 1998;14(13):1187-1198.

[39] Matano T, Shibata R, Siemon C, Connors M, Lane HC, Martin MA. Administration of an anti-CD8 monoclonal antibody interferes with the clearance of chimeric simian/human immunodeficiency virus during primary infections of rhesus macaques. J Virol. 1998;72(1):164-169.

[40] Cao J, McNevin J, Malhotra U, McElrath MJ. Evolution of CD8+ T cell immunity and viral escape following acute HIV-1 infection. J Immunol. 2003;171(7):3837-3846.

[41] Pantaleo G, Demarest JF, Soudeyns H, Graziosi C, Denis F, Adelsberger JW, *et al*. Major expansion of CD8+ T cells with a predominant V beta usage during the primary immune response to HIV. Nature. 1994;370(6489):463-467.

[42] Koup RA, Safrit JT, Cao Y, Andrews CA, McLeod G, Borkowsky W, *et al*. Temporal association of cellular immune responses with the initial control of viremia in primary human immunodeficiency virus type 1 syndrome. J Virol. 1994;68(7):4650-4655.

[43] Yang OO, Kalams SA, Trocha A, Cao H, Luster A, Johnson RP, *et al*. Suppression of human immunodeficiency virus type 1 replication by CD8+ cells: evidence for HLA class I-restricted triggering of cytolytic and noncytolytic mechanisms. J Virol. 1997;71(4):3120-3128.

[44] Rosenberg ES, Billingsley JM, Caliendo AM, Boswell SL, Sax PE, Kalams SA, *et al.* Vigorous HIV-1-specific CD4+ T cell responses associated with control of viremia. Science. 1997;278(5342):1447-1450.

[45] Zaunders JJ, Dyer WB, Wang B, Munier ML, Miranda-Saksena M, Newton R, *et al.* Identification of circulating antigen-specific CD4+ T lymphocytes with a CCR5+, cytotoxic phenotype in an HIV-1 long-term nonprogressor and in CMV infection. Blood. 2004;103(6):2238-2247.

[46] Draenert R, Verrill CL, Tang Y, Allen TM, Wurcel AG, Boczanowski M, *et al.* Persistent recognition of autologous virus by high-avidity CD8 T cells in chronic, progressive human immunodeficiency virus type 1 infection. J Virol. 2004;78(2):630-641.

[47] Migueles SA, Laborico AC, Shupert WL, Sabbaghian MS, Rabin R, Hallahan CW, *et al.* HIV-specific CD8+ T cell proliferation is coupled to perforin expression and is maintained in nonprogressors. Nat Immunol. 2002;3(11):1061-1068.

[48] Lieberman J, Shankar P, Manjunath N, Andersson J. Dressed to kill? A review of why antiviral CD8 T lymphocytes fail to prevent progressive immunodeficiency in HIV-1 infection. Blood. 2001;98(6):1667-1677.

[49] Barouch DH, Kunstman J, Kuroda MJ, Schmitz JE, Santra S, Peyerl FW, *et al.* Eventual AIDS vaccine failure in a rhesus monkey by viral escape from cytotoxic T lymphocytes. Nature. 2002;415(6869):335-339.

[50] Lange CG, Lederman MM, Madero JS, Medvik K, Asaad R, Pacheko C, *et al.* Impact of suppression of viral replication by highly active antiretroviral therapy on immune function and phenotype in chronic HIV-1 infection. J Acquir Immune Defic Syndr. 2002;30(1):33-40.

[51] Walker CM, Levy JA. A diffusible lymphokine produced by CD8+ T lymphocytes suppresses HIV replication. Immunology. 1989;66(4):628-630.

[52] Mackewicz CE, Blackbourn DJ, Levy JA. CD8+ T cells suppress human immunodeficiency virus replication by inhibiting viral transcription. Proc Natl Acad Sci USA. 1995;92(6):2308-2312.

[53] Mackewicz CE, Patterson BK, Lee SA, Levy JA. CD8(+) cell noncytotoxic anti-human immunodeficiency virus response inhibits expression of viral RNA but not reverse transcription or provirus integration. J Gen Virol. 2000;81(Pt 5):1261-1264.

[54] Chang TL, Mosoian A, Pine R, Klotman ME, Moore JP. A soluble factor(s) secreted from CD8(+) T lymphocytes inhibits human immunodeficiency virus type 1 replication through STAT1 activation. J Virol. 2002;76(2):569-581.

[55] Tumne A, Prasad VS, Chen Y, Stolz DB, Saha K, Ratner DM, *et al.* Noncytotoxic Suppression of HIV-1Transcription by Exosomes Secreted from CD8+ T Cells. J Virol. 2009.

[56] Wada M, Wada NA, Shirono H, Taniguchi K, Tsuchie H, Koga J. Amino-terminal fragment of urokinase-type plasminogen activator inhibits HIV-1 replication. Biochem Biophys Res Commun. 2001;284(2):346-351.

[57] Alfano M, Mariani SA, Elia C, Pardi R, Blasi F, Poli G. Ligand-engaged urokinase-type plasminogen activator receptor and activation of the CD11b/CD18 integrin inhibit late events of HIV expression in monocytic cells. Blood. 2009;113(8):1699-1709.

[58] Mackewicz CE, Craik CS, Levy JA. The CD8+ cell noncytotoxic anti-HIV response can be blocked by protease inhibitors. Proc Natl Acad Sci USA. 2003;100(6):3433-3438.

[59] Alfano M, Sidenius N, Panzeri B, Blasi F, Poli G. Urokinase-urokinase receptor interaction mediates an inhibitory signal for HIV-1 replication. Proc Natl Acad Sci USA. 2002;99(13):8862-8867.

[60] Chang TL, Francois F, Mosoian A, Klotman ME. CAF-mediated human immunodeficiency virus (HIV) type 1 transcriptional inhibition is distinct from alpha-defensin-1 HIV inhibition. J Virol. 2003;77(12):6777-6784.

[61] Furci L, Sironi F, Tolazzi M, Vassena L, Lusso P. Alpha-defensins block the early steps of HIV-1 infection: interference with the binding of gp120 to CD4. Blood. 2007;109(7):2928-2935.

[62] Cocchi F, DeVico AL, Garzino-Demo A, Arya SK, Gallo RC, Lusso P. Identification of RANTES, MIP-1 alpha, and MIP-1 beta as the major HIV-suppressive factors produced by CD8+ T cells. Science. 1995;270(5243):1811-1815.

[63] Brinchmann JE, Gaudernack G, Vartdal F. CD8+ T cells inhibit HIV replication in naturally infected CD4+ T cells. Evidence for a soluble inhibitor. J Immunol. 1990;144(8):2961-2966.

[64] Le Borgne S, Fevrier M, Callebaut C, Lee SP, Riviere Y. CD8(+)-Cell antiviral factor activity is not restricted to human immunodeficiency virus (HIV)-specific T cells and can block HIV replication after initiation of reverse transcription. J Virol. 2000;74(10):4456-4464.

[65] Geiben-Lynn R, Kursar M, Brown NV, Kerr EL, Luster AD, Walker BD. Noncytolytic inhibition of X4 virus by bulk CD8(+) cells from human immunodeficiency virus type 1 (HIV-1)-infected persons and HIV-1-specific cytotoxic T lymphocytes is not mediated by beta-chemokines. J Virol. 2001;75(17):8306-8316.

[66] Steinman RM, Granelli-Piperno A, Pope M, Trumpfheller C, Ignatius R, Arrode G, *et al.* The interaction of immunodeficiency viruses with dendritic cells. Curr Top Microbiol Immunol. 2003;276:1-30.

[67]   Castelli J, Thomas EK, Gilliet M, Liu YJ, Levy JA. Mature dendritic cells can enhance CD8+ cell noncytotoxic anti-HIV responses: the role of IL-15. Blood. 2004;103(7):2699-2704.

[68]   Wilkinson J, Zaunders JJ, Carr A, Cooper DA. CD8+ anti-human immunodeficiency virus suppressor activity (CASA) in response to antiretroviral therapy: loss of CASA is associated with loss of viremia. J Infect Dis. 1999;180(1):68-75.

[69]   Wilkinson J, Zaunders JJ, Carr A, Guillemin G, Cooper DA. Characterization of the phenotypic and lymphokine profile associated with strong CD8+ anti-HIV-1 suppressor activity (CASA). Clin Exp Immunol. 2002;127(1):145-150.

[70]   Gray CM, Schapiro JM, Winters MA, Merigan TC. Changes in CD4+ and CD8+ T cell subsets in response to highly active antiretroviral therapy in HIV type 1-infected patients with prior protease inhibitor experience. AIDS Res Hum Retroviruses. 1998;14(7):561-569.

[71]   Stranford SA, Ong JC, Martinez-Marino B, Busch M, Hecht FM, Kahn J, *et al*. Reduction in CD8+ cell noncytotoxic anti-HIV activity in individuals receiving highly active antiretroviral therapy during primary infection. Proc Natl Acad Sci USA. 2001;98(2):597-602.

[72]   Ogg GS, Jin X, Bonhoeffer S, Dunbar PR, Nowak MA, Monard S, *et al*. Quantitation of HIV-1-specific cytotoxic T lymphocytes and plasma load of viral RNA. Science. 1998;279(5359):2103-2106.

[73]   Torres KJ, Gutierrez F, Espinosa E, Mackewicz C, Regalado J, Reyes-Teran G. CD8+ cell noncytotoxic anti-HIV response: restoration by HAART in the late stage of infection. AIDS Res Hum Retroviruses. 2006;22(2):144-152.

[74]   McCune JM. The dynamics of CD4+ T-cell depletion in HIV disease. Nature. 2001;410(6831):974-979.

[75]   McCune JM. HIV-1: the infective process in vivo. Cell. 1991;64(2):351-363.

[76]   Haase AT. Population biology of HIV-1 infection: viral and CD4+ T cell demographics and dynamics in lymphatic tissues. Annu Rev Immunol. 1999;17:625-656.

[77]   Imami N, Gotch F. Mechanisms of loss of HIV-1-specific T-cell responses. J HIV Ther. 2002;7(2):30-34.

[78]   Bennett SR, Carbone FR, Karamalis F, Miller JF, Heath WR. Induction of a CD8+ cytotoxic T lymphocyte response by cross-priming requires cognate CD4+ T cell help. J Exp Med. 1997;186(1):65-70.

[79]   Keene JA, Forman J. Helper activity is required for the in vivo generation of cytotoxic T lymphocytes. J Exp Med. 1982;155(3):768-782.

[80]   Ridge JP, Di Rosa F, Matzinger P. A conditioned dendritic cell can be a temporal bridge between a CD4+ T-helper and a T-killer cell. Nature. 1998;393(6684):474-478.

[81]   Schoenberger SP, Toes RE, van der Voort EI, Offringa R, Melief CJ. T-cell help for cytotoxic T lymphocytes is mediated by CD40-CD40L interactions. Nature. 1998;393(6684):480-483.

[82]   Spiegel HM, Ogg GS, DeFalcon E, Sheehy ME, Monard S, Haslett PA, *et al*. Human immunodeficiency virus type 1- and cytomegalovirus-specific cytotoxic T lymphocytes can persist at high frequency for prolonged periods in the absence of circulating peripheral CD4(+) T cells. J Virol. 2000;74(2):1018-1022.

[83]   Kalams SA, Buchbinder SP, Rosenberg ES, Billingsley JM, Colbert DS, Jones NG, *et al*. Association between virus-specific cytotoxic T-lymphocyte and helper responses in human immunodeficiency virus type 1 infection. J Virol. 1999;73(8):6715-6720.

[84]   Cardin RD, Brooks JW, Sarawar SR, Doherty PC. Progressive loss of CD8+ T cell-mediated control of a gamma-herpesvirus in the absence of CD4+ T cells. J Exp Med. 1996;184(3):863-871.

[85]   Bourgeois C, Rocha B, Tanchot C. A role for CD40 expression on CD8+ T cells in the generation of CD8+ T cell memory. Science. 2002;297(5589):2060-2063.

[86]   Janssen EM, Lemmens EE, Wolfe T, Christen U, von Herrath MG, Schoenberger SP. CD4+ T cells are required for secondary expansion and memory in CD8+ T lymphocytes. Nature. 2003;421(6925):852-856.

[87]   Lichterfeld M, Kaufmann DE, Yu XG, Mui SK, Addo MM, Johnston MN, *et al*. Loss of HIV-1-specific CD8+ T cell proliferation after acute HIV-1 infection and restoration by vaccine-induced HIV-1-specific CD4+ T cells. J Exp Med. 2004;200(6):701-712.

[88]   Kahn JO, Walker BD. Acute human immunodeficiency virus type 1 infection. N Engl J Med. 1998;339(1):33-39.

[89]   Borrow P, Lewicki H, Hahn BH, Shaw GM, Oldstone MB. Virus-specific CD8+ cytotoxic T-lymphocyte activity associated with control of viremia in primary human immunodeficiency virus type 1 infection. J Virol. 1994;68(9):6103-6110.

[90]   Addo MM, Yu XG, Rathod A, Cohen D, Eldridge RL, Strick D, *et al*. Comprehensive epitope analysis of human immunodeficiency virus type 1 (HIV-1)-specific T-cell responses directed against the entire expressed HIV-1 genome demonstrate broadly directed responses, but no correlation to viral load. J Virol. 2003;77(3):2081-2092.

[91]   Betts MR, Ambrozak DR, Douek DC, Bonhoeffer S, Brenchley JM, Casazza JP, *et al*. Analysis of total human immunodeficiency virus (HIV)-specific CD4(+) and CD8(+) T-cell responses: relationship to viral load in untreated HIV infection. J Virol. 2001;75(24):11983-11991.

[92] Hazenberg MD, Stuart JW, Otto SA, Borleffs JC, Boucher CA, de Boer RJ, *et al*. T-cell division in human immunodeficiency virus (HIV)-1 infection is mainly due to immune activation: a longitudinal analysis in patients before and during highly active antiretroviral therapy (HAART). Blood. 2000;95(1):249-255.

[93] Lieberman J, Trimble LA, Friedman RS, Lisziewicz J, Lori F, Shankar P, *et al*. Expansion of CD57 and CD62L-CD45RA+ CD8 T lymphocytes correlates with reduced viral plasma RNA after primary HIV infection. AIDS. 1999;13(8):891-899.

[94] Trimble LA, Lieberman J. Circulating CD8 T lymphocytes in human immunodeficiency virus-infected individuals have impaired function and downmodulate CD3 zeta, the signaling chain of the T-cell receptor complex. Blood. 1998;91(2):585-594.

[95] Shankar P, Russo M, Harnisch B, Patterson M, Skolnik P, Lieberman J. Impaired function of circulating HIV-specific CD8(+) T cells in chronic human immunodeficiency virus infection. Blood. 2000;96(9):3094-3101.

[96] Shankar P, Xu Z, Lieberman J. Viral-specific cytotoxic T lymphocytes lyse human immunodeficiency virus-infected primary T lymphocytes by the granule exocytosis pathway. Blood. 1999;94(9):3084-3093.

[97] Salerno-Goncalves R, Lu W, Andrieu JM. Quantitative analysis of the antiviral activity of CD8(+) T cells from human immunodeficiency virus-positive asymptomatic patients with different rates of CD4(+) T-cell decrease. J Virol. 2000;74(14):6648-6651.

[98] Dioszeghy V, Benlhassan-Chahour K, Delache B, Dereuddre-Bosquet N, Aubenque C, Gras G, *et al*. Changes in soluble factor-mediated CD8+ cell-derived antiviral activity in cynomolgus macaques infected with simian immunodeficiency virus SIVmac251: relationship to biological markers of progression. J Virol. 2006;80(1):236-245.

[99] Giri MS, Nebozhyn M, Showe L, Montaner LJ. Microarray data on gene modulation by HIV-1 in immune cells: 2000-2006. J Leukoc Biol. 2006;80(5):1031-1043.

[100] Ryo A, Suzuki Y, Ichiyama K, Wakatsuki T, Kondoh N, Hada A, *et al*. Serial analysis of gene expression in HIV-1-infected T cell lines. FEBS Lett. 1999;462(1-2):182-186.

[101] Diaz LS, Stone MR, Mackewicz CE, Levy JA. Differential gene expression in CD8+ cells exhibiting noncytotoxic anti-HIV activity. Virology. 2003;311(2):400-409.

[102] Martinez-Marino B, Foster H, Hao Y, Levy JA. Differential gene expression in CD8(+) cells from HIV-1-infected subjects showing suppression of HIV replication. Virology. 2007;362(1):217-225.

[103] Hyrcza MD, Kovacs C, Loutfy M, Halpenny R, Heisler L, Yang S, *et al*. Distinct transcriptional profiles in ex vivo CD4+ and CD8+ T cells are established early in human immunodeficiency virus type 1 infection and are characterized by a chronic interferon response as well as extensive transcriptional changes in CD8+ T cells. J Virol. 2007;81(7):3477-3486.

[104] Wu JQ, Wang B, Belov L, Chrisp J, Learmont J, Dyer WB, *et al*. Antibody microarray analysis of cell surface antigens on CD4+ and CD8+ T cells from HIV+ individuals correlates with disease stages. Retrovirology. 2007;4:83.

[105] Wu JQ, Dwyer DE, Dyer WB, Yang YH, Wang B, Saksena NK. Transcriptional profiles in CD8+ T cells from HIV+ progressors on HAART are characterized by coordinated up-regulation of oxidative phosphorylation enzymes and interferon responses. Virology. 2008;380(1):124-135.

CHAPTER 2

Cytokines and HIV Infection

Massimo Alfano[1,*] and Guido Poli[1,2].

[1]*AIDS Immunopathogenesis Unit, Division of Immunology, Transplantation and Infectious Diseases, San Raffaele Scientific Institute, Milan, Italy;* [2]*Vita-Salute San Raffaele University, School of Medicine, Milan, Italy*

Abstract: HIV is the ethiological agent of the Acquired Immunodeficiency Syndrome (AIDS). HIV infects mostly CD4[+] immune cells, such as T lymphocytes, mononuclear phagocytes and myeloid dendritic cells and induces a progressive and deadly state of immunodeficiency if untreated with potent combinations of antiretroviral agents. The immunodeficient status of the host allows the development of several opportunistic infections as well as "opportunistic" tumors such as Kaposis' sarcoma and B cell lymphomas. In addition, the ability of HIV-1 infected immune cells to localize in various tissues leads to tissue specific HIV-associated pathology, such as AIDS dementia, interstitial lung disease, nephropathy, enteropathy, and wasting syndrome. Of note, all these processes involve the upregulation or modulation of cytokines, soluble factors that regulate the immune responses and inflammation in addition to hematopoiesis. Due to space limitation and to the extent of informations about HIV and cytokines, this chapter will not discuss topics such as interactions between intracellular signalings by cytokines and HIV or the effect of the single viral proteins, such as gp120 Env, Tat and Nef, for which updated reviews/book chapters are available. In this chapter, we describe the general activities of cytokines and their role in modulating HIV infection, both in vitro and in vivo, animal models and human tissues such as gut and lymphoid tissue, and finally ways to which cytokines have been used as immunotherapy, either alone or in combination with anti-retrovirals.

CYTOKINES OVERVIEW

Cytokines are low molecular weight (15-25 kDa) and soluble proteins, produced by both immune and non-immune cells, such as leukocytes and endothelial cells, which play fundamental roles for allowing communication between different cell types. Cytokines are soluble factors, characterized by peculiar features, such as:

- different cytokines inducing similar effects, redundancy,

- many cell types producing the same cytokine, pleiotropy,

- cytokines have short half-life and act as "autacoids", i.e. as factors released locally and acting on cells in close proximity to their release, influencing the physiology of the cells in their microenvironmen. this paracrine mode of action of cytokines is often associated to autocrine effects (i.e. the released cytokine interacts with specific receptors on the surface of the secreting cell) frequently aimed at curtailing its effect to the local microenvironment, Overproduction of cytokines (or their therapeutic administration) may exceptionally lead to their systemic dissemination as observed during sepsis,

- cytokines act via specific receptors as well as intracellular signalings, tuning tissue development, haematopoiesis, inflammation and immune responses [1]. Cytokine receptors add a further level of complexity. Frequently, a single cytokine or chemokine can interact with more than a single receptor on the surface of target cells; receptors are often released from the cells by proteolytic cleavage and act as buffering systems limiting the effect of the cognate cytokine. Some receptors act as "decoys" (for example, type II receptors for interleukin-1, IL-1) by sequestering the cytokine and thus impeding its interaction with functional receptors [2]. Chemokine receptors may accomplish a similar role still remaining expressed at the plasma membrane uncoupled from the transducing elements interacting with their cytoplasmic tails [2],

*****Address Correspondence to this Author Dr. Massimo Alfano at:** AIDS Immunopathogenesis Unit, Division of Immunology, Transplantation and Infectious Diseases, San Raffaele Scientific Institute, Via Olgettina, 58, 20132 Milan, Italy. E-mail: massimo.alfano@hsr.it

- analogues of cytokines and cytokine receptors are expresses by DNA viruses such as Poxviruses; these virus-encoded molecules favor virus capacity to infect cells by shutting-off inflammatory responses [3].

On the other hand, HIV proteins such as Tat Nef and Vpr, owns cytokine-like characteristics. Indeed, Tat induces the expression and release of cytokines from infected cells or upon being uptake by uninfected neighboring cells. On the other side, HIV accessory proteins Nef and VpR are internalized in infected cells only by virions [4]. Depending on the cell type, receptor engagement (In the case of extracellular Tat), the effect of these viral proteins is variable, but often involves modulation of cytokines or cytokine receptors.

All physiological and pathological processes are tuned by multiple interactions involving cellular phenotypes and soluble factors, also involving the complex network of cytokines and their receptors. Thus, cytokines levels in peripheral circulation are very low [5] but drastically increased in response to pathologies. On the other hand, solube cytokines receptors (sIL-1r, sIL-2r, sIL-6r) can be easily detected in serum or other biological fluids even in healthy individuals [5], likely in order to prevent systemic effects of cytokines thus limiting their action at athe autocrine/paracrine levels.

Cytokines control both innate and specific immune responses, including the on-off state of inflammatory processes [6], and specific immune responses. They can also exert mitogenic activity or promote growth arrest, cell differentiation and, in some case, trigger apoptotic pathways [7]. Cytokines are conventionally subdivided into pro- and anti-inflammatory molecules, whereas some of them exert predominant immunoregolatory effects, for example in terms of polarization towards Th1 (cellular immune response, phagocyte-dependent), Th2 (humoral immune response, phagocyte-independent) [8] and, more recently, T regulatory (Treg) [9] and Th17 inflamamtory cells [10].

Due to their fundamental role in the above processes, chronic dysregulation of cytokines production or action is thought to have a central role in the development of pathological processes, such as autoimmunity [11], tumor development and metastasis, AIDS pathogenesis, as well as. to modulate the expression of multi-drug receptors, such as P-gp [12], thus influencing the bioavailability of drugs.

Cytokines are among the very first molecules released during inflammatory processes, either of bacterial or viral origin, independently of antigen specificity. Acute inflammation represents the first line of defense towards pathogens, and is characterized by a very fast and finely chronologically controlled expression of cytokines. In fact, in the case of bacterial infection inflammatory cytokines are secreted within 4-8 hours (with the production of TNF-α, followed by IL-1 and IL-6) after tissue localization of the pathogen. Inflammatory cytokines produced by resident macrophages enhances endothelial permeability (TNF-α and IL-1), favors recruitment of leukocytes (IL-8 and chemokines) to the site of inflammation, as well as to induce the cytotoxic mechanisms (via IL-12 induced secretion of INF-γ by T cells) of the recruited leukocytes (i.e., neutrophils and monocytes). The release of inflammatory cytokines is then followed by production of anti-inflammatory cytokines, such as IL-4, IL-10, IL-13 and TGF-β, and cytokine decoy receptors.

CLASS I IFNs

(IFN-α and IFN-β). In peripheral blood mononuclear cells (PBMC) IFN-α is mainly produced by monocytes and plasmacytoid dendritic cells (PDC). IFN-α influences antibody (Ab) production, cell cytotoxicity by T and NK cells, activity of T suppressor/regulatory cells, and anti-tumor activity [13]. Regarding HIV, both IFN-α and IFN-β have the ability to influence many steps of the virus life cycle, either pre- or post-integration, including steps involved in virion maturation [14].

Indded, IFN-α has shown the capacity to inhibit both reverse transcription and viral expression from integrated provirus in acutely infected primary cells [15], HIV replication in primary monocyte-derived macrophages (MDM) [16] and virion release from chronically infected cell lines [17]. Indeed, in the last year another anti-HIV mechanism attributed to IFN-α has been shown in many primary cells, such as human macrophages [18], PDC [19], resting but not activated CD4+ T cells [20] and brain microvascular endothelial cells [21]. This mechanism relies on the ability of IFN-α to induce oversexpression of active form of apolipoprotein B m-RNA-editing enzyme-catalytic polypeptide-like (APOBEC) family members, such as APOBEC-3G and 3F, 3A and 3C, thus preventing the reverse transcription of incoming virus [22].

HIV infection has been reported to influence IFN-α expression dependending on the cell type. In fact, in HIV+ individuals DC are chracterized by decresed levels of IFN-αexpression [23], whereas expression by PDC is inversely correlated with viral load [24]. Indeed, HIV+ individuals on highly active anti-retroviral therapy (HAART) were characterized by decreased plasma viremia, and increased number of IFN-αproducing PDC [25]. However, other reports did not show influence of viral load and HAART on the capacity of PDC to produce IFN-α [26]. In another anatomical compartment, such as the cerebrospinal fluid, levels of IFN-α have been positively associated with viral load and the staging of AIDS dementia complex [27].

IFN-γ

T and NK cells represent the cellular source of IFN-γ. In HIV individuals, levels of IFN-γ have been found elevated both in the peripheral blood compartment and in the germinal centers of lymph nodes (LN) [28].

IFN-γ can mediate either suppressive [29] or upregulatory effects on HIV replication as a function of whether cells are acutely or chronically infected by HIV and whether other stimuli are present. In chronically HIV infected promonocytic U1 cells IFN-γ has been reported to induced viral expression [30], either by itself or with TNF-α [31]. Similar findings have also been reported in primary cells, demonstrating reduced viral replication in IL-2 stimulated PBMC infected *in vitro* in which IFN-γ has been neutralized [32]. On the other side, IFN-γ stimulation of infected monocytic cells may lead to the redirection of the primary site of virion budding from the plasma membrane to Golgi-derived intracytoplasmic vacuoles [30], today recognized belonging to multivesicular bodies (MVB), and resembling morphological features typical of brain macrophages of individuals with HIV encephalitis [33,34]. Of interest is the fact that signaling generated by IFN-γ unrelated molecules, including CCL2/MCP-1 [35], and urokinase/urokinase receptor [36], may induce similar features in infected and differentiated monocytic cells. These observation suggest the existence of a common target of diverse signaling pathways that can influence the "choice" of the virion assembly machinery to target either the plasma membrane or endosomal membranes [37]. Of interest, this seems to be restricted to mononuclear phagocytes, although inactivation of VpU results in similar features in T lymphocytes [38].

IFN-γ, as well as IL-10, production increased during the interaction of infected DC and T cells leading to HIV spreading [39]. In particular, the HIV matrix protein p17 Gag upregulated the secretion of IFN-γ and TNF-α in human NK cells stimulated with IL-12 and IL-15 [40].

Concerning the interaction between the cytokine network and the virus in animal models, it has been shown that IFN-γ mRNA expression in PBMC, LN, bronchoalveolar mononuclear cells [41-43], and in intestinal lamina propria lymphocytes [44] is increased during primary SIV infection of macaques. At later time points, IFN-γexpression decreased in SIV infected macaques receiving IL-12 vs. controls [45] as also observed in SIV-infected PBMC stimulated [44]. During primary SIV infection of macaques, upregulation of IFN-γmRNA expression in PBMC, LN, bronchoalveolar mononuclear cells [41-43], and intestinal lamina propria lymphocytes [44] has been associated with the containment of viral replication.

PRO-INFLAMMATORY CYTOKINES IN HIV INFECTION

Pro-inflammatory cytokines, including TNF-α, IL-1β, and IL-6 have been associated to increased levels of HIV replication *in vivo* and *in vitro*. At the molecular level, both NF-kB and AP-1 can mediate transcriptional activation of HIV expression either by a direct interaction with DNA binding sites in the HIV LTR or, in the case of AP-1, via binding to an intragenic enhancer [46]. However, additional post-transcriptional control of virus replication is likely to play an important role in cytokine-mediated upregulation of virus replication, as discussed in the case of IL-4, IL-6 and IL-13 [47-50].

IL-2 is a central regulator of T cell function and survival produced by activated T lymphocytes and, very recently, also by microbial stimulation of DC [51,52]. IL-2 induces proliferation and activation of both CD4$^+$

and CD8[+] T cells [53], potentiates the cytotoxicity of CD8[+] T lymphocytes and NK cells and stimulates B cell function, therefore playing a major role in the containment of viral infections and in the elimination of intracellular organism [54]. IL-2 expression in LN is barely detectable at all stages of HIV infection in both adults [55] and children [56], although increased expression of this cytokine has been associated with reduction of plasma viremia [57]. In one study, overexpression of IL-2 was observed in HIV infected tonsils [58], whereas a modest inhibition of cytokine expression has been independently reported in the intestinal mucosa [59]. IL-2 mRNA expression in LN of rhesus macaques has been correlated to SIV replication early after infection [41]. PHA-stimulated lymphocytes of SIV infected monkeys, as well as of HIV-infected chimpanzees, showed decreased IL-2 transcription and cell proliferation [42,60].

IL-2 production is deficient in HIV infected individuals as well as after *in vitro* infection of PBMC, a defect that has been correlated to an increased production of IL-4 and IL-10 [61]. IL-2 expression in LN is barely detectable at all stages of HIV infection in both adults [62] and childrens [56]. In macaques, IL-2 mRNA expression in LN early after infection has been correlated to SIV replication [41]. Increased IL-2 expression was found in HIV infected tonsil [58] and LN [63] following HAART, concomitantly with reduction of plasma viremia [57]. *In vitro,* IL-2 strongly synergized with IL-4, causing viral production from *in vitro* infected mature thymocytes [64], an effect associated with increased expression of CCR5 and CXCR4 [65].

IL-6 is produced by CD4+ T-cells, mast cells, monocytes, macrophages, fibroblasts, and endothelial cells [66], and is a multifunctional cytokine in that it participates in growth and differentiation of B- and T-cell effectors, and hematopoetic precursors, as well as by inducing a pyretic acute phase reaction, and promoting tumor growth and angiogenesis [66].

IL-6 expression has been reported increased in HIV-infected thymocytes [67], thymic epithelial cells [68], and in LN of both HIV-infected individuals [69] and rhesus macaques infected with SIV. Furthermore, IL-6 expression has been correlated to viral replication [41], although other studies did not support this observation [70]. Together with IL-6, IL-1β expression was also found elevated in both HIV and SIV infected LN [41] and thymocytes [67]. HAART has been shown to decrease both IL-1β and IL-6 expression in LN, followed by a decrease of the number of LN-associated T lymphocytes with concomitant increase in peripheral blood [71].

IL-7. Thymic epithelial cells represent the main cellular source of IL-7. As validated by studies in immunodeficient individuals [72], IL-7 plays a master role for T cell development and homeostasis [73]

Related to HIV infection, it has been demonstrated that in the thymus IL-7 is crucial for inducing HIV replication [74] and protecting thymocytes from apoptosis by superinduction of Bcl-2 expression [75]. On the other hand, apoptosis by IL-7 has been observed in both astrocytes and neuronal cell line [76] and primary naïve and memory T cells [77]. Moreover IL-7, as well as IL-2, IL-15 and IL-21, has recently been reported to induce expression of programmed death (PD) pathway in memory T cells and monocytes/macrophages in PBMC, in both healthy and HIV+ individuals receiving IL-2 immunotherapy [78]; these findings have been interpreted as that IL-7 could reduce the immune-mediated damage of the host induced TCR engagement. Both IL-7 and IL-15 have been reported to increase the function of NK cells from infected individuals, with the latter being more potent [79]. The two cytokines activated different cytolytic mechanisms, namely Fas and TRAIL mediated, respectively, resulting in the *ex vivo* depletion of HIV-infected PBMC isolated from infected individuals [79].

In both HIV+ individuals [80,81] and uninfected children born from HIV[+] mothers [82] elevated levels of IL-7 have been reported, thus suggesting that exposure to HIV or HIV proteins across the placenta may perturb thymopoiesis.

In support of the above findings, a correlation between i) circulating levels of IL-7, ii) CD4[+] T cells loss, and iii) plasma viremia has been demonstrated [83].

Indeed, it has been reported that IL-7 levels before therapy are predictive of virological but not immunological response to ART in both HIV+ children and adults [80,84]. On the other hand, a correlation between plasma levels of IL-7 and increased CXCR4 expression by peripheral blood mononuclear cells (PBMC) has been observed in children infected with X4 viruses, while reversion of their viral phenotype to CCR5 use induced by highly active antiretroviral therapy (HAART) was associated with reduced plasmatic levels of both viremia and IL-7 [85,86]. Although a positive correlation was observed between CXCR4 levels and the identification of X4 viruses [87], the levels of circulating IL-7 were not found correlated to those of CXCR4 on PBMC of infected adults [85,86]. Independently, a decrease of cells expressing the IL-7 receptor has been observed in PBMC and lymphoid tissues of macaques infected with SIV as a function of disease progression [88], likely explaining why elevated levels of IL-7 are not sufficient to maintain T cell homeostasis in this animal model [89].

IL-7 was early investigated in the context of HIV infection, replication and cell depletion in the thymus [75]. This effect at has been recently linked to a skewed enhancement of CXCR4-dependent (X4) virus replication in mature thymocytes concomitantly with an increased expression of CXCR4 [87]. In addition, IL-7 has been shown to upregulate CXCR4 expression in both naïve T cells [90], PBMC and thymocytes [87,91], an effect that has been correlated with the emergence of X4 HIV-1 variants in peripheral blood [92]. This hypothesis was supported by the observation of increased plasma levels of both IL-7 and CXCL12 and upregulated expression of CXCR4 and plasma viremia [93].

When *ex vivo* CD8-depleted PBMC of infected individuals under effective HAART were incubated with various stimuli, IL-7 was identified as the most effective HIV-inductive cytokine in terms of reactivation of latent proviral DNA, while IL-2 alone was ineffective unless combined with the mitogen phytohemagglutinin (PHA) [94]. Furthermore, the analysis of the viral quasispecies induced by IL-7 vs. PHA+IL-2 suggested the possibility that segregated pools of latently infected cells were activated by the two stimuli [94]. However, more recent studies did not observe an inductive effect of IL-7 on latent HIV-infected CD8-depleted cells of infected individuals [95], and synergistic anti-viral effects have been reported by incubating these cells in combination with IFN-α [95].

On the other hand, IL-7 was early documented to increase HIV replication in CD8-depleted PBMC of infected individuals stimulated with anti-CD3 Ab [96,97], to enhance HIV replication in resting naïve CD4$^+$ T lymphocytes, an effect that was correlated to the autocrine/paracrine release of other cytokines, such as IFN-γ, but also IL-4 and IL-10 [98], and been reported to synergize with TNF-α in sustaining HIV spreading in single CD4$^+$ thymocytes by inducing the upregulation of the p75 TNF receptor [74]. Finally, NFAT and not NF-kB was identified as molecular effector of IL-7 induced upregulation of HIV replication [98].

Concerning the potential role of IL-7 in the modulation of infection of macrophages, both inhibition [99] and enhancement of virus replication [100] have been reported almost simultaneously. In the latter study, HIV infection or cell stimulation with extracellular Tat upregulated the levels of expression of the IL-7Rα, increasing cellular responsiveness to the related cytokine [100].

In spite of its potentiation of HIV replication, IL-7 remains a potentially important cytokine for the immunologic reconstitution of HIV infected individuals, given its ability to contribute to CTL development [101], and by the fact that in HIV$^+$ individuals and children HAART+IL-2 treatment induced significant increase of CD4$^+$ cells and plasma levels of IL-7 [102,103], and increased expression of IL-7 receptor (CD127) on CD8$^+$ T cells [104].

IL-12 is a heterodimeric cytokine produced by macrophages and DC upon the encounter with the pathogen [105]. It is the most potent inducers of Th1 cell polarization and IFN-γ production, although it also induces proliferation and stimulatory activity on T and NK cells, and CTL maturation [106].

Decreased levels of IL-12 production have been reported from from PBMC of HIV$^+$ individuals [107] or SIV$_{mac251}$ infected macaques [108,109]. However, even on HIV chronically infected cell lines, cells of HIV infected individuals or SIV infected animals, IL-12 was shown to rescue i) proliferation of T and NK cells, ii) IFN-γ production by T and NK cells, iii) Ag presentation and accessory functions of macrophages and DC, and iv) the cytolytic capacity of CTL and NK cells [107-112]. On the other side, IL-12 has been reported to influence HIV replication, either by enhancing [113], or inhibiting virus replication [114]. The inhibitory effect was correlated to CCR5 down-regulation [115] as consequence of cells stimulation with the cytokine before infection.

Despite the reported decreased production of IL-12 from PBMC of HIV$^+$ individuals or SIV$_{mac251}$ infected macaques, expression of IL-12 in LN was found to be upregulated during acute SIV infection and this was correlated to the extent of viral replication [41,42].

IL-15 is secreted by macrophages and NK cells and not by activated T cells (like IL-2) and is a Th1 cytokine [116] sharing with IL-2 the βγ chains of the receptor complex produced by MP, thus sharing with IL-2 many activities, such as the ability to induce T cell proliferation and activation [117].

On the other hand, IL-15 is more potent than IL-2 in stimulating both NK cell maturation, differentiation [118] and survival, and NK cells function in HIV+ individuals [117], including the growth and survival of naïve rather than memory T cells [118], secretion of IFN-γ and of CCR5-binding chemokines [119]. In fact, in one study, IL-15 stimulation of PBMC enhanced both HIV replication and secretion of CCR5-binding chemokines; however, IL-15 induced levels of CC chemokines (<10 ng/ml) were likely insufficient for inhibiting HIV infection and replication [120]. Thus, IL-15 was shown to enhance HIV replication in acutely infected PBMC or T cells with a predilection for R5 HIV strains [32,113,121,122]; as previously shown for IL-2 [32], this effect was caused by the induction of pro-inflammatory cytokines including TNF-α, IFN-γ, and IL1-β and by the up-regulation of CCR5. However, IL-15 levels did not correlate with HIV replication in *in vitro* infected PBMC [117].

In vitro, recombinant HIV-1 gp120 Env induced a 2-7 fold increase of IL-15 production from chimpanzees whole blood [123]. IL-15 has been reported to inhibit *in vitro* HIV-1 infection of activated PBMC [79], likely as a consequent of its capacity of inducing expression of IFNs and CCR5-binding chemokines from NK cells [79].

In contrast to these studies, others have observed that IL-15 either did not affect HIV replication *in vitro* or *ex vivo* (3) or that it enhanced it in both primary unfractionated PBMC [113,124], CD4$^+$ T lymphocytes [125] and T cell lines [113,124]. This latter effect has been linked to the capacity of IL-15 to induce expression of apolipoprotein B mRNA-editing enzyme catalytic polypeptide-like 3G (APOBEC3G) (29) and to promote its shift from an active (anti-HIV) to an inactive high molecular weight form in primary T cells [126].

Ex vivo increased levels of IL-15 were detected in histocultures established from lymph nodes of both HIV$^+$ individuals [127] and macaques infected with SIV [88]. In addition, IL-15 reduced the spontaneous apoptosis of both PBMC [128] and HIV-specific CD8$^+$ T cells [129] isolated from acutely HIV infected individuals. Moreover, IL-15 induced the chemotaxis and potentiated the fungicidal activity of neutrophils from HIV$^+$ individuals [130].

Low levels of circulating IL-15, that increased in response to effective HAART, have been observed in primary HIV infection (PHI) [131,132] and during disease progression [133]. Furthermore, IL-15 levels are reported decreased in both therapy-naïve patients in advanced stage of disease [132,134,135] and in HIV$^+$ individuals failing HAART [132], suggesting that either antiretroviral agents or their consequence on the immunological reconstitution of infected individuals may influence its secretion.

IL-17. Due to the recent findings about the selective depletion of CD4+ Th17 cells in the gut of HIV+ individuals [136,137] and SIV+ macaques [138], several authors have recently investigated the role of IL-17 in the modulation of HIV replication as well as its levels in infected individuals.

Indeed, serum levels of IL-17 are inversely correlated to levels of viremia, both in SIV-infected macaques [138] and HIV infected children [139]. In macaques and human this correlation is, at least in part, consequence of the fact that Th17 are infectable with SIV [138] and HIV [137], respectively; however, other authors mentioned that human Th17 are probably not infectable by HIV because CCR5 negative [139]. On the other an existing relationship (either direct or indirect, via cytokines or viral products) between viremia and levels of Th17 cells has also been proven by the fact that individuals on HAART partially accumulated Th17 cells in the gut mucosa [136].

Other findings in support of the relationship between viremia/IL-7 levels are from authors that reported that frequency of Th17 cells upon PMA/ionomycin stimulation is lower in HIV infected children with viremia levels higher than 50, versus either infected children with undetectable viremia or HIV negative. Nevertheless, Th17 are completely depleted in chronic infected individuals and animals, thus explaining the increased bacteremia (i.e., bacterial dissemination from the intestinal mucosa) observed in infected individuals and animals [140]. In fact, it has been proposed that because the lack of Th17 in the gut, thus lacking also recruitment of neutrophils.

On the other side, other authors were not able to show any correlation between viremia and levels of serum IL-17 [141], and even showed that upon SEB stimulation up to 2% of CD4+ T cells were able to express IL-17 [141]; however, this was a characteristic mostly of "early-infected individuals (less than 1 year of infection)", and not revealed in the other populations tested (i.e., chronic infection, LTNP, HAART treated individuals) [141]. These data are in partial agreement with those earlier reported, showing a significant increase in the constitutive production of IL-17 from peripheral CD4$^+$ T cells of asymptomatic HIV+ and treatment naïve individuals, further inducible by PMA/ionomycin stimulation [142]. However, these two last reports do not agree with the ones reported above.

IL-18 is a pro-inflammatory/Th1 cytokine produced by activated PBMC and epidermal cells that induces the production of IFN-γ from NK cells [143] and enhances the cytolytic potential of both NK cells and of CD8$^+$ cytotoxic T lymphocytes [143]. In virtue of its ability to induce Th1 response, IL-18 has been used as an adjuvant either in mice vaccinated with DNA expressing HIV-1 Nef, Gag/Tat/Nef, or Env [144]. As predicted, IL-18 treated animals showed an enhanced cellular response and decreased Ab production [145,146].

In vitro, both acute HIV infection or incubation of the THP-1 cell line with the accessory viral protein Nef induced expression of IL-18 [147]. As most pro-inflammatory cytokines, IL-18 induced HIV expression in chronically infected monocytic [148] and T cell lines [149] via induction of the release of endogenous TNF-α and IL-6 [148], as previously reported for PMA [150]. In contrast, other studies have indicated that IL-18 inhibited the acute *in vitro* infection of PBMC infection consequently to its capacity of inducing CD4 downmodulation and release of IFN-γ [151], as previously reported for the otherwise HIV-inductive cytokines TNF-α and IFN-γ [152]. These apparent discrepancies are mostly accounted for by the experimental design in that incubation of cells with high concentrations of these cytokines does result in a downregulation of different cell surface receptors, including CD4 and chemokine receptors, whereas stimulation of already infected cells (or lower concentrations of the same cytokines) results in the opposite effect of increasing virus expression, as previously discussed [153].

In vivo, increased serum levels of IL-18 have been observed during PHI/early infection in association with high levels of IFN-γ and reduced expression of CXCR4 from the surface of CD4+ T cells [154]. Although serum levels of IL-18 were found comparable in LTNP and HIV progressors [155], other studies indicated that they were higher in symptomatic *vs.* asymptomatic HIV$^+$ individuals, including children, or healthy individuals [155-159] and that they were correlated to disease progression [158,160]. Similar results were reported in macaques infected with pathogenic vs. non-pathogenic strains of simian HIV (SHIV) [161]. In partial contrast, a reduced capacity of secreting IL-18 from *ex vivo* stimulated PBMC was observed in those individuals characterized by high circulating levels of this cytokine [157,162,163]. This apparent discrepancy, in addition to a functional exhaustion of PBMC, could be explained by the fact that IL-18 can be secreted by activated platelets [164] as well as by the adipose tissue[165]. Indeed, higher levels of IL-18 have been observed in HIV+ individuals affected by lipodistrophy compared to those without lipodistrophy [165,166] as well as in HIV+ individuals with hypertriglyceridemia [167]. Successful HAART has been linked to reduction of IL-18 circulating levels [155,156,158,160]. In addition, increased IL-18 concentrations have been observed in the cerebrospinal fluid (CSF) of HIV$^+$ individuals with opportunistic infections, although not in those with HIV-associated dementia (HAD) [159].

IL-21 is mostly secreted by activated CD4+ T cells, including Th17 cells on which acts as an amplifier of their function [168], and targets several immune cells belonging to both lymphocytic and myelomonocytic lineages, as reviews elsewhere [169]. In fact, it has recently been reported that serum levels of IL-21 are significantly reduced in AIDS individuals and correlate with CD4+ T cell counts [170]. Concerning HIV infection, IL-21 has been shown to augment NK effector functions, such as perforin expression, in chronically HIV+ individuals [171]. Moreover, IL-21 has been shown to enhance CD8+ T cell function, including secretion of IFN-γ [172,173] and expression of perforin without inducing broad cellular activation or proliferation, in HIV+ individuals [174]. Furthermore, IL-21 has been shown to promote the expansion of HIV-specific CD8+ memory T cells [172,173] as well as the Ab-dependent cellular cytotoxicity (ADCC) and Complement-mediated lysis of antigen-expressing cells in synergy with IL-15 [172,173]. Therefore, IL-21 owns the potential for either immunotherapy or as a vaccine adjuvant. In fact, it has recently reported that, both alone and in combination with IL-15, IL-21 increased the magnitude of the response of mice vaccinated with DNA vaccine expressing the HIV-1 Env glycoprotein providing evidence of resistance to viral transmission [172].

IL-27. As for IL-12 and IL-23, IL-27 is also primarily produced by macrophages, monocytes, and DCs following their activation by pathogen recognized through Toll-like receptors (TLRs) [175,176]. In fact, IL-27 belongs to the IL-6/IL-12 family and can exert both pro- and anti-inflammatory effects as well as affecting T helper cell commitment, T cell proliferation and cytotoxic activity [177,178]. In fact, as for IL-12 and IL-23, IL-27 induces IFN-γ production by naive T cells and NK cells [175,176,179] and promotes Th commitment toward Th1 cell differentiation and proliferation [175,180,181]. In addition, it has been shown to affect the maturation of the Ab response by inducing isotype switching in B cells [182].

The potential role of IL-27 in HIV infection has been thus far investigated in the context of DC and antigen presentation. When DC derived from IFN-α stimulation were compared to those generated in mice immunized with CD40L and IL-4 they were found to be superior in inducing in vitro cross-priming of HIV-specific CD8+ T cells. Of interest is the fact that this effect was correlated to an enhanced expression of both IL-23 and IL-27 [183]. Furthermore, binding of human papilloma virus (HPV)-like particles (VLPs) to DC and induce the expression of IFN-α, IFN-γ and IL-10 and suppress the replication of both X4 and R5 HIV-1 without affecting the expression of HIV receptors and co-receptors. In addition, these VLPs induced the expression of IL-27 that inhibited HIV-1 replication in activated PBMCs, CD4+ T cells, and macrophages. However, very recently it has been shown that IL-27 inhibits in vitro HIV infection mainly of monocyte-derived macrophages, independently of the expression of IFNs [184].

TNF-α is released in its mature form as a trimer, and is produced by a wide variety of cells including T cells, macrophages [185] and dendritic cells [186]. In macrophages and DC, TNF synthesis can be induced by various pathogens including viruses, parasites, bacteria, LPS and as well as by cytokines (IL-1, IL-2, IFN-γ, GM-CSF, M-CSF, and TNF itself). On the other hand, TNF inhibits interferon-γ priming for production of high levels of IL-12 by macrophages [187]. Thus, by blocking TH1 cytokine production, TNF might limit the extent and duration of inflammatory response in vivo. Thus, chronic TNF exposure suppresses the response of both TH1 and TH2 subsets and attenuates T-cell receptor signalling [188]. TNF is produced in small quantities in quiescent cells, but becomes one of the major factors secreted in activated cells [185]. Thus chronic TNF stimulation suppresses T-cell function in vivo and might have important implications for understanding pathogenesis of chronic inflammatory diseases [188], such as represented by the HIV infection. Anti-inflammatory cytokines, such as TGF-β, IL-4 and IL-10 inhibits TNF-α production in macrophages

The multiple activities of TNF are mediated through two receptors; type 1 TNFR and type 2 TNFR with molecular masses of 60 and 80 kDa, respectively. Both TNFR are type I transmembrane glycoproteins and are present virtually on all cell but red blood cells, although TNFR1 is more ubiquitous, and TNFR2 is often more abundant on endothelial cells and cells of hematopoietic lineage.

TNFR1 is the major mediator of TNF biological functions including the effects on apoptosis and cytotoxicity. On the other hand, TNFR2 signaling appears to be mainly confined to cells of the immune system, and is involved in the proliferation of thymocytes [189], proliferative response of human mononuclear cells [190], in the induction of GM-CSF secretion, in the inhibition of early hematopoiesis [191], and in downregulating activated T cells by inducing apoptosis [192]. Indeed, the biological response to TNF is believed to be a result of the balance of multiple signals delivered via both TNFR1 and TNFR2. In fact, in latently HIV-infected lymphocytic cells (ACH-2), the TNFR1 plays a major role in stimulation of HIV production [193]. In contrast, when both TNFR are activated simultaneously by agonistic antibodies or co-culture with cells expressing a noncleavable membrane form of TNF, HIV production is downregulated, and cell death is enhanced [193].

HIV infection is characterized by a progressive depletion of $CD4^+$ T cells resulting in cellular immunodeficiency [194] and chronic status of inflammation, as highlighted by the increases in both cellular and soluble markers of immune activation, such as cellular markers (CD38, HLA-DR, CD44) and levels of neopterin, ß2 microglobulin, soluble CD30, TNF and the soluble form of TNFR2 [195].

In vitro, it has been shown that TNF modulates the viral cycle of HIV-1, in both T cells and macrophages, by targeting two main steps of the viral life cycle such as viral entry and transcription.

TNF has been shown to inhibit entry (either membrane fusion or viral uncoating, but preceeding reverse transcription) of R5 HIV-1 strain into macrophages [152]. On the other hand, both CD4 and CCR5 are downregulated on the cell surface by TNF [196,197], that might result from increased CCR5-binding chemokine production following TNF treatment [198]. Another explanation is that TNF triggers the release of GM-CSF, that has been shown to downregulate CCR5 and subsequently block entry of R5 viruses into macrophages [199].

The second viral step influence by TNF is the viral transactivation. In fact, recombinant TNF stimulates HIV-1 replication in chronically infected U1 and ACH-2 cell lines through activation of NF-κB and subsequent transactivation of the proviral LTR [150]. Stimulation with TNF of HIV-1 replication in U1 cell lines is mediated by engagement of TNFR1 [200] and activation of NF-kB. Moreover, even HIV expression by the phorbol esters such as phorbol-myristate-acetate (PMA), a broadly used chemical agent that activates protein kinase C, also induced viral transcription and expression in U1 and ACH2 cell lines at least in part by triggering an autocrine pathway mediated by endogenous TNF-α [150]. In addition to cell lines, TNF-α sustains HIV replication also in primary MDM and PBMC [32]. Of note, even TNF-β (also known as lymphotoxin-α, LT-α) a molecule that utilizes the same receptors of TNF-α, showed a similar effects than TNF-α, at least in the chronically infected cells lines [201].

The relevance of TNF-a/b inducing HIV expression via NF-kB is stressed by the fact that clade B HIV-1 possesses two binding sites for NF-kB in close proximity of the transcription start site, whereas clade C virus, spreading in Sub-Saharan Africa, displays three binding regions, and thus express higher levels of virions upon TNF-α stimulation, than clade B or A (1 NF-kB binding site) [202]. Of interest, HIV-2, a related AIDS causing virus characterized by slower disease progression and inefficient vertical transmission from mother to child as well as its closely related SIV have only one NF-kB binding site [203].

Moreover, TNF-α increases HIV replication by inducing NF-kB activation [204]. In tonsil and lymph node, HIV does not influence TNF-α expression [205], although enhances virion trapping [206]. In SIV infection of rhesus macaques strongly correlates with TNF-α expression in lymph nodes [41], whereasTNF-α, induced SIV production from simian alveolar macrophages [207].

Monocytes and tissue macrophages are amongst the major cell sources of this cytokine and their stimulation by bacterial products, such as lipopolysaccharide (LPS), or other microbial agents such as *P. falciparum* [208], may increase both cytokine expression and HIV replication [209]. In vivo, TNF-α may increase HIV replication at both mucosal [210,211] and systemic [212-214] levels, as well as in HIV spreading in the central nervous system (CNS) [215,216]. However, because the ability of TNF also to inhibit HIV entry, into macrophages, LPS/bacterial infections might result in a controlled viral production within infected macrophages that could be critical to avoid macrophage death and to optimize viral production.

Conversely, at least some HIV strains and/or their gp120 Env [10,31] can upregulate TNF-α secretion from macrophages as well as from T and B lymphocytes [217].

In vivo, a positive correlation between viral replication and the increased levels of TNF-α in the sera [218] LN [41,219], PBMC [220,221], bronchoalveolar lavage mononuclear cells [219], and microglial cells [221] has been shown in macaques infected with SIV. Moreover, high levels of TNF-α[219,222,223] has also been reported in vaginal mucosa, favoring infection of HIV clade C [224-227], possibly in virtue of the transcription binding sites (3 sites for NF-kB and 1 site for AP1) forming its LTR promoter [202]. Converserly, no substantial up- or down modulation of TNF-αexpression was observed in tonsils and LN of infected individuals [205], although an enhanced virion trapping has been correlated with the expression of this cytokine during primary infection [206].

ANTI-INFLAMMATORY CYTOKINES IN HIV INFECTION

Anti-inflammatory cytokines, like IL-4, IL-10, IL-13, IL-19, IL-20 and TGF-β appear later than inflammatory cytokines and increase the expression of decoy receptors, limit the production of pro-inflammatory cytokines and chemokines (mandatory for leukocyte recruitment) and cytotoxic processes. Regarding HIV infection, anti-inflammatory cytokines have been reported to either activate or inhibit HIV replication, depending on different experimental conditions and models of infection, making difficult to assign them a precise role in the balance between virus replication and latency.

IL-4 and IL-10 are the prototypic anti-inflammatory cytokines that downregulate tissue inflammation by switching off pro-inflammatory effects of Th1 cytokines such as IFN-α and TNF.

IL-4 is produced by CD4+ Th cells, mast cells [228] and macrophages upon recognition of extracellular pathogens [229]. Upon TLR-mediated activation of DC, naïve T cells release IL-4 serving as growth factor for the expansion and activation of Th2 cells [230] secreting IL-4, IL-5 and IL-6 [231]. Th2 cytokines inhibit the development of Th1 cells and, consequently, cell-mediated immune responses [232]. On the other side, IL-4 has also been reported to induce over-expression of DC-SIGN on in vitro differentiated DC [233], thus boosting both the ability of DC to interact with pathogens and the above described mechanism.

Concerning HIV infection, IL-4 can up-regulate CXCR4 and down-regulate CCR5, thus potentially playing a role in the so called "phenotypic switch" from R5 to X4 HIV-1 strains, an event occurring at late stage of disease in approximately 50% of individuals infected with clade B HIV-1 [234-239]. *In vitro*, IL-4 has been reported to induce virus replication on freshly isolated monocytes but to inhibit in MDM, depending on its ability to inhibit the levels of pro-inflammatory cytokines in the two cellular systems [240].

IL-10 is secreted by DC and Th2 cells [241]. This cytokine shuts off T cell activation because of its ability to inhibit the production of pro-inflammatory cytokines and chemokines, as well as the expression of DC-costimulatory molecules [242].

IL-10 has been reported to upregulate *in vitro* CXCR4 expression and X4 HIV infection of DC [243]. However, this effect did not alter the efficiency of viral transmission to autologous CD4$^+$ T cells, since this process involves DC-SIGN and not conventional viral receptors, such as CXCR4 [243]. In a similar way, IL-10 has been founf to enhance CCR5 expression on freshly isolated monocytes and thus their susceptibility to R5 infection [234]. However, other reports have shown that IL-10 inhibits in vitro HIV infection in macrophages [244,245].

As reported for other cytokines, depending on the cellular models and experimental conditions (in particular levels of exogenously added IL-10) both inhibitory and inductive effects on HIV replication have been reported. Indeed, in MDM inhibition of viral replication was correlated to the prevention of the synthesis and release of endogenous pro-inflammatory cytokines, such as TNF-α and IL-6 [246], whereas lower concentrations of IL-10 induced HIV replication, an effect that has been correlated to the cooperation with the released TNF-α and IL-6, as demonstrated in the chronically infected U1 cells [247-249].

IL-10 levels has been found elevated in lymph nodes of HIV-infected individuals [55,250,251], although progression to AIDS is characterized by decreased expression an event that has been correlated with the expression of an IL-10 promoter variant [252]. In SCID mice reconstituted with human cells, such as hu-PBL-SCID and thy/liv-SCID-hu-mice, IL-10 levels have been correlated to the activation state of human cells [253]. However, IL-10 has been shown to induce up-regulation of MHC-I on CD4+CD8+ human thymocytes [254] and to inhibit IFN-γ production and HIV replication [244,255].

IL-13 is produced by mononuclear phagocytes and its decreased plasma levels in HIV+ individuals have been associated with the progression of disease [256]. In fact, effective antiretroviral therapy, such as HAART+IL-2 increased IL-13 plasma levels [257]. Unfortunately, side-effect such as intestinal epithelial atrophy has been reported in SIV-infected macaques treated with IL-13 [258].

IL-13 has been reported to inhibit HIV replication via indirect mechanisms, such as downregulation of CD4 [259], CCR5 [238,259] and CXCR4 [238,256,259-261] in MDM or HIV expression by induction of an endogenous IL-1β/IL-1 receptor antagonist balance in favor of the latter in chronically infected U1 cells stimulated with LPS and GM-CSF [262]. On the other hand, IL-13 did not inhibit HIV replication in activated T cells [48,263].

Finally, IL-13 has been reported to upregulated DC-SIGN expression on monocytes [264,265], although it did influence the ability of monocytes to transmit the virus T cells [264].

IL-19 and *IL-20* belong to the anti-inflammatory cytokines of the IL-10 family, and are produced mostly by monocytes during inflammation [266]. They act predominantly on non immunological tissue and organs, such as the skin, lungs and various internal organs, including reproductive organs [266]. No information is available on their potential involvement in HIV infection, although upregulated expression of both cytokines has been reported following stimulation of mammary and amniotic epithelial cells with extracellular Tat [267].

TGF-β is a potent anti-inflammatory cytokine, secreted by hemopoietic, endothelial, and connective tissue cells. Different from other cytokines, TGF-β is produced as inactive cytokine and it became activated by proteolytic cleavage once secreted [268]. Active TGF-β influences cell cycle, differentiation, wound healing, angiogenesis and apoptosis, and its potency and multiple activities are likely also due to the fact that it is stored by the extracellular matrix. Enhanced TGF-β expression has been postulated to suppress macrophages as well as T and B lymphocyte function [269,270].

In vivo, increased levels of TGF-β have been reported in the sera of AIDS patients with <50 CD4$^+$ T lymphocytes/μl [271] and in the brain tissue of HIV$^+$ individuals with HIV encephalitis [272], and cerebro-spinal fluid (CSF). Indeed, increased levels of TGF-β mRNA has been reported reported in i) mononuclear cells infiltrating the kidney in patients with HIV-associated renal disease [273], ii) both infected and non infected cells resident in the brain of HIV infected individuals [274] and iii) PBMC of AIDS patients [275]. These findings have also been confirmed in *ex vivo* infected PBMC, shown produce increased levels of TGF-β upon stimulation.

According to the above *in vivo* findings, such as overexpression of TGF-β from uninfected cells in HIV+ individuals, stimulation with exogenous Tat or gp120 Env proteins can upregulate TGF-β expression in PBMC [276], monocytes [277], NK cells [278], bone marrow-derived macrophages [279], chondrocytes [280], CD8$^+$ T cells [281], and CNS cells [282]. In fact, *in vitro* HIV infection of human PBMC, macrophages and astrocytes increase TGF-β expression [274,283].

It has also been reported that TGF-β induces HIV replication , either by NF-kB-dependent viral transcription in cell lines [284] or by upregulating CCR5 and CXCR4 expression in MDM [285]. However, different studies indicated that TGF-β could either induce or suppress HIV transcription and replication in MDM as a function of whether the cells were stimulated with the cytokine before or after infection [286-290]. Of note, increased levels of TGF-β in CSF were found inversely correlated with both viral load and the severity of AIDS-dementia complex [291].

ROLE OF CYTOKINES ON HIV REPLICATION IN THE GUT AND LYMPHOID TISSUES

Evaluation of plasma viremia and CD4$^+$ T cell count in peripheral blood are the two main parameters tested in order to evaluate progression of HIV infection. However, these two parameters are the consequence of what happened into tissues. In fact, crucial events of HIV pathogenesis occur in lymphoid tissue [292], CNS [293], and gut and vaginal mucosa [294]. Discussed below are the main anatomical sites such as the lymphoid tissue resident in the gut and vaginal mucosae, at at which HIV gain the entry into the host, and the secondary lymphoid organs (i.e., tonsils) that favor viral spreading. Of note, not only after sexual intercourse but even after virus inoculation via contaminated blood/blood products and ingestion of milk from HIV+ mothers [295] the gut mucosa and gut-associated lymphoid tissue (GALT) are highly infected [296]. Thus lymphoid tissue resident in the gut and vaginal mucosa represent the primary site of infection and CD4$^+$ T cells depletion during HIV acute infection, as first reported in 1989 [297] and more recently emphasized [298].

Gut. Activated memory T cells have been shown to be the preferential target of HIV [299], and GALT is highly prone to HIV infection because it contains 60% of total CD4+ T cells [300], mainly of memory phenotype expressing activation markers [301] as well as high levels of IL-2 and IL-2R [302]. Related to the cellular phenotype, it has been shown that higher percentage of CD4+ cells resident in the gut mucosa express the chemokine receptor CCR5, and even at greater levels, than those present in blood [303,304] and tonsil [305], whereas no differences (both in the percentage and levels of expression) were observed for CXCR4 [304]. Thus, gut mucosa appears to provide a cellular environment highly susceptible to HIV infection, in particular for R5 strains. In fact, in vitro R5 infection of gut mucosa resulted in increased replication when compared to either PBMC [304] or tonsils [305]. On the other hand, it is of note that CD4+ cells resident in the gut mucosa are also infectable in vitro with the HIV-1 X4 strain [303-305], whereas no data about in vivo X4 infection are available [306]. In fact, this tissue probably represent the main barrier preventing X4 but favouring R5 infection [307]. Thus, it could be argued that other factors independently of cellular phenotype are involved.

In fact, over the cellular phenotype the extracellular environment and in particular the cytokine/chemokine milieu exerts a profound effect on HIV infection and replication. In fact, the cytokine microenvironment in GALT and vagina mucosa influence HIV subtype localization; high levels of IL-2, IL-7 and IL-15 in GALT [308] and of TNF-α[223] in vaginal mucosa favor infection of HIV clade C [224], possibly in virtue of the transcription binding sites (3 sites for NF-kB and 1 site for AP1) forming its LTR promoter.

Regarding cytokines, gut and viral pathogenesis many findings have been reported either in SIV infected animal and HIV+ individuals. Although the time points at which biopsies are collected are very different in the two systems (i.e., primary infection in SIV infected animals, chronic infection in HIV+ individuals), most of the findings reported in SIV infected animals have then been reproduced in humans. Regarding cytokines and SIV infection, it has been demonstrated that upon SIV infection viral replication and cytokines expression occurs at the same time points [223,309] in the different tissues, although with different levels of cytokine expression [223]. In particular, that mucosal tissue of genital tract express highest levels than systemic lymphoid tissues, and the gut even less IFN-I than LN [223]. In particular, it has been reported that the pro-inflammatory cytokines (TNF-α, MIP-1α, IL-6, CXCL8/IL-8 and CCL5/RANTES) [223,309] are associated with the peak of viral expression from mucosa, whereas expression of IFNs occurs at later time points [223]. Of note, IFN-γ expression is particularly enhanced in vagina and gut mucosae, than lymph nodes [223] (vagina>colon>lymph nodes), whereas CXCL8/IL-8 in colon more than in vagina (colon>vagina), whereas IL-12 was more expressed in lymph nodes than gut (lymph nodes>gut). The above findings also suggest that the i) cytokine milieu present in colon (i.e., high levels of pro-inflammatory cytokines, low levels of IFNs) and ii) kinetic of cytokines expression is in favor of viral replication. Moreover, that TNF-α, IFN-γ and CXCL8/IL-8 favor apoptosis of infected and non-infected cells, thus leading to the consistent lymphocyte depletion of gut. On this latter point, it has also been shown that both CD4+ and CD8+ T cells in lymphoid tissues, gut and vaginal tract express lower levels of IL-7R [310], thus preventing/counter-acting the positive effect of enhanced levels of IL-7 [310] on cellular proliferation.

Similarly to SIV, colon biopsy of chronically infected and under antiretroviral treatment HIV+ individuals (compared to healthy controls) were characterize to have higher levels of chemokine receptors CCR5 and CXCR4 [311], as well as of CCL5/RANTES, CCL3/MIP-1α and CCL4/MIP-1β [311,312], IL-2 [312], TNF-α [312], IL-12 [312], IL-4 [312], IFN-γ [312], CXCL10 [313] and IL-1α [313]. Another similitude with SIV+ animals was the fact that high levels of CCL5/RANTES in gut were associated with high viral loads [311], suggesting that b-chemokines are not an in vivo correlate of immune-protection. In this regard, CCR5 ligands can stimulate the replication of X4 viruses in activated primary T cells [314,315], as well as other chemokines of both the CC (such as CCL2/MCP-1) [315,316] and CXC (for example CXCL8/IL-8 and CXCL1/Gro-α) families can stimulate HIV replication in both T cells and MDM [49,50]. In addition, it is unclear whether physiological levels of these molecules may ultimately exert a positive preventive role in natural infection or whether they would ultimately favor viral spreading by recruiting T cells at the site of virus infection.

In the last years an in vitro system for the culture of gut biopsy/explant has been developed [305], providing important clues about acute HIV infection of this tissue. In fact, it has been shown that GALT supports very well infection with both R5 and X4 strains [305]. On the other hand, GALT does not express b-chemokines upon HIV infection, as otherwise observed in tonsils [305]. However, several immunomodulatory cytokines were upregulated upon HIV infection, such as GM-CSF, TGF-β, IL-16, IP-10, MIG, IL-10 [305]. These information suggest that in GALT acute HIV infection (at least in this in vitro system) does not increase the expression of CCR5-binding chemokines, thus explaining, at least in part, why gut mucosa is more prone than tonsillar tissue to R5 infection [305]. In conclusion, the cellular phenotype (activated memory T cells), the high percentage of CD4+ T positive for CCR5 expression, the high levels of CCR5 and the inability of HIV to induce CCR5-binding chemokines may explain why GALT is highly prone to R5 infection; these characteristics are then translated in the high cellular depletions observed after R5 infection in the gut, not/poorly observed in lymphoid tissues [305]. The above characteristics do not explain why acute X4 infection in vivo normally does not show up, a finding reported also in vitro by using intestinal lamina propria isolated mononuclear cells stimulated with CD2/CD28 showing no productive infection with X4 strain [317]. Probably other additional mechanisms may serve as gatekeepers restricting X4 infection *in vivo* [307]. Related to the pattern of induced cytokines it is also important to observe that the fold of induction of GM-CSF, TGF-β, IL-16, IP-10, MIG, IL-10 is always much higher that those observed in lymphoid tissue[305]; this characteristic may be important for explaining the high percentage of CD4+ cell depletion observed in gut [305,318], exceeding the number of infected cells [305]. Moreover, GM-CSF plays a role as T cells and monocyte-macrophage activator, whereas IL-10 and TGF-β are potent immunosuppressor factors, possibly contributing to cell depletion. On the other side, GM-CSF, TGF-β, IL-16, IP-10, MIG, IL-10 also have direct role in the control of viral replication [153]. Of note it is the fact that most of the chemokines induced in the gut of HIV+ individuals are also characteristic of chronic inflammations, such as ulcerative colitis and Chrohn's disease (i.e., CCL2/MCP-1, CCL3/MIP-1α, Eotaxin, IP-10, IL-8) [319], characterized by recruitment from blood of leukocytes infiltrating the intestinal mucosa [319]. Thus, a superimposable mechanism might also be present in HIV infected individuals, leading to the continous recruitment of target cells after the acute phase (at which time point most of the resident CD4+ cells are depleted) and thus contributing to the steady-state level of viremia. Although an important innate immune response is evident during the acute HIV infection in the gut, it is also important to note that this immunoresponse is not properly functional, as evidenced by the lack of perforin expression from resident CTL [312].

During the last years many new information became available about HIV infection of GALT and vagina, shifting the scientific interest on the primary and chronic infection of mucosae. The above reports clearly show that either SIV or HIV infection induce a broad and early immune activation in the gut mucosae. Therefore, therapeutical strategies reducing inflammation (i.e., glucocorticoids and antioxidants) at mucosae must be evaluate in the regimen of anti-HIV therapies. The study of this approach is facilitated by the existence of in vitro system for the culture of gut biopsy/explant [305], recently used to evaluate toxicity and efficacy of microbicides [301,320]. Moreover, gut mucosa, as well as vaginal tissue, represent also an important anatomical site where to induce immunological responses, then translated to the systemic immunity.

Lymphoid tissue. Over GALT, the primary site of infection and CD4$^+$ T cells depletion during acute HIV infection [321], draining lymph nodes represent the main reservoir of HIV infection, with the virus carried by

DC [322]. Virions released via the lymphatic system spread the infection throughtout the body, whereas into the lymph node virions bind to follicular dendritic cells (FDC) [292]. Highlitghtin the relevance of virus-bearing FDC is the fact that these cells have been proposed to be responsible of the second-phase of the biphasic plasma viral decay [323].

Another lymphoid organ targeted by HIV is thymus. Altered thymopoiesis is due to direct infection thymocytes [324], as well as indirect cytopathic mechanisms. This latter mechanism is mediated by the aktered cytokine milieu in the stromal of thymus. This cytokine milieu derives from apoptosis of uninfected cells [324] and mediates disruption of stromal architecture and thymocytes depletion [325]. The impairment of thymic function ends in a diminished capacity of replenish the lymphocyte pool, therefore contributing to the $CD4^+$ T cells depletion observed during the disease progression [326]. In fact, the immune restoration observed in HIV^+ children under HAART [327] or HIV^+ adults under HAART plus IL-2 [328] has been described to be in part thymus dependent.

CLINICAL USE OF CYTOKINES IN HIV INFECTION

IFN-α/β has shown potent antiviral activity in *in vitro* and *ex-vivo* infected cells, animal models of HIV infection as well as in vivo. In HIV-infected SCID mice reconstituted with human cells or tissues IFN-α, provided by i) continuos infusion or either expressed by ii) U937 cells or iii) CD4+ T cells containing a retroviral vector expressing the cytokine, strongly reduced infection and protected from HIV-induced $CD4^+$ T cell depletion [329]. The anti-viral mechanism of IFN-α observed in the animal model has been associated with trapping of new progeny virions within cells, resulting in anti-HIV potency and protection from virus-induced depletion of CD4+ T cells higher than what observed with AZT [329].

In vivo, administration of IFN-α as a therapeutic agent has been proven to have beneficial effects in either AIDS patient either Kaposi'sarcoma and high (>500 cells/µl) $CD4^+$ T cell counts [330,331], or in individuals with HIV-associated progressive multifocal leukoencephalopathy. Moreover, the polyethilen-glycol (PEG) conjugated form of IFN-α, characterized by a prolonged half-life, has been shown to enhance lytic activity along with increased concentrations of perforin and granzyme A expression in NK cells were demonstrated in HIV^+ individuals [332].

IL-2. As observed in SCID-hu mice [333], expression of IL-2 by a vaccinia virus vector or by means of DNA vaccination did not alter viral replication, but proved to represent a good adjuvant [334]. Due to the short half-life of IL-2, a chimeric IL-2/Ig fusion protein has been developed and has shown to increase the efficacy of DNA vaccination also in terms of CD4+ T cells activation and proliferation [335-337]. In addition, IL-2 has been shown to prevent depletion of immature CD4+CD8+ and CD5+CD1+ thymocytes in the HIV-infected thymus of SCID mice implanted with human fetal thymus and liver tissues without increasing viral load [333]. In addition, IL-2 administration in humans has been shown to induce HIV peptide-specific and non-specific IFN-γ producing cells [338], and both naïve [257], memory T cells [339] and NK cells [340].

IL-2 did not increase viral production, but strongly synergized with IL-4 in cultures of infected mature thymocytes [64]. IL-2 and IL-4 induced over-expression of CCR5 and CXCR4 [91], and increased viral replication also in HIV-infected tonsils [65]. In thy/liv-SCID-hu mice, exogenous administration of IL-2 was demonstrated to maintain alive an immature thymocyte subset without increasing viral load [341]. Furthermore, IL-2 prevented the outgrowth of human Epstein-Barr virus (EBV)-induced lymphoproliferative disease (an opportunistic cancer typical of AIDS patients) in hu-PBL-SCID mice engrafted with human PBL from healthy EBVseropositive donors [342]. In this regard, IL-2 has been successfully used in humans to prevent EBV disease [343,344].

IL-2 plus HAART reduced the state of immune activation and, in some studies, the HIV DNA content of PBMC, likely as a consequence of the numerical expansion of circulating $CD4^+$ T cells [345]. In addition, administration of IL-2 without antiretrovirals has not resulted in the expression of a previously silent quasispecies [346]. Administration of intermittent IL-2 induced "blips" of virus replication without inducing an increase in steady-state viremia, even in the absence of a full suppression of HIV replication by HAART [347].

Unique among all cytokines, IL-2 has been evaluated in phase III clinical trials (ESPRIT and SILCAAT) for its potential therapeutic effect when administered with anti-retroviral therapy to stably increase the levels of circulating $CD4^+$ T cells [348]. In spite of promising conclusions of phase II studies and of their metaanalysis, these trials have recently unequivocally demonstrated the lack of efficacy of intermittent IL-2 administration in terms of protection from AIDS-related deaths and events defining AIDS progression in the face of significantly increased levels of peripheral CD4+ T cell counts [349,350]. Furthermore, increased cardiovascular pathologies, were linked to IL-2 administration [351]. The reasons for this unexpected clear-cut failure of this promising form of immunotherapy are unclear and will be throroughly investigated in the next years.

It is likely that the net effect of cytokines and chemokines in *in vivo* infection will result not only from a direct effect on the infected cells, but also, and perhaps even more importantly, from the indirect activation of other effectors, such as $CD8^+$ T and NK cells, which may contribute and even take advantage of transiently increased expression of viral proteins to eliminate infected cells. These concepts are currently explored in experimental protocols aimed at eradicating infection from latent reservoirs, including resting memory T cells [352,353] and monocytes [354,355].

Finally, IL-2 has also been used to ameliorate clinical side-effects induced by HAART (see paragraph about IRIS).

IL-12 administration did not induce substantial changes in plasma viremia and viral load in PBMC of rhesus macaques chronically infected with SIV [45]. However, an increased proliferative response of T cells to multiple HIV Ag was noted in chimpanzees vaccinated with HIV DNA plus IL-12 [356]. Administration of exogenous IL-12 did not affect either the virus load or the frequency of circulating infected lymphocytes in chronically SIV-infected rhesus monkeys [45], although it increased the proliferative response to multiple HIV Ags in chimpanzee vaccinated with a DNA-based vaccine [357]. IL-12 administration to either SIV-infected macaques [45] or HIV-infected individuals [356] at an early stage of infection increased the frequency and activity of circulating NK cells in contrast to an earlier report indicated a paradoxical decrease of NK cell activities in IL-12 treated HIV^+ individuals [358].

IL-15 has been shown to exert number of immunorestorating functions, including the up-regulation of Ab-dependent cellular cytotoxicity from PBMC and several polymorphonuclear phagocyte functions in HIV^+ individuals [116,130]. In addition, IL-15 induced virus-specific CTL in primates infected with SIV and in humans [359]. Exogenous IL-15 restored the deficient IL-12 production from *ex-vivo* infected PBMC [117]; in contrast, neither IL-15 nor IL-12 reversed the functional anergy of $\gamma\delta$ T cells isolated from infected individuals [360]. IL-15 stimulation of NK cells, from both HIV^+ or HIV seronegative individuals, induced their proliferation and cytokine production [40,117,120,361-363]. These effects, together with the IL-15 ability to boost NK cell functions and PBMC proliferation in response to a number of Ag in synergy with IL-2 [364], renders this cytokine of great interest for clinical exploitation.

IL-15 has been also combined to IL-21 resulting in a synergistic expansion and functional enhancement of $CD8^+$ T cells both *in vitro* and *in vivo* in mice [172,173], as well as on CD8+ T cells harvested from HIV^+ individuals [174]. For the above reasons, IL-15 has been tested as a vaccine adjuvant for experimental SIV infection with contrasting results. Early reports indicated that IL-15 enhanced cell-mediated and humoral immune responses in chronically SIV-infected macaques [365] as well as in macaques immunized with SIV_{gag} DNA resulting in an ameliorated clinical outcome after virus challenge [366]. In contrast, recent studies indicated that IL-15 did not ameliorate the immune responses of macaques immunized with ALVAC-SIV-*gpe* expressing the *gag*, *pol*, and *env* genes of SIV_{mac251} [367] and even abrogated the vaccine-induced decrease of the viral set point [367] while not influencing the levels of viremia in chronically infected macaques [365].

TNF-α. Because TNF-α/β are able to inhibit R5 HIV entry and because of their ability to kill preferentially cells infected by several viruses, particularly in combination with IFN-γ [368,369], TNF-α/β were originally considered potential anti-viral agents. TNF-α may indeed play a protective role on uninfected cells by enhancing the capacity of NK/LAK cells to kill cells chronically infected with HIV [370], although stimulation of MDM after infection confirmed that up-regulation of viral expression occurred [152]. In contrast, TNF-α induced the expression of CXCR4 and replication of X4 viruses in both U937 cell clones [371] and PBMC stimulated with anti-CD3 plus anti-CD28 Ab [372]. These observations suggest that the increased levels of TNF-α/β observed in the advanced stages of infection may play a role in the emergence of CXCR4-using viruses.

IMMUNE RECONSTITUTION INFLAMMATORY SYNDROME (IRIS)

Represent a manifestation of clinical phenomena that mainly occur in immunodeficient individuals upon reconstitution of immune responses [373]. In fact, in the last years IRIS has frequently been observed in HIV+ individuals responding to HAART, thus characterized by undetectable viremia and partial restoration of immunological functions, such as increased levels of memory (CD45RO) CD4+ T cells, due to redistribution from lymphoid tissue, followed by a steady rise of naïve (CD45RA) lymphocytes as consequent of restoration of thymic activity [374]. In fact, during IRIS is commonly observed reconstitution of cellular and humoral responses against different pathogens, such as expansion of Tubercolosis specific IFN-γ secreting CD4+ T cells [375] and decrease of cytomegalovirus (CMV) viremia associated with enhanced levels of anti-CMV antibodies [376].

However, due to the fact that HAART must be maintained for ever, secondary to the rapid HAART induced immunological reconstitution and restoration of pathogen-specific immunity [377] IRIS is common and due to a marked inflammatory reaction (necessary for the initial immunological responses). In the case of HIV+ individuals, where many opportunistic infections (OIs) can take place or latent infections be re-activated, IRIS can also be associated with active replication of mycobacterial and cryptococcal infections, fungi and herpes viruses [375,378,379]. Thus, due to the characteristic of HIV (i.e., integration into host DNA and presence of latent viral reservoirs, thus making HAART a life-long treatment) and the immunodeficient status of HIV+ individuals, IRIS is a consequence of immunodeficiency, in which only partial and inadequate immune reconstitution is obtained, and the life-long anti-retroviral treatment.

On the other side, IRIS can be fight by using anti-inflammatory molecules, as recently proposed (i.e., glucocorticoids and corticosteroids [377,378]) or by using HAART in combination with administration of cytokines. Indeed, it has been reported that combination of HAART with IL-2 and GM-CSF is beneficial over HAART alone, in that the combination results in a better clearance of *Mycobacterium avium* [379]. The better clinical outcome due to two cytokines is due to a boost the T cell response, also probably associated with proliferative sinalings to immature thymocytes and/or rescue of anergic CD4 T cells, thus generating functional T cell response [379]. Moreover, due to the effect of GM-CSF in inducing maturation of macrophages in can also be ruled in the possibility that this cytokine enhances the degradation on intracellular pathogens in macrophages [379].

In conclusion, the usage of cytokines in combination with HAART might represent a combination therapy aimed to a better control of HIV infection and of the immune system in immunodeficient individuals, thus providing an adequate clearance of OIs.

ACKNOWLEDGMENTS

This work has been partially supported by Europrise and NEAT Network of Excellence (EC-FP6).

REFERENCES

[1]   Hofmann SR, Ettinger R, Zhou YJ, Gadina M, Lipsky P, Siegel R, et al. Cytokines and their role in lymphoid development, differentiation and homeostasis. Curr Opin Allergy Clin Immunol. 2002 Dec;2(6):495-506.

[2]   Mantovani A, Locati M, Vecchi A, Sozzani S, Allavena P. Decoy receptors: a strategy to regulate inflammatory cytokines and chemokines. Trends Immunol. 2001 Jun;22(6):328-36.

[3]   Lusso P. Chemokines and viruses: the dearest enemies. Virology. 2000 Aug 1;273(2):228-40.

[4]   Frankel AD, Young JA. HIV-1: fifteen proteins and an RNA. Annual review of biochemistry. 1998;67:1-25.

[5]   Daniel V, Huber W, Bauer K, Suesal C, Conradt C, Opelz G. Associations of blood levels of PCB, HCHS, and HCB with numbers of lymphocyte subpopulations, in vitro lymphocyte response, plasma cytokine levels, and immunoglobulin autoantibodies. Environmental health perspectives. 2001 Feb;109(2):173-8.

[6]   Slifka MK, Whitton JL. Clinical implications of dysregulated cytokine production. J Mol Med. 2000;78(2):74-80.

[7]   Refaeli Y, Van Parijs L, London CA, Tschopp J, Abbas AK. Biochemical mechanisms of IL-2-regulated Fas-mediated T cell apoptosis. Immunity. 1998;8(5):615-23.

[8]   O'Garra A, Murphy K. Role of cytokines in development of Th1 and Th2 cells. Chem Immunol. 1996;63:1-13.

[9]   Hansen W, Westendorf AM, Buer J. Regulatory T cells as targets for immunotherapy of autoimmunity and inflammation. Inflammation & allergy drug targets. 2008 Dec;7(4):217-23.

[10]   Kitani A, Xu L. Regulatory T cells and the induction of IL-17. Mucosal immunology. 2008 Nov;1 Suppl 1:S43-6.

[11]   O'Shea JJ, Ma A, Lipsky P. Cytokines and autoimmunity. Nat Rev Immunol. 2002 Jan;2(1):37-45.

[12]   Fernandez C, Buyse M, German-Fattal M, Gimenez F. Influence of the pro-inflammatory cytokines on P-glycoprotein expression and functionality. J Pharm Pharm Sci. 2004 Nov 17;7(3):359-71.

[13]   Belardelli F, Ferrantini M, Proietti E, Kirkwood JM. Interferon-alpha in tumor immunity and immunotherapy. Cytokine Growth Factor Rev. 2002 Apr;13(2):119-34.

[14]   Pitha PM. Multiple effects of interferon on the replication of human immunodeficiency virus type 1. Antiviral Res. 1994 Jul;24(2-3):205-19.

[15]   Popik W, Pitha PM. Exploitation of cellular signaling by HIV-1: unwelcome guests with master keys that signal their entry. Virology. 2000 Oct 10;276(1):1-6.

[16]   Weiden M, Tanaka N, Qiao Y, Zhao BY, Honda Y, Nakata K, et al. Differentiation of monocytes to macrophages switches the Mycobacterium tuberculosis effect on HIV-1 replication from stimulation to inhibition: modulation of interferon response and CCAAT/enhancer binding protein beta expression. J Immunol. 2000 Aug 15;165(4):2028-39.

[17]   Poli G, Orenstein JM, Kinter A, Folks TM, Fauci AS. Interferon-alpha but not AZT suppresses HIV expression in chronically infected cell lines. Science. 1989 May 5;244(4904):575-7.

[18]   Peng G, Lei KJ, Jin W, Greenwell-Wild T, Wahl SM. Induction of APOBEC3 family proteins, a defensive maneuver underlying interferon-induced anti-HIV-1 activity. The Journal of experimental medicine. 2006 Jan 23;203(1):41-6.

[19]   Wang FX, Huang J, Zhang H, Ma X, Zhang H. APOBEC3G upregulation by alpha interferon restricts human immunodeficiency virus type 1 infection in human peripheral plasmacytoid dendritic cells. The Journal of general virology. 2008 Mar;89(Pt 3):722-30.

[20]   Chen K, Huang J, Zhang C, Huang S, Nunnari G, Wang FX, et al. Alpha interferon potently enhances the anti-human immunodeficiency virus type 1 activity of APOBEC3G in resting primary CD4 T cells. Journal of virology. 2006 Aug;80(15):7645-57.

[21]   Argyris EG, Acheampong E, Wang F, Huang J, Chen K, Mukhtar M, et al. The interferon-induced expression of APOBEC3G in human blood-brain barrier exerts a potent intrinsic immunity to block HIV-1 entry to central nervous system. Virology. 2007 Oct 25;367(2):440-51.

[22]   Aguiar RS, Peterlin BM. APOBEC3 proteins and reverse transcription. Virus research. 2008 Jun;134(1-2):74-85.

[23]   Ferbas J, Navratil J, Logar A, Rinaldo C. Selective decrease in human immunodeficiency virus type 1 (HIV-1)-induced alpha interferon production by peripheral blood mononuclear cells during HIV-1 infection. Clin Diagn Lab Immunol. 1995 Mar;2(2):138-42.

[24]   Feldman S, Stein D, Amrute S, Denny T, Garcia Z, Kloser P, et al. Decreased interferon-alpha production in HIV-infected patients correlates with numerical and functional deficiencies in circulating type 2 dendritic cell precursors. Clin Immunol. 2001 Nov;101(2):201-10.

[25]   Servet C, Zitvogel L, Hosmalin A. Dendritic cells in innate immune responses against HIV. Curr Mol Med. 2002 Dec;2(8):739-56.

[26]   Chehimi J, Campbell DE, Azzoni L, Bacheller D, Papasavvas E, Jerandi G, et al. Persistent decreases in blood plasmacytoid dendritic cell number and function despite effective highly active antiretroviral therapy and increased blood myeloid dendritic cells in HIV-infected individuals. J Immunol. 2002 May 1;168(9):4796-801.

[27]   Krivine A, Force G, Servan J, Cabee A, Rozenberg F, Dighiero L, et al. Measuring HIV-1 RNA and interferon-alpha in the cerebrospinal fluid of AIDS patients: insights into the pathogenesis of AIDS Dementia Complex. J Neurovirol. 1999 Oct;5(5):500-6.

[28] Poli G, Biswas P, Fauci AS. Interferons in the pathogenesis and treatment of human immunodeficiency virus infection. Antiviral Res. 1994 Jul;24(2-3):221-33.

[29] Bovolenta C, Lorini AL, Mantelli B, Camorali L, Novelli F, Biswas P, et al. A selective defect of IFN-gamma- but not of IFN-alpha-induced JAK/STAT pathway in a subset of U937 clones prevents the antiretroviral effect of IFN-gamma against HIV-1. J Immunol. 1999;162(1):323-30.

[30] Biswas P, Poli G, Kinter AL, Justement JS, Stanley SK, Maury WJ, et al. Interferon gamma induces the expression of human immunodeficiency virus in persistently infected promonocytic cells (U1) and redirects the production of virions to intracytoplasmic vacuoles in phorbol myristate acetate-differentiated U1 cells. J Exp Med. 1992 Sep 1;176(3):739-50.

[31] Biswas P, Poli G, Orenstein JM, Fauci AS. Cytokine-mediated induction of human immunodeficiency virus (HIV) expression and cell death in chronically infected U1 cells: do tumor necrosis factor alpha and gamma interferon selectively kill HIV- infected cells? J Virol. 1994;68(4):2598-604.

[32] Kinter AL, Poli G, Fox L, Hardy E, Fauci AS. HIV replication in IL-2-stimulated peripheral blood mononuclear cells is driven in an autocrine/paracrine manner by endogenous cytokines. J Immunol. 1995 Mar 1;154(5):2448-59.

[33] Koenig S, Gendelman HE, Orenstein JM, Dal Canto MC, Pezeshkpour GH, Yungbluth M, et al. Detection of AIDS virus in macrophages in brain tissue from AIDS patients with encephalopathy. Science. 1986;223:1089-93.

[34] Orenstein JM, Jannotta F. Human immunodeficiency virus and papovavirus infections in acquired immunodeficiency syndrome: an ultrastructural study of three cases. Hum Pathol. 1988;19:350-61.

[35] Fantuzzi L, Spadaro F, Vallanti G, Canini I, Ramoni C, Vicenzi E, et al. Endogenous CCL2 (monocyte chemotactic protein-1) modulates human immunodeficiency virus type-1 replication and affects cytoskeleton organization in human monocyte-derived macrophages. Blood. 2003 Jun 12.

[36] Alfano M, Sidenius N, Panzeri B, Blasi F, Poli G. Urokinase-urokinase receptor interaction mediates an inhibitory signal for HIV-1 replication. Proc Natl Acad Sci U S A. 2002;99:8862-7.

[37] Pelchen-Matthews A, Kramer B, Marsh M. Infectious HIV-1 assembles in late endosomes in primary macrophages. J Cell Biol. 2003 Aug 4;162(3):443-55.

[38] Klimkait T, Strebel K, Hoggan MD, Martin MA, Orenstein JM. The human immunodeficiency virus type 1-specific protein vpu is required for efficient virus maturation and release. J Virol. 1990 Feb;64(2):621-9.

[39] Ludewig B, Gelderblom HR, Becker Y, Schafer A, Pauli G. Transmission of HIV-1 from productively infected mature Langerhans cells to primary CD4+ T lymphocytes results in altered T cell responses with enhanced production of IFN-gamma and IL-10. Virology. 1996 Jan 1;215(1):51-60.

[40] Vitale M, Caruso A, De Francesco MA, Rodella L, Bozzo L, Garrafa E, et al. HIV-1 matrix protein p17 enhances the proliferative activity of natural killer cells and increases their ability to secrete proinflammatory cytokines. Br J Haematol. 2003 Jan;120(2):337-43.

[41] Khatissian E, Chakrabarti L, Hurtrel B. Cytokine patterns and viral load in lymph nodes during the early stages of SIV infection. Res Virol. 1996 Mar-Jun;147(2-3):181-9.

[42] Villinger F, Brar SS, Brice GT, Chikkala NF, Novembre FJ, Mayne AE, et al. Immune and hematopoietic parameters in HIV-1-infected chimpanzees during clinical progression toward AIDS. J Med Primatol. 1997 Feb-Apr;26(1-2):11-8.

[43] Cheret A, Le Grand R, Caufour P, Neildez O, Matheux F, Theodoro F, et al. RANTES, IFN-gamma, CCR1, and CCR5 mRNA expression in peripheral blood, lymph node, and bronchoalveolar lavage mononuclear cells during primary simian immunodeficiency virus infection of macaques. Virology. 1999 Mar 15;255(2):285-93.

[44] Smit-McBride Z, Mattapallil JJ, McChesney M, Ferrick D, Dandekar S. Gastrointestinal T lymphocytes retain high potential for cytokine responses but have severe CD4(+) T-cell depletion at all stages of simian immunodeficiency virus infection compared to peripheral lymphocytes. Journal of virology. 1998 Aug;72(8):6646-56.

[45] Villinger F, Bucur S, Chikkala NF, Brar SS, Bostik P, Mayne AE, et al. In vitro and in vivo responses to interleukin 12 are maintained until the late SIV infection stage but lost during AIDS. AIDS Res Hum Retroviruses. 2000 May 20;16(8):751-63.

[46] Van Lint C, Ghysdael J, Paras P, Jr., Burny A, Verdin E. A transcriptional regulatory element is associated with a nuclease- hypersensitive site in the pol gene of human immunodeficiency virus type 1. J Virol. 1994;68(4):2632-48.

[47] Poli G, Bressler P, Kinter A, Duh E, Timmer WC, Rabson A, et al. Interleukin 6 induces human immunodeficiency virus expression in infected monocytic cells alone and in synergy with tumor necrosis factor alpha by transcriptional and post-transcriptional mechanisms. J Exp Med. 1990;172(1):151-8.

[48] Montaner LJ, Bailer RT, Gordon S. IL-13 acts on macrophages to block the completion of reverse transcription, inhibit virus production, and reduce virus infectivity. J Leukoc Biol. 1997;62(1):126-32.

[49] Lane BR, Lore K, Bock PJ, Andersson J, Coffey MJ, Strieter RM, et al. Interleukin-8 stimulates human immunodeficiency virus type 1 replication and is a potential new target for antiretroviral therapy. J Virol. 2001;75:8195-202.

[50] Lane BR, Strieter RM, Coffey MJ, Markovitz DM. Human immunodeficiency virus type 1 (HIV-1)-induced GRO-alpha production stimulates HIV-1 replication in macrophages and T lymphocytes. J Virol. 2001;75:5812-22.

[51] Granucci F, Zanoni I, Feau S, Ricciardi-Castagnoli P. Dendritic cell regulation of immune responses: a new role for interleukin 2 at the intersection of innate and adaptive immunity. Embo J. 2003 Jun 2;22(11):2546-51.

[52] Granucci F, Vizzardelli C, Pavelka N, Feau S, Persico M, Virzi E, et al. Inducible IL-2 production by dendritic cells revealed by global gene expression analysis. Nat Immunol. 2001 Sep;2(9):882-8.

[53] Waldmann TA. T-cell receptors for cytokines: targets for immunotherapy of leukemia/lymphoma. Ann Oncol. 2000;11 Suppl 1:101-6.

[54] Napolitano LA. Approaches to immune reconstitution in HIV infection. Top HIV Med. 2003 Sep-Oct;11(5):160-3.

[55] Graziosi C, Pantaleo G, Gantt KR, Fortin JP, Demarest JF, Cohen OJ, et al. Lack of evidence for the dichotomy of TH1 and TH2 predominance in HIV-infected individuals. Science. 1994 Jul 8;265(5169):248-52.

[56] Airoldi I, Saverino D, Favre A, Ghiotto F, Tacchetti C, Facchetti P, et al. Cytokine gene expression and T-cell proliferative responses in lymph node mononuclear cells from children with early stage human immunodeficiency virus infection. Haematologica. 2000 Dec;85(12):1237-47.

[57] Sei S, Akiyoshi H, Bernard J, Venzon DJ, Fox CH, Schwartzentruber DJ, et al. Dynamics of virus versus host interaction in children with human immunodeficiency virus type 1 infection. J Infect Dis. 1996 Jun;173(6):1485-90.

[58] Andersson J, Fehniger TE, Patterson BK, Pottage J, Agnoli M, Jones P, et al. Early reduction of immune activation in lymphoid tissue following highly active HIV therapy. AIDS (London, England). 1998 Jul 30;12(11):F123-9.

[59] McGowan I, Radford-Smith G, Jewell DP. Cytokine gene expression in HIV-infected intestinal mucosa. AIDS (London, England). 1994 Nov;8(11):1569-75.

[60] Spring M, Bodemer W, Stahl-Hennig C, Nisslein T, Hunsmann G, Dittmer U. Impaired mitogen-driven proliferation and cytokine transcription of lymphocytes from macaques early after simian immunodeficiency virus (SIV) infection. Viral immunology. 1997;10(2):65-72.

[61] Klein SA, Dobmeyer JM, Dobmeyer TS, Pape M, Ottmann OG, Helm EB, et al. Demonstration of the Th1 to Th2 cytokine shift during the course of HIV-1 infection using cytoplasmic cytokine detection on single cell level by flow cytometry. AIDS (London, England). 1997 Jul 15;11(9):1111-8.

[62] Koopman G, Niphuis H, Newman W, Kishimoto TK, Maino VC, Heeney JL. Decreased expression of IL-2 in central and effector CD4 memory cells during progression to AIDS in rhesus macaques. AIDS (London, England). 2001 Dec 7;15(18):2359-69.

[63] Gray CM, Morris L, Murray J, Keeton J, Shalekoff S, Lyons SF, et al. Identification of cell subsets expressing intracytoplasmic cytokines within HIV-1-infected lymph nodes. Aids. 1996 Nov;10(13):1467-75.

[64] Hays EF, Uittenbogaart CH, Brewer JC, Vollger LW, Zack JA. In vitro studies of HIV-1 expression in thymocytes from infants and children. AIDS (London, England). 1992 Mar;6(3):265-72.

[65] Glushakova S, Grivel JC, Suryanarayana K, Meylan P, Lifson JD, Desrosiers R, et al. Nef enhances human immunodeficiency virus replication and responsiveness to interleukin-2 in human lymphoid tissue ex vivo. Journal of virology. 1999 May;73(5):3968-74.

[66] Van Snick J. Interleukin-6: an overview. Annual review of immunology. 1990;8:253-78.

[67] Rothe M, Chene L, Nugeyre MT, Braun J, Barre-Sinoussi F, Israel N. Contact with thymic epithelial cells as a prerequisite for cytokine-enhanced human immunodeficiency virus type 1 replication in thymocytes. Journal of virology. 1998 Jul;72(7):5852-61.

[68] Ramarli D, Reina S, Merola M, Scupoli MT, Poffe O, Riviera AP, et al. HTLV type IIIB infection of human thymic epithelial cells: viral expression correlates with the induction of NF-kappa B-binding activity in cells activated by cell adhesion. AIDS research and human retroviruses. 1996 Sep 1;12(13):1217-25.

[69] Devergne O, Peuchmaur M, Humbert M, Navratil E, Leger-Ravet MB, Crevon MC, et al. In vivo expression of IL-1 beta and IL-6 genes during viral infections in human. Eur Cytokine Netw. 1991 May-Jun;2(3):183-94.

[70] Sandborg CI, Imfeld KL, Zaldivar F, Jr., Berman MA. HIV type 1 induction of interleukin 1 and 6 production by human thymic cells. AIDS research and human retroviruses. 1994 Oct;10(10):1221-9.

[71] Bucy RP, Hockett RD, Derdeyn CA, Saag MS, Squires K, Sillers M, et al. Initial increase in blood CD4(+) lymphocytes after HIV antiretroviral therapy reflects redistribution from lymphoid tissues. The Journal of clinical investigation. 1999 May 15;103(10):1391-8.

[72] Ruiz-Mateos E, de la Rosa R, Franco JM, Martinez-Moya M, Rubio A, Soriano N, et al. Endogenous IL-7 is associated with increased thymic volume in adult HIV-infected patients under highly active antiretroviral therapy. AIDS (London, England). 2003 May 2;17(7):947-54.

[73] Fry TJ, Mackall CL. Interleukin-7: master regulator of peripheral T-cell homeostasis? Trends Immunol. 2001 Oct;22(10):564-71.

[74] Chene L, Nugeyre MT, Guillemard E, Moulian N, Barre-Sinoussi F, Israel N. Thymocyte-thymic epithelial cell interaction leads to high-level replication of human immunodeficiency virus exclusively in mature CD4(+) CD8(-) CD3(+) thymocytes: a critical role for tumor necrosis factor and interleukin-7. Journal of virology. 1999 Sep;73(9):7533-42.

[75] Guillemard E, Nugeyre MT, Chene L, Schmitt N, Jacquemot C, Barre-Sinoussi F, et al. Interleukin-7 and infection itself by human immunodeficiency virus 1 favor virus persistence in mature CD4(+)CD8(-)CD3(+) thymocytes through sustained induction of Bcl-2. Blood. 2001 Oct 1;98(7):2166-74.

[76] Nunnari G, Xu Y, Acheampong EA, Fang J, Daniel R, Zhang C, et al. Exogenous IL-7 induces Fas-mediated human neuronal apoptosis: potential effects during human immunodeficiency virus type 1 infection. Journal of neurovirology. 2005 Aug;11(4):319-28.

[77] Fluur C, De Milito A, Fry TJ, Vivar N, Eidsmo L, Atlas A, et al. Potential role for IL-7 in Fas-mediated T cell apoptosis during HIV infection. J Immunol. 2007 Apr 15;178(8):5340-50.

[78] Kinter AL, Godbout EJ, McNally JP, Sereti I, Roby GA, O'Shea MA, et al. The common gamma-chain cytokines IL-2, IL-7, IL-15, and IL-21 induce the expression of programmed death-1 and its ligands. J Immunol. 2008 Nov 15;181(10):6738-46.

[79] Lum JJ, Schnepple DJ, Nie Z, Sanchez-Dardon J, Mbisa GL, Mihowich J, et al. Differential effects of interleukin-7 and interleukin-15 on NK cell anti-human immunodeficiency virus activity. Journal of virology. 2004 Jun;78(11):6033-42.

[80] Boulassel MR, Smith GH, Gilmore N, Klein M, Murphy T, MacLeod J, et al. Interleukin-7 levels may predict virological response in advanced HIV-1-infected patients receiving lopinavir/ritonavir-based therapy. HIV Med. 2003 Oct;4(4):315-20.

[81] Chiappini E, Galli L, Azzari C, de Martino M. Interleukin-7 and immunologic failure despite treatment with highly active antiretroviral therapy in children perinatally infected with HIV-1. J Acquir Immune Defic Syndr. 2003 Aug 15;33(5):601-4.

[82] Clerici M, Saresella M, Colombo F, Fossati S, Sala N, Bricalli D, et al. T-lymphocyte maturation abnormalities in uninfected newborns and children with vertical exposure to HIV. Blood. 2000 Dec 1;96(12):3866-71.

[83] Napolitano LA, Grant RM, Deeks SG, Schmidt D, De Rosa SC, Herzenberg LA, et al. Increased production of IL-7 accompanies HIV-1-mediated T-cell depletion: implications for T-cell homeostasis. Nat Med. 2001 Jan;7(1):73-9.

[84] Boulassel MR, Samson J, Khammy A, Lapointe N, Soudeyns H, Routy JP. Predictive value of interleukin-7 levels for virological response to treatment in HIV-1-infected children. Viral immunology. 2007 Dec;20(4):649-56.

[85] Resino S, Galan I, Correa R, Pajuelo L, Bellon JM, Munoz-Fernandez MA. Homeostatic role of IL-7 in HIV-1 infected children on HAART: association with immunological and virological parameters. Acta Paediatr. 2005 Feb;94(2):170-7.

[86] Resino S, Perez A, Leon JA, Gurbindo MD, Munoz-Fernandez MA. Interleukin-7 levels before highly active antiretroviral therapy may predict CD4+ T-cell recovery and virological failure in HIV-infected children. J Antimicrob Chemother. 2006 Apr;57(4):798-800.

[87] Schmitt N, Chene L, Boutolleau D, Nugeyre MT, Guillemard E, Versmisse P, et al. Positive regulation of CXCR4 expression and signaling by interleukin-7 in CD4+ mature thymocytes correlates with their capacity to favor human immunodeficiency X4 virus replication. Journal of virology. 2003 May;77(10):5784-93.

[88] Caufour P, Le Grand R, Cheret A, Neildez O, Thiebot H, Theodoro F, et al. Longitudinal analysis of CD8(+) T-cell phenotype and IL-7, IL-15 and IL-16 mRNA expression in different tissues during primary simian immunodeficiency virus infection. Microbes and infection / Institut Pasteur. 2001 Mar;3(3):181-91.

[89] Muthukumar A, Wozniakowski A, Gauduin MC, Paiardini M, McClure HM, Johnson RP, et al. Elevated interleukin-7 levels not sufficient to maintain T-cell homeostasis during simian immunodeficiency virus-induced disease progression. Blood. 2004 Feb 1;103(3):973-9.

[90] Ducrey-Rundquist O, Guyader M, Trono D. Modalities of interleukin-7-induced human immunodeficiency virus permissiveness in quiescent T lymphocytes. J Virol. 2002 Sep;76(18):9103-11.

[91] Pedroza-Martins L, Gurney KB, Torbett BE, Uittenbogaart CH. Differential tropism and replication kinetics of human immunodeficiency virus type 1 isolates in thymocytes: coreceptor expression allows viral entry, but productive infection of distinct subsets is determined at the postentry level. J Virol. 1998 Dec;72(12):9441-52.

[92]   Llano A, Barretina J, Gutierrez A, Blanco J, Cabrera C, Clotet B, et al. Interleukin-7 in plasma correlates with CD4 T-cell depletion and may be associated with emergence of syncytium-inducing variants in human immunodeficiency virus type 1-positive individuals. Journal of virology. 2001 Nov;75(21):10319-25.

[93]   Shalekoff S, Tiemessen CT. Circulating levels of stromal cell-derived factor 1alpha and interleukin 7 in HIV type 1 infection and pulmonary tuberculosis are reciprocally related to CXCR4 expression on peripheral blood leukocytes. AIDS Res Hum Retroviruses. 2003 Jun;19(6):461-8.

[94]   Wang FX, Xu Y, Sullivan J, Souder E, Argyris EG, Acheampong EA, et al. IL-7 is a potent and proviral strain-specific inducer of latent HIV-1 cellular reservoirs of infected individuals on virally suppressive HAART. The Journal of clinical investigation. 2005 Jan;115(1):128-37.

[95]   Audige A, Schlaepfer E, Joller H, Speck RF. Uncoupled anti-HIV and immune-enhancing effects when combining IFN-alpha and IL-7. J Immunol. 2005 Sep 15;175(6):3724-36.

[96]   Smithgall MD, Wong JG, Critchett KE, Haffar OK. IL-7 up-regulates HIV-1 replication in naturally infected peripheral blood mononuclear cells. J Immunol. 1996 Mar 15;156(6):2324-30.

[97]   Moran PA, Diegel ML, Sias JC, Ledbetter JA, Zarling JM. Regulation of HIV production by blood mononuclear cells from HIV-infected donors: I. Lack of correlation between HIV-1 production and T cell activation. AIDS Res Hum Retroviruses. 1993 May;9(5):455-64.

[98]   Managlia EZ, Landay A, Al-Harthi L. Interleukin-7 induces HIV replication in primary naive T cells through a nuclear factor of activated T cell (NFAT)-dependent pathway. Virology. 2006 Jul 5;350(2):443-52.

[99]   Song H, Nakayama EE, Shioda T. Effects of human interleukin 7 on HIV-1 replication in monocyte-derived human macrophages. AIDS (London, England). 2006 Apr 4;20(6):937-9.

[100] Zhang M, Drenkow J, Lankford CS, Frucht DM, Rabin RL, Gingeras TR, et al. HIV regulation of the IL-7R: a viral mechanism for enhancing HIV-1 replication in human macrophages in vitro. Journal of leukocyte biology. 2006 Jun;79(6):1328-38.

[101] Kim JH, Loveland JE, Sitz KV, Ratto Kim S, McLinden RJ, Tencer K, et al. Expansion of restricted cellular immune responses to HIV-1 envelope by vaccination: IL-7 and IL-12 differentially augment cellular proliferative responses to HIV-1. Clinical and experimental immunology. 1997 May;108(2):243-50.

[102] Marchetti G, Meroni L, Varchetta S, Terzieva V, Bandera A, Manganaro D, et al. Low-dose prolonged intermittent interleukin-2 adjuvant therapy: results of a randomized trial among human immunodeficiency virus-positive patients with advanced immune impairment. J Infect Dis. 2002 Sep 1;186(5):606-16.

[103] Correa R, Resino S, Munoz-Fernandez MA. Increased interleukin-7 plasma levels are associated with recovery of CD4+ T cells in HIV-infected children. J Clin Immunol. 2003 Sep;23(5):401-6.

[104] MacPherson PA, Fex C, Sanchez-Dardon J, Hawley-Foss N, Angel JB. Interleukin-7 receptor expression on CD8(+) T cells is reduced in HIV infection and partially restored with effective antiretroviral therapy. J Acquir Immune Defic Syndr. 2001 Dec 15;28(5):454-7.

[105] Trinchieri G. Proinflammatory and immunoregulatory functions of interleukin-12. Int Rev Immunol. 1998;16(3-4):365-96.

[106] Sartori A, Ma X, Gri G, Showe L, Benjamin D, Trinchieri G. Interleukin-12: an immunoregulatory cytokine produced by B cells and antigen-presenting cells. Methods. 1997 Jan;11(1):116-27.

[107] Marshall JD, Chehimi J, Gri G, Kostman JR, Montaner LJ, Trinchieri G. The interleukin-12-mediated pathway of immune events is dysfunctional in human immunodeficiency virus-infected individuals. Blood. 1999 Aug 1;94(3):1003-11.

[108] Poaty-Mavoungou V, Toure FS, Tevi-Benissan C, Mavoungou E. Enhancement of natural killer cell activation and antibody-dependent cellular cytotoxicity by interferon-alpha and interleukin-12 in vaginal mucosae Sivmac251-infected Macaca fascicularis. Viral Immunol. 2002;15(1):197-212.

[109] Chehimi J, Starr SE, Frank I, D'Andrea A, Ma X, MacGregor RR, et al. Impaired interleukin 12 production in human immunodeficiency virus-infected patients. J Exp Med. 1994 Apr 1;179(4):1361-6.

[110] Chehimi J, Valiante NM, D'Andrea A, Rengaraju M, Rosado Z, Kobayashi M, et al. Enhancing effect of natural killer cell stimulatory factor (NKSF/interleukin-12) on cell-mediated cytotoxicity against tumor-derived and virus-infected cells. Eur J Immunol. 1993 Aug;23(8):1826-30.

[111] Clerici M, Lucey DR, Berzofsky JA, Pinto LA, Wynn TA, Blatt SP, et al. Restoration of HIV-specific cell-mediated immune responses by interleukin-12 in vitro. Science. 1993 Dec 10;262(5140):1721-4.

[112] Sirianni MC, Ansotegui IJ, Aiuti F, Wigzell H. Natural killer cell stimulatory factor (NKSF)/IL-12 and cytolytic activities of PBL/NK cells from human immunodeficiency virus type-1 infected patients. Scand J Immunol. 1994 Jul;40(1):83-6.

[113] Al-Harthi L, Roebuck KA, Landay A. Induction of HIV-1 replication by type 1-like cytokines, interleukin (IL)-12 and IL-15: effect on viral transcriptional activation, cellular proliferation, and endogenous cytokine production. J Clin Immunol. 1998 Mar;18(2):124-31.

[114] Akridge RE, Reed SG. Interleukin-12 decreases human immunodeficiency virus type 1 replication in human macrophage cultures reconstituted with autologous peripheral blood mononuclear cells. J Infect Dis. 1996 Mar;173(3):559-64.

[115] Wang J, Guan E, Roderiquez G, Norcross MA. Inhibition of CCR5 expression by IL-12 through induction of beta-chemokines in human T lymphocytes. J Immunol. 1999 Dec 1;163(11):5763-9.

[116] Loubeau M, Ahmad A, Toma E, Menezes J. Enhancement of natural killer and antibody-dependent cytolytic activities of the peripheral blood mononuclear cells of HIV-infected patients by recombinant IL-15. J Acquir Immune Defic Syndr Hum Retrovirol. 1997 Nov 1;16(3):137-45.

[117] Chehimi J, Marshall JD, Salvucci O, Frank I, Chehimi S, Kawecki S, et al. IL-15 enhances immune functions during HIV infection. J Immunol. 1997 Jun 15;158(12):5978-87.

[118] Waldmann TA, Tagaya Y. The multifaceted regulation of interleukin-15 expression and the role of this cytokine in NK cell differentiation and host response to intracellular pathogens. Annu Rev Immunol. 1999;17:19-49.

[119] d'Ettorre G, Andreotti M, Carnevalini M, Andreoni C, Zaffiri L, Vullo V, et al. Interleukin-15 enhances the secretion of IFN-gamma and CC chemokines by natural killer cells from HIV viremic and aviremic patients. Immunology letters. 2006 Mar 15;103(2):192-5.

[120] Chang KH, Kim JM, Yoo NC, Kim WH, Park JH, Choi IH, et al. Restoration of P-glycoprotein function is involved in the increase of natural killer activity with exogenous interleukin-15 in human immunodeficiency virus-infected individuals. Yonsei Med J. 2000 Oct;41(5):600-6.

[121] Kinter AL, Bende SM, Hardy EC, Jackson R, Fauci AS. Interleukin 2 induces CD8+ T cell-mediated suppression of human immunodeficiency virus replication in CD4+ T cells and this effect overrides its ability to stimulate virus expression. Proc Natl Acad Sci U S A. 1995 Nov 21;92(24):10985-9.

[122] Patki AH, Quinones-Mateu ME, Dorazio D, Yen-Lieberman B, Boom WH, Thomas EK, et al. Activation of antigen-induced lymphocyte proliferation by interleukin-15 without the mitogenic effect of interleukin-2 that may induce human immunodeficiency virus-1 expression. J Clin Invest. 1996 Aug 1;98(3):616-21.

[123] Rodriguez AR, Arulanandam BP, Hodara VL, McClure HM, Cobb EK, Salas MT, et al. Influence of interleukin-15 on CD8+ natural killer cells in human immunodeficiency virus type 1-infected chimpanzees. The Journal of general virology. 2007 Feb;88(Pt 2):641-51.

[124] Bayard-McNeeley M, Doo H, He S, Hafner A, Johnson WD, Jr., Ho JL. Differential effects of interleukin-12, interleukin-15, and interleukin-2 on human immunodeficiency virus type 1 replication in vitro. Clinical and diagnostic laboratory immunology. 1996 Sep;3(5):547-53.

[125] Perera LP, Goldman CK, Waldmann TA. IL-15 induces the expression of chemokines and their receptors in T lymphocytes. J Immunol. 1999 Mar 1;162(5):2606-12.

[126] Stopak KS, Chiu YL, Kropp J, Grant RM, Greene WC. Distinct patterns of cytokine regulation of APOBEC3G expression and activity in primary lymphocytes, macrophages, and dendritic cells. The Journal of biological chemistry. 2007 Feb 9;282(6):3539-46.

[127] Biancotto A, Grivel JC, Iglehart SJ, Vanpouille C, Lisco A, Sieg SF, et al. Abnormal activation and cytokine spectra in lymph nodes of people chronically infected with HIV-1. Blood. 2007 May 15;109(10):4272-9.

[128] Zaunders JJ, Moutouh-de Parseval L, Kitada S, Reed JC, Rought S, Genini D, et al. Polyclonal proliferation and apoptosis of CCR5+ T lymphocytes during primary human immunodeficiency virus type 1 infection: regulation by interleukin (IL)-2, IL-15, and Bcl-2. The Journal of infectious diseases. 2003 Jun 1;187(11):1735-47.

[129] Mueller YM, Bojczuk PM, Halstead ES, Kim AH, Witek J, Altman JD, et al. IL-15 enhances survival and function of HIV-specific CD8+ T cells. Blood. 2003 Feb 1;101(3):1024-9.

[130] Mastroianni CM, d'Ettorre G, Forcina G, Lichtner M, Mengoni F, D'Agostino C, et al. Interleukin-15 enhances neutrophil functional activity in patients with human immunodeficiency virus infection. Blood. 2000 Sep 1;96(5):1979-84.

[131] Boulassel MR, Young M, Routy JP, Sekaly RP, Tremblay C, Rouleau D. Circulating levels of IL-7 but not IL-15, IGF-1, and TGF-beta are elevated during primary HIV-1 infection. HIV Clin Trials. 2004 Sep-Oct;5(5):357-9.

[132] d'Ettorre G, Forcina G, Lichtner M, Mengoni F, D'Agostino C, Massetti AP, et al. Interleukin-15 in HIV infection: immunological and virological interactions in antiretroviral-naive and -treated patients. AIDS (London, England). 2002 Jan 25;16(2):181-8.

[133] Kacani L, Stoiber H, Dierich MP. Role of IL-15 in HIV-1-associated hypergammaglobulinaemia. Clinical and experimental immunology. 1997 Apr;108(1):14-8.

[134] Forcina G, D'Ettorre G, Mastroianni CM, Carnevalini M, Scorzolini L, Ceccarelli G, et al. Interleukin-15 modulates interferon-gamma and beta-chemokine production in patients with HIV infection: implications for immune-based therapy. Cytokine. 2004 Mar 21;25(6):283-90.

[135] Ahmad R, Sindhu ST, Toma E, Morisset R, Ahmad A. Studies on the production of IL-15 in HIV-infected/AIDS patients. Journal of clinical immunology. 2003 Mar;23(2):81-90.

[136] Macal M, Sankaran S, Chun TW, Reay E, Flamm J, Prindiville TJ, et al. Effective CD4+ T-cell restoration in gut-associated lymphoid tissue of HIV-infected patients is associated with enhanced Th17 cells and polyfunctional HIV-specific T-cell responses. Mucosal Immunol. 2008 Nov;1(6):475-88.

[137] Brenchley JM, Paiardini M, Knox KS, Asher AI, Cervasi B, Asher TE, et al. Differential Th17 CD4 T-cell depletion in pathogenic and nonpathogenic lentiviral infections. Blood. 2008 Oct 1;112(7):2826-35.

[138] Cecchinato V, Trindade CJ, Laurence A, Heraud JM, Brenchley JM, Ferrari MG, et al. Altered balance between Th17 and Th1 cells at mucosal sites predicts AIDS progression in simian immunodeficiency virus-infected macaques. Mucosal Immunol. 2008 Jul;1(4):279-88.

[139] Ndhlovu LC, Chapman JM, Jha AR, Snyder-Cappione JE, Pagan M, Leal FE, et al. Suppression of HIV-1 plasma viral load below detection preserves IL-17 producing T cells in HIV-1 infection. AIDS (London, England). 2008 May 11;22(8):990-2.

[140] Raffatellu M, Santos RL, Verhoeven DE, George MD, Wilson RP, Winter SE, et al. Simian immunodeficiency virus-induced mucosal interleukin-17 deficiency promotes Salmonella dissemination from the gut. Nature medicine. 2008 Apr;14(4):421-8.

[141] Yue FY, Merchant A, Kovacs CM, Loutfy M, Persad D, Ostrowski MA. Virus-specific interleukin-17-producing CD4+ T cells are detectable in early human immunodeficiency virus type 1 infection. Journal of virology. 2008 Jul;82(13):6767-71.

[142] Maek ANW, Buranapraditkun S, Klaewsongkram J, Ruxrungtham K. Increased interleukin-17 production both in helper T cell subset Th17 and CD4-negative T cells in human immunodeficiency virus infection. Viral Immunol. 2007 Spring;20(1):66-75.

[143] Kohno K, Kataoka J, Ohtsuki T, Suemoto Y, Okamoto I, Usui M, et al. IFN-gamma-inducing factor (IGIF) is a costimulatory factor on the activation of Th1 but not Th2 cells and exerts its effect independently of IL-12. J Immunol. 1997 Feb 15;158(4):1541-50.

[144] Bradney CP, Sempowski GD, Liao HX, Haynes BF, Staats HF. Cytokines as adjuvants for the induction of anti-human immunodeficiency virus peptide immunoglobulin G (IgG) and IgA antibodies in serum and mucosal secretions after nasal immunization. Journal of virology. 2002 Jan;76(2):517-24.

[145] Billaut-Mulot O, Idziorek T, Ban E, Kremer L, Dupre L, Loyens M, et al. Interleukin-18 modulates immune responses induced by HIV-1 Nef DNA prime/protein boost vaccine. Vaccine. 2000 Aug 15;19(1):95-102.

[146] Billaut-Mulot O, Idziorek T, Loyens M, Capron A, Bahr GM. Modulation of cellular and humoral immune responses to a multiepitopic HIV-1 DNA vaccine by interleukin-18 DNA immunization/viral protein boost. Vaccine. 2001 Apr 6;19(20-22):2803-11.

[147] Pugliese A, Vidotto V, Beltramo T, Torre D. Regulation of interleukin-18 by THP-1 monocytoid cells stimulated with HIV-1 and Nef viral protein. European cytokine network. 2005 Sep;16(3):186-90.

[148] Shapiro L, Puren AJ, Barton HA, Novick D, Peskind RL, Shenkar R, et al. Interleukin 18 stimulates HIV type 1 in monocytic cells. Proceedings of the National Academy of Sciences of the United States of America. 1998 Oct 13;95(21):12550-5.

[149] Torre D, Pugliese A, Speranza F, Martegani R, Tambini R. Role of interleukin-18 in human immunodeficiency virus type 1 infection. The Journal of infectious diseases. 2002 Apr 1;185(7):998; author reply -9.

[150] Poli G, Kinter A, Justement JS, Kehrl JH, Bressler P, Stanley S, et al. Tumor necrosis factor alpha functions in an autocrine manner in the induction of human immunodeficiency virus expression. Proceedings of the National Academy of Sciences of the United States of America. 1990 Jan;87(2):782-5.

[151] Choi HJ, Dinarello CA, Shapiro L. Interleukin-18 inhibits human immunodeficiency virus type 1 production in peripheral blood mononuclear cells. The Journal of infectious diseases. 2001 Sep 1;184(5):560-8.

[152] Herbein G, Montaner LJ, Gordon S. Tumor necrosis factor alpha inhibits entry of human immunodeficiency virus type 1 into primary human macrophages: a selective role for the 75-kilodalton receptor. Journal of virology. 1996 Nov;70(11):7388-97.

[153] Alfano M, Poli G. Role of cytokines and chemokines in the regulation of innate immunity and HIV infection. Molecular immunology. 2005 Feb;42(2):161-82.

[154] Sailer CA, Pott GB, Dinarello CA, Whinney SM, Forster JE, Larson-Duran JK, et al. Whole-blood interleukin-18 level during early HIV-1 infection is associated with reduced CXCR4 coreceptor expression and interferon- gamma levels. The Journal of infectious diseases. 2007 Mar 1;195(5):734-8.

[155] Tornero C, Alberola J, Tamarit A, Navarro D. Effect of highly active anti-retroviral therapy and hepatitis C virus co-infection on serum levels of pro-inflammatory and immunoregulatory cytokines in human immunodeficiency virus-1-infected individuals. Clin Microbiol Infect. 2006 Jun;12(6):555-60.

[156] Torre D, Speranza F, Martegani R, Pugliese A, Castelli F, Basilico C, et al. Circulating levels of IL-18 in adult and paediatric patients with HIV-1 infection. AIDS (London, England). 2000 Sep 29;14(14):2211-2.

[157] Ahmad R, Sindhu ST, Toma E, Morisset R, Ahmad A. Elevated levels of circulating interleukin-18 in human immunodeficiency virus-infected individuals: role of peripheral blood mononuclear cells and implications for AIDS pathogenesis. Journal of virology. 2002 Dec;76(24):12448-56.

[158] Wiercinska-Drapalo A, Jaroszewicz J, Flisiak R, Prokopowicz D. Plasma interleukin-18 is associated with viral load and disease progression in HIV-1-infected patients. Microbes and infection / Institut Pasteur. 2004 Nov;6(14):1273-7.

[159] von Giesen HJ, Jander S, Koller H, Arendt G. Serum and cerebrospinal fluid levels of interleukin-18 in human immunodeficiency virus type 1-associated central nervous system disease. Journal of neurovirology. 2004 Dec;10(6):383-6.

[160] Stylianou E, Bjerkeli V, Yndestad A, Heggelund L, Waehre T, Damas JK, et al. Raised serum levels of interleukin-18 is associated with disease progression and may contribute to virological treatment failure in HIV-1-infected patients. Clinical and experimental immunology. 2003 Jun;132(3):462-6.

[161] Kaizu M, Ami Y, Nakasone T, Sasaki Y, Izumi Y, Sato H, et al. Higher levels of IL-18 circulate during primary infection of monkeys with a pathogenic SHIV than with a nonpathogenic SHIV. Virology. 2003 Aug 15;313(1):8-12.

[162] David D, Chevrier D, Treilhou MP, Joussemet M, Dupont B, Theze J, et al. IL-18 underexpression reduces IL-2 levels during HIV infection: a critical step towards the faulty cell-mediated immunity? AIDS (London, England). 2000 Sep 29;14(14):2212-4.

[163] He L, Terunuma H, Hanabusa H, Iwamoto A, Oka S, Tanabe F, et al. Interleukin 18 and interleukin 1beta production is decreased in HIV type 1-seropositive hemophiliacs but not in HIV type 1-seropositive nonhemophiliacs. AIDS research and human retroviruses. 2000 Mar 1;16(4):345-53.

[164] Ahmad R, Iannello A, Samarani S, Morisset R, Toma E, Grosley M, et al. Contribution of platelet activation to plasma IL-18 concentrations in HIV-infected AIDS patients. AIDS (London, England). 2006 Sep 11;20(14):1907-9.

[165] Lindegaard B, Hansen AB, Pilegaard H, Keller P, Gerstoft J, Pedersen BK. Adipose tissue expression of IL-18 and HIV-associated lipodystrophy. AIDS (London, England). 2004 Sep 24;18(14):1956-8.

[166] Lindegaard B, Hansen AB, Gerstoft J, Pedersen BK. High plasma level of interleukin-18 in HIV-infected subjects with lipodystrophy. Journal of acquired immune deficiency syndromes (1999). 2004 May 1;36(1):588-93.

[167] Falasca K, Manigrasso MR, Racciatti D, Zingariello P, Dalessandro M, Ucciferri C, et al. Associations between hypertriglyceridemia and serum ghrelin, adiponectin, and IL-18 levels in HIV-infected patients. Annals of clinical and laboratory science. 2006 Winter;36(1):59-66.

[168] Bettelli E, Korn T, Kuchroo VK. Th17: the third member of the effector T cell trilogy. Current opinion in immunology. 2007 Dec;19(6):652-7.

[169] Brandt K, Singh PB, Bulfone-Paus S, Ruckert R. Interleukin-21: a new modulator of immunity, infection, and cancer. Cytokine Growth Factor Rev. 2007 Jun-Aug;18(3-4):223-32.

[170] Iannello A, Tremblay C, Routy JP, Boulassel MR, Toma E, Ahmad A. Decreased levels of circulating IL-21 in HIV-infected AIDS patients: correlation with CD4+ T-cell counts. Viral immunology. 2008 Sep;21(3):385-8.

[171] Strbo N, de Armas L, Liu H, Kolber MA, Lichtenheld M, Pahwa S. IL-21 augments natural killer effector functions in chronically HIV-infected individuals. AIDS (London, England). 2008 Aug 20;22(13):1551-60.

[172] Bolesta E, Kowalczyk A, Wierzbicki A, Eppolito C, Kaneko Y, Takiguchi M, et al. Increased level and longevity of protective immune responses induced by DNA vaccine expressing the HIV-1 Env glycoprotein when combined with IL-21 and IL-15 gene delivery. J Immunol. 2006 Jul 1;177(1):177-91.

[173] Zeng R, Spolski R, Finkelstein SE, Oh S, Kovanen PE, Hinrichs CS, et al. Synergy of IL-21 and IL-15 in regulating CD8+ T cell expansion and function. The Journal of experimental medicine. 2005 Jan 3;201(1):139-48.

[174] White L, Krishnan S, Strbo N, Liu H, Kolber MA, Lichtenheld MG, et al. Differential effects of IL-21 and IL-15 on perforin expression, lysosomal degranulation, and proliferation in CD8 T cells of patients with human immunodeficiency virus-1 (HIV). Blood. 2007 May 1;109(9):3873-80.

[175] Pflanz S, Timans JC, Cheung J, Rosales R, Kanzler H, Gilbert J, et al. IL-27, a heterodimeric cytokine composed of EBI3 and p28 protein, induces proliferation of naive CD4(+) T cells. Immunity. 2002 Jun;16(6):779-90.

[176] Hibbert L, Pflanz S, De Waal Malefyt R, Kastelein RA. IL-27 and IFN-alpha signal via Stat1 and Stat3 and induce T-Bet and IL-12Rbeta2 in naive T cells. J Interferon Cytokine Res. 2003 Sep;23(9):513-22.

[177] Batten M, Ghilardi N. The biology and therapeutic potential of interleukin 27. J Mol Med. 2007 Jul;85(7):661-72.

[178] Morishima N, Owaki T, Asakawa M, Kamiya S, Mizuguchi J, Yoshimoto T. Augmentation of effector CD8+ T cell generation with enhanced granzyme B expression by IL-27. J Immunol. 2005 Aug 1;175(3):1686-93.

[179] Takeda A, Hamano S, Yamanaka A, Hanada T, Ishibashi T, Mak TW, et al. Cutting edge: role of IL-27/WSX-1 signaling for induction of T-bet through activation of STAT1 during initial Th1 commitment. J Immunol. 2003 May 15;170(10):4886-90.

[180] Collison LW, Vignali DA. Interleukin-35: odd one out or part of the family? Immunological reviews. 2008 Dec;226:248-62.

[181] Oppmann B, Lesley R, Blom B, Timans JC, Xu Y, Hunte B, et al. Novel p19 protein engages IL-12p40 to form a cytokine, IL-23, with biological activities similar as well as distinct from IL-12. Immunity. 2000 Nov;13(5):715-25.

[182] Boumendjel A, Tawk L, Malefijt Rde W, Boulay V, Yssel H, Pene J. IL-27 induces the production of IgG1 by human B cells. European cytokine network. 2006 Dec;17(4):281-9.

[183] Fakruddin JM, Lempicki RA, Gorelick RJ, Yang J, Adelsberger JW, Garcia-Pineres AJ, et al. Noninfectious papilloma virus-like particles inhibit HIV-1 replication: implications for immune control of HIV-1 infection by IL-27. Blood. 2007 Mar 1;109(5):1841-9.

[184] Imamichi T, Yang J, Huang DW, Brann TW, Fullmer BA, Adelsberger JW, et al. IL-27, a novel anti-HIV cytokine, activates multiple interferon-inducible genes in macrophages. AIDS (London, England). 2008 Jan 2;22(1):39-45.

[185] Beutler B, Greenwald D, Hulmes JD, Chang M, Pan YC, Mathison J, et al. Identity of tumour necrosis factor and the macrophage-secreted factor cachectin. Nature. 1985 Aug 8-14;316(6028):552-4.

[186] Foti M, Granucci F, Aggujaro D, Liboi E, Luini W, Minardi S, et al. Upon dendritic cell (DC) activation chemokines and chemokine receptor expression are rapidly regulated for recruitment and maintenance of DC at the inflammatory site. International immunology. 1999 Jun;11(6):979-86.

[187] Hodge-Dufour J, Marino MW, Horton MR, Jungbluth A, Burdick MD, Strieter RM, et al. Inhibition of interferon gamma induced interleukin 12 production: a potential mechanism for the anti-inflammatory activities of tumor necrosis factor. Proceedings of the National Academy of Sciences of the United States of America. 1998 Nov 10;95(23):13806-11.

[188] Cope AP, Liblau RS, Yang XD, Congia M, Laudanna C, Schreiber RD, et al. Chronic tumor necrosis factor alters T cell responses by attenuating T cell receptor signaling. The Journal of experimental medicine. 1997 May 5;185(9):1573-84.

[189] Grell M, Becke FM, Wajant H, Mannel DN, Scheurich P. TNF receptor type 2 mediates thymocyte proliferation independently of TNF receptor type 1. European journal of immunology. 1998 Jan;28(1):257-63.

[190] Gehr G, Gentz R, Brockhaus M, Loetscher H, Lesslauer W. Both tumor necrosis factor receptor types mediate proliferative signals in human mononuclear cell activation. J Immunol. 1992 Aug 1;149(3):911-7.

[191] Jacobsen FW, Rothe M, Rusten L, Goeddel DV, Smeland EB, Veiby OP, et al. Role of the 75-kDa tumor necrosis factor receptor: inhibition of early hematopoiesis. Proceedings of the National Academy of Sciences of the United States of America. 1994 Oct 25;91(22):10695-9.

[192] Zheng L, Fisher G, Miller RE, Peschon J, Lynch DH, Lenardo MJ. Induction of apoptosis in mature T cells by tumour necrosis factor. Nature. 1995 Sep 28;377(6547):348-51.

[193] Lazdins JK, Grell M, Walker MR, Woods-Cook K, Scheurich P, Pfizenmaier K. Membrane tumor necrosis factor (TNF) induced cooperative signaling of TNFR60 and TNFR80 favors induction of cell death rather than virus production in HIV-infected T cells. The Journal of experimental medicine. 1997 Jan 6;185(1):81-90.

[194] Fauci AS. Multifactorial nature of human immunodeficiency virus disease: implications for therapy. Science. 1993 Nov 12;262(5136):1011-8.

[195] Lahdevirta J, Maury CP, Teppo AM, Repo H. Elevated levels of circulating cachectin/tumor necrosis factor in patients with acquired immunodeficiency syndrome. Am J Med. 1988 Sep;85(3):289-91.

[196] Karsten V, Gordon S, Kirn A, Herbein G. HIV-1 envelope glycoprotein gp120 down-regulates CD4 expression in primary human macrophages through induction of endogenous tumour necrosis factor-alpha. Immunology. 1996 May;88(1):55-60.

[197] Herbein G, Doyle AG, Montaner LJ, Gordon S. Lipopolysaccharide (LPS) down-regulates CD4 expression in primary human macrophages through induction of endogenous tumour necrosis factor (TNF) and IL-1 beta. Clinical and experimental immunology. 1995 Nov;102(2):430-7.

[198] Schmidtmayerova H, Nottet HS, Nuovo G, Raabe T, Flanagan CR, Dubrovsky L, et al. Human immunodeficiency virus type 1 infection alters chemokine beta peptide expression in human monocytes: implications for recruitment of leukocytes into brain and lymph nodes. Proceedings of the National Academy of Sciences of the United States of America. 1996 Jan 23;93(2):700-4.

[199] Di Marzio P, Tse J, Landau NR. Chemokine receptor regulation and HIV type 1 tropism in monocyte-macrophages. AIDS research and human retroviruses. 1998 Jan 20;14(2):129-38.

[200] Herbein G, Gordon S. 55- and 75-kilodalton tumor necrosis factor receptors mediate distinct actions in regard to human immunodeficiency virus type 1 replication in primary human macrophages. Journal of virology. 1997 May;71(5):4150-6.

[201] Folks TM, Clouse KA, Justement J, Rabson A, Duh E, Kehrl JH, et al. Tumor necrosis factor alpha induces expression of human immunodeficiency virus in a chronically infected T-cell clone. Proceedings of the National Academy of Sciences of the United States of America. 1989 Apr;86(7):2365-8.

[202] Jeeninga RE, Hoogenkamp M, Armand-Ugon M, de Baar M, Verhoef K, Berkhout B. Functional differences between the long terminal repeat transcriptional promoters of human immunodeficiency virus type 1 subtypes A through G. Journal of virology. 2000 Apr;74(8):3740-51.

[203] Blackard JT, Renjifo BR, Mwakagile D, Montano MA, Fawzi WW, Essex M. Transmission of human immunodeficiency type 1 viruses with intersubtype recombinant long terminal repeat sequences. Virology. 1999 Feb 15;254(2):220-5.

[204] Israel A. The IKK complex: an integrator of all signals that activate NF-kappaB? Trends Cell Biol. 2000 Apr;10(4):129-33.

[205] Li Q, Gebhard K, Schacker T, Henry K, Haase AT. The relationship between tumor necrosis factor and human immunodeficiency virus gene expression in lymphoid tissue. Journal of virology. 1997 Sep;71(9):7080-2.

[206] Knuchel MC, Speck RF, Schlaepfer E, Kuster H, Ott P, Gunthard HF, et al. Impact of TNFalpha, LTalpha, Fc gammaRII and complement receptor on HIV-1 trapping in lymphoid tissue from HIV-infected patients. AIDS (London, England). 2000 Dec 1;14(17):2661-9.

[207] Walsh DG, Horvath CJ, Hansen-Moosa A, MacKey JJ, Sehgal PK, Daniel MD, et al. Cytokine influence on simian immunodeficiency virus replication within primary macrophages. TNF-alpha, but not GMCSF, enhances viral replication on a per-cell basis. The American journal of pathology. 1991 Oct;139(4):877-87.

[208] Xiao L, Owen SM, Rudolph DL, Lal RB, Lal AA. Plasmodium falciparum antigen-induced human immunodeficiency virus type 1 replication is mediated through induction of tumor necrosis factor-alpha. The Journal of infectious diseases. 1998 Feb;177(2):437-45.

[209] da Silva B, Singer W, Fong IW, Ottaway CA. In vivo cytokine and neuroendocrine responses to endotoxin in human immunodeficiency virus-infected subjects. The Journal of infectious diseases. 1999 Jul;180(1):106-15.

[210] Lawn SD, Shattock RJ, Acheampong JW, Lal RB, Folks TM, Griffin GE, et al. Sustained plasma TNF-alpha and HIV-1 load despite resolution of other parameters of immune activation during treatment of tuberculosis in Africans. AIDS (London, England). 1999 Nov 12;13(16):2231-7.

[211] Sturm-Ramirez K, Gaye-Diallo A, Eisen G, Mboup S, Kanki PJ. High levels of tumor necrosis factor-alpha and interleukin-1beta in bacterial vaginosis may increase susceptibility to human immunodeficiency virus. The Journal of infectious diseases. 2000 Aug;182(2):467-73.

[212] Sulkowski MS, Chaisson RE, Karp CL, Moore RD, Margolick JB, Quinn TC. The effect of acute infectious illnesses on plasma human immunodeficiency virus (HIV) type 1 load and the expression of serologic markers of immune activation among HIV-infected adults. The Journal of infectious diseases. 1998 Dec;178(6):1642-8.

[213] Vigano A, Bricalli D, Trabattoni D, Salvaggio A, Ruzzante S, Barbi M, et al. Immunization with both T cell-dependent and T cell-independent vaccines augments HIV viral load secondarily to stimulation of tumor necrosis factor alpha. AIDS research and human retroviruses. 1998 Jun 10;14(9):727-34.

[214] Lawn SD, Subbarao S, Wright TC, Jr., Evans-Strickfaden T, Ellerbrock TV, Lennox JL, et al. Correlation between human immunodeficiency virus type 1 RNA levels in the female genital tract and immune activation associated with ulceration of the cervix. The Journal of infectious diseases. 2000 Jun;181(6):1950-6.

[215] Obregon E, Punzon C, Fernandez-Cruz E, Fresno M, Munoz-Fernandez MA. HIV-1 infection induces differentiation of immature neural cells through autocrine tumor necrosis factor and nitric oxide production. Virology. 1999 Sep 1;261(2):193-204.

[216] Cota M, Kleinschmidt A, Ceccherini-Silberstein F, Aloisi F, Mengozzi M, Mantovani A, et al. Upregulated expression of interleukin-8, RANTES and chemokine receptors in human astrocytic cells infected with HIV-1. Journal of neurovirology. 2000 Feb;6(1):75-83.

[217] Rieckmann P, Poli G, Kehrl JH, Fauci AS. Activated B lymphocytes from human immunodeficiency virus-infected individuals induce virus expression in infected T cells and a promonocytic cell line, U1. The Journal of experimental medicine. 1991 Jan 1;173(1):1-5.

[218] Clayette P, Le Grand R, Noack O, Vaslin B, Le Naour R, Benveniste O, et al. Tumor necrosis factor-alpha in serum of macaques during SIVmac251 acute infection. J Med Primatol. 1995 Feb;24(2):94-100.

[219] Cheret A, Le Grand R, Caufour P, Dereuddre-Bosquet N, Matheux F, Neildez O, et al. Cytokine mRNA expression in mononuclear cells from different tissues during acute SIVmac251 infection of macaques. AIDS research and human retroviruses. 1996 Sep 1;12(13):1263-72.

[220] Benveniste O, Vaslin B, Le Grand R, Fouchet P, Omessa V, Theodoro F, et al. Interleukin 1 beta, interleukin 6, tumor necrosis factor alpha, and interleukin 10 responses in peripheral blood mononuclear cells of cynomolgus macaques during acute infection with SIVmac251. AIDS research and human retroviruses. 1996 Feb 10;12(3):241-50.

[221] Sopper S, Demuth M, Stahl-Hennig C, Hunsmann G, Plesker R, Coulibaly C, et al. The effect of simian immunodeficiency virus infection in vitro and in vivo on the cytokine production of isolated microglia and peripheral macrophages from rhesus monkey. Virology. 1996 Jun 15;220(2):320-9.

[222] Belec L, Gherardi R, Payan C, Prazuck T, Malkin JE, Tevi-Benissan C, et al. Proinflammatory cytokine expression in cervicovaginal secretions of normal and HIV-infected women. Cytokine. 1995 Aug;7(6):568-74.

[223] Abel K, Rocke DM, Chohan B, Fritts L, Miller CJ. Temporal and anatomic relationship between virus replication and cytokine gene expression after vaginal simian immunodeficiency virus infection. Journal of virology. 2005 Oct;79(19):12164-72.

[224] Centlivre M, Sommer P, Michel M, Fang RH, Gofflo S, Valladeau J, et al. HIV-1 clade promoters strongly influence spatial and temporal dynamics of viral replication in vivo. The Journal of clinical investigation. 2005 Feb;115(2):348-58.

[225] Montano MA, Nixon CP, Ndung'u T, Bussmann H, Novitsky VA, Dickman D, et al. Elevated tumor necrosis factor-alpha activation of human immunodeficiency virus type 1 subtype C in Southern Africa is associated with an NF-kappaB enhancer gain-of-function. The Journal of infectious diseases. 2000 Jan;181(1):76-81.

[226] Centlivre M, Sommer P, Michel M, Ho Tsong Fang R, Gofflo S, Valladeau J, et al. The HIV-1 clade C promoter is particularly well adapted to replication in the gut in primary infection. AIDS (London, England). 2006 Mar 21;20(5):657-66.

[227] van der Hoek L, Sol CJ, Snijders F, Bartelsman JF, Boom R, Goudsmit J. Human immunodeficiency virus type 1 RNA populations in faeces with higher homology to intestinal populations than to blood populations. The Journal of general virology. 1996 Oct;77 (Pt 10):2415-25.

[228] Lucey DR, Clerici M, Shearer GM. Type 1 and type 2 cytokine dysregulation in human infectious, neoplastic, and inflammatory diseases. Clinical microbiology reviews. 1996 Oct;9(4):532-62.

[229] Schroeter M, Jander S. T-cell cytokines in injury-induced neural damage and repair. Neuromolecular medicine. 2005;7(3):183-95.

[230] von der Weid T, Beebe AM, Roopenian DC, Coffman RL. Early production of IL-4 and induction of Th2 responses in the lymph node originate from an MHC class I-independent CD4+NK1.1- T cell population. J Immunol. 1996 Nov 15;157(10):4421-7.

[231] Paul WE. Interleukin 4: signalling mechanisms and control of T cell differentiation. Ciba Found Symp. 1997;204:208-16; discussion 16-9.

[232] O'Garra A. Cytokines induce the development of functionally heterogeneous T helper cell subsets. Immunity. 1998 Mar;8(3):275-83.

[233] Relloso M, Puig-Kroger A, Pello OM, Rodriguez-Fernandez JL, de la Rosa G, Longo N, et al. DC-SIGN (CD209) expression is IL-4 dependent and is negatively regulated by IFN, TGF-beta, and anti-inflammatory agents. J Immunol. 2002 Mar 15;168(6):2634-43.

[234] Sozzani S, Ghezzi S, Iannolo G, Luini W, Borsatti A, Polentarutti N, et al. Interleukin 10 increases CCR5 expression and HIV infection in human monocytes. J Exp Med. 1998 Feb 2;187(3):439-44.

[235] Valentin A, Lu W, Rosati M, Schneider R, Albert J, Karlsson A, et al. Dual effect of interleukin 4 on HIV-1 expression: implications for viral phenotypic switch and disease progression. Proc Natl Acad Sci U S A. 1998 Jul 21;95(15):8886-91.

[236] Galli G, Annunziato F, Mavilia C, Romagnani P, Cosmi L, Manetti R, et al. Enhanced HIV expression during Th2-oriented responses explained by the opposite regulatory effect of IL-4 and IFN-gamma of fusin/CXCR4. Eur J Immunol. 1998 Oct;28(10):3280-90.

[237] Jourdan P, Abbal C, Noraz N, Hori T, Uchiyama T, Vendrell JP, et al. IL-4 induces functional cell-surface expression of CXCR4 on human T cells. J Immunol. 1998 May 1;160(9):4153-7.

[238] Wang J, Roderiquez G, Oravecz T, Norcross MA. Cytokine regulation of human immunodeficiency virus type 1 entry and replication in human monocytes/macrophages through modulation of CCR5 expression. J Virol. 1998 Sep;72(9):7642-7.

[239] Houle M, Thivierge M, Le Gouill C, Stankova J, Rola-Pleszczynski M. IL-10 up-regulates CCR5 gene expression in human monocytes. Inflammation. 1999 Jun;23(3):241-51.

[240] Kedzierska K, Crowe SM, Turville S, Cunningham AL. The influence of cytokines, chemokines and their receptors on HIV-1 replication in monocytes and macrophages. Rev Med Virol. 2003 Jan-Feb;13(1):39-56.

[241] Banchereau J, Paczesny S, Blanco P, Bennett L, Pascual V, Fay J, et al. Dendritic cells: controllers of the immune system and a new promise for immunotherapy. Ann N Y Acad Sci. 2003 Apr;987:180-7.

[242] Moore KW, de Waal Malefyt R, Coffman RL, O'Garra A. Interleukin-10 and the interleukin-10 receptor. Annu Rev Immunol. 2001;19:683-765.

[243] Ancuta P, Bakri Y, Chomont N, Hocini H, Gabuzda D, Haeffner-Cavaillon N. Opposite effects of IL-10 on the ability of dendritic cells and macrophages to replicate primary CXCR4-dependent HIV-1 strains. J Immunol. 2001 Mar 15;166(6):4244-53.

[244] Kollmann TR, Pettoello-Mantovani M, Katopodis NF, Hachamovitch M, Rubinstein A, Kim A, et al. Inhibition of acute in vivo human immunodeficiency virus infection by human interleukin 10 treatment of SCID mice implanted with human fetal thymus and liver. Proc Natl Acad Sci U S A. 1996 Apr 2;93(7):3126-31.

[245] Schols D, De Clercq E. Human immunodeficiency virus type 1 gp120 induces anergy in human peripheral blood lymphocytes by inducing interleukin-10 production. J Virol. 1996 Aug;70(8):4953-60.

[246] Weissman D, Poli G, Fauci AS. Interleukin 10 blocks HIV replication in macrophages by inhibiting the autocrine loop of tumor necrosis factor alpha and interleukin 6 induction of virus. AIDS Res Hum Retroviruses. 1994 Oct;10(10):1199-206.

[247] Weissman D, Poli G, Fauci AS. IL-10 synergizes with multiple cytokines in enhancing HIV production in cells of monocytic lineage. J Acquir Immune Defic Syndr Hum Retrovirol. 1995 Aug 15;9(5):442-9.

[248] Barcellini W, Rizzardi GP, Marriott JB, Fain C, Shattock RJ, Meroni PL, et al. Interleukin-10-induced HIV-1 expression is mediated by induction of both membrane-bound tumour necrosis factor (TNF)-alpha and TNF receptor type 1 in a promonocytic cell line. Aids. 1996 Jul;10(8):835-42.

[249] Rabbi MF, Finnegan A, Al-Harthi L, Song S, Roebuck KA. Interleukin-10 enhances tumor necrosis factor-alpha activation of HIV-1 transcription in latently infected T cells. J Acquir Immune Defic Syndr Hum Retrovirol. 1998 Dec 1;19(4):321-31.

[250] Graziosi C, Gantt KR, Vaccarezza M, Demarest JF, Daucher M, Saag MS, et al. Kinetics of cytokine expression during primary human immunodeficiency virus type 1 infection. Proc Natl Acad Sci U S A. 1996 Apr 30;93(9):4386-91.

[251] Fakoya A, Matear PM, Filley E, Rook GA, Stanford J, Gilson RJ, et al. HIV infection alters the production of both type 1 and 2 cytokines but does not induce a polarized type 1 or 2 state. Aids. 1997 Oct;11(12):1445-52.

[252] Shin HD, Winkler C, Stephens JC, Bream J, Young H, Goedert JJ, et al. Genetic restriction of HIV-1 pathogenesis to AIDS by promoter alleles of IL10. Proc Natl Acad Sci U S A. 2000 Dec 19;97(26):14467-72.

[253] Rizza P, Santini SM, Logozzi MA, Lapenta C, Sestili P, Gherardi G, et al. T-cell dysfunctions in hu-PBL-SCID mice infected with human immunodeficiency virus (HIV) shortly after reconstitution: in vivo effects of HIV on highly activated human immune cells. Journal of virology. 1996 Nov;70(11):7958-64.

[254] Kovalev G, Duus K, Wang L, Lee R, Bonyhadi M, Ho D, et al. Induction of MHC class I expression on immature thymocytes in HIV-1-infected SCID-hu Thy/Liv mice: evidence of indirect mechanisms. J Immunol. 1999 Jun 15;162(12):7555-62.

[255] Goldstein H, Pettoello-Mantovani M, Katopodis NF, Kim A, Yurasov S, Kollmann TR. SCID-hu mice: a model for studying disseminated HIV infection. Seminars in immunology. 1996 Aug;8(4):223-31.

[256] Bailer RT, Holloway A, Sun J, Margolick JB, Martin M, Kostman J, et al. IL-13 and IFN-gamma secretion by activated T cells in HIV-1 infection associated with viral suppression and a lack of disease progression. J Immunol. 1999 Jun 15;162(12):7534-42.

[257] Zanussi S, Simonelli C, Bortolin MT, D'Andrea M, Crepaldi C, Vaccher E, et al. Immunological changes in peripheral blood and in lymphoid tissue after treatment of HIV-infected subjects with highly active anti-retroviral therapy (HAART) or HAART + IL-2. Clin Exp Immunol. 1999 Jun;116(3):486-92.

[258] Zou W, Coulomb A, Venet A, Foussat A, Berrebi D, Beyer C, et al. Administration of interleukin 13 to simian immunodeficiency virus-infected macaques: induction of intestinal epithelial atrophy. AIDS Res Hum Retroviruses. 1998 Jun 10;14(9):775-83.

[259] Bailer RT, Lee B, Montaner LJ. IL-13 and TNF-alpha inhibit dual-tropic HIV-1 in primary macrophages by reduction of surface expression of CD4, chemokine receptors CCR5, CXCR4 and post-entry viral gene expression. Eur J Immunol. 2000 May;30(5):1340-9.

[260] Kedzierska K, Crowe SM. Cytokines and HIV-1: interactions and clinical implications. Antivir Chem Chemother. 2001 May;12(3):133-50.

[261] Wang J, Guan E, Roderiquez G, Calvert V, Alvarez R, Norcross MA. Role of tyrosine phosphorylation in ligand-independent sequestration of CXCR4 in human primary monocytes-macrophages. J Biol Chem. 2001 Dec 28;276(52):49236-43.

[262] Goletti D, Kinter AL, Hardy EC, Poli G, Fauci AS. Modulation of endogenous IL-1 beta and IL-1 receptor antagonist results in opposing effects on HIV expression in chronically infected monocytic cells. J Immunol. 1996 May 1;156(9):3501-8.

[263] Montaner LJ, Doyle AG, Collin M, Herbein G, Illei P, James W, et al. Interleukin 13 inhibits human immunodeficiency virus type 1 production in primary blood-derived human macrophages in vitro. J Exp Med. 1993 Aug 1;178(2):743-7.

[264] Chehimi J, Luo Q, Azzoni L, Shawver L, Ngoubilly N, June R, et al. HIV-1 transmission and cytokine-induced expression of DC-SIGN in human monocyte-derived macrophages. J Leukoc Biol. 2003 Nov;74(5):757-63.

[265] Soilleux EJ, Morris LS, Leslie G, Chehimi J, Luo Q, Levroney E, et al. Constitutive and induced expression of DC-SIGN on dendritic cell and macrophage subpopulations in situ and in vitro. J Leukoc Biol. 2002 Mar;71(3):445-57.

[266] Sabat R, Wallace E, Endesfelder S, Wolk K. IL-19 and IL-20: two novel cytokines with importance in inflammatory diseases. Expert Opin Ther Targets. 2007 May;11(5):601-12.

[267] Bettaccini AA, Baj A, Accolla RS, Basolo F, Toniolo AQ. Proliferative activity of extracellular HIV-1 Tat protein in human epithelial cells: expression profile of pathogenetically relevant genes. BMC Microbiol. 2005;5:20.

[268] Blobe GC, Schiemann WP, Lodish HF. Role of transforming growth factor beta in human disease. N Engl J Med. 2000 May 4;342(18):1350-8.

[269] Sousa AE, Chaves AF, Doroana M, Antunes F, Victorino RM. Kinetics of the changes of lymphocyte subsets defined by cytokine production at single cell level during highly active antiretroviral therapy for HIV-1 infection. J Immunol. 1999 Mar 15;162(6):3718-26.

[270] Valdez H, Lederman MM. Cytokines and cytokine therapies in HIV infection. AIDS Clin Rev. 1997:187-228.

[271] Alonso K, Pontiggia P, Medenica R, Rizzo S. Cytokine patterns in adults with AIDS. Immunol Invest. 1997 Apr;26(3):341-50.

[272] Johnson MD, Gold LI. Distribution of transforming growth factor-beta isoforms in human immunodeficiency virus-1 encephalitis. Hum Pathol. 1996 Jul;27(7):643-9.

[273] Bodi I, Kimmel PL, Abraham AA, Svetkey LP, Klotman PE, Kopp JB. Renal TGF-beta in HIV-associated kidney diseases. Kidney Int. 1997 May;51(5):1568-77.

[274] Wahl SM, Allen JB, McCartney-Francis N, Morganti-Kossmann MC, Kossmann T, Ellingsworth L, et al. Macrophage- and astrocyte-derived transforming growth factor beta as a mediator of central nervous system dysfunction in acquired immune deficiency syndrome. J Exp Med. 1991 Apr 1;173(4):981-91.

[275] Navikas V, Link J, Wahren B, Persson C, Link H. Increased levels of interferon-gamma (IFN-gamma), IL-4 and transforming growth factor-beta (TGF-beta) mRNA expressing blood mononuclear cells in human HIV infection. Clin Exp Immunol. 1994 Apr;96(1):59-63.

[276] Hu R, Oyaizu N, Than S, Kalyanaraman VS, Wang XP, Pahwa S. HIV-1 gp160 induces transforming growth factor-beta production in human PBMC. Clin Immunol Immunopathol. 1996 Sep;80(3 Pt 1):283-9.

[277] Gibellini D, Zauli G, Re MC, Milani D, Furlini G, Caramelli E, et al. Recombinant human immunodeficiency virus type-1 (HIV-1) Tat protein sequentially up-regulates IL-6 and TGF-beta 1 mRNA expression and protein synthesis in peripheral blood monocytes. Br J Haematol. 1994 Oct;88(2):261-7.

[278] Rubartelli A, Poggi A, Sitia R, Zocchi MR. HIV-I Tat: a polypeptide for all seasons. Immunol Today. 1998 Dec;19(12):543-5.

[279] Zauli G, Davis BR, Re MC, Visani G, Furlini G, La Placa M. tat protein stimulates production of transforming growth factor-beta 1 by marrow macrophages: a potential mechanism for human immunodeficiency virus-1-induced hematopoietic suppression. Blood. 1992 Dec 15;80(12):3036-43.

[280] Lotz M, Clark-Lewis I, Ganu V. HIV-1 transactivator protein Tat induces proliferation and TGF beta expression in human articular chondrocytes. J Cell Biol. 1994 Feb;124(3):365-71.

[281] Garba ML, Pilcher CD, Bingham AL, Eron J, Frelinger JA. HIV antigens can induce TGF-beta(1)-producing immunoregulatory CD8+ T cells. J Immunol. 2002 Mar 1;168(5):2247-54.

[282] Sawaya BE, Thatikunta P, Denisova L, Brady J, Khalili K, Amini S. Regulation of TNFalpha and TGFbeta-1 gene transcription by HIV-1 Tat in CNS cells. J Neuroimmunol. 1998 Jul 1;87(1-2):33-42.

[283] Hori K, Burd PR, Kutza J, Weih KA, Clouse KA. Human astrocytes inhibit HIV-1 expression in monocyte-derived macrophages by secreted factors. Aids. 1999 May 7;13(7):751-8.

[284] Li JM, Shen X, Hu PP, Wang XF. Transforming growth factor beta stimulates the human immunodeficiency virus 1 enhancer and requires NF-kappaB activity. Mol Cell Biol. 1998 Jan;18(1):110-21.

[285] Wang J, Guan E, Roderiquez G, Norcross MA. Synergistic induction of apoptosis in primary CD4(+) T cells by macrophage-tropic HIV-1 and TGF-beta1. J Immunol. 2001 Sep 15;167(6):3360-6.

[286] Lazdins JK, Klimkait T, Alteri E, Walker M, Woods-Cook K, Cox D, et al. TGF-beta: upregulator of HIV replication in macrophages. Res Virol. 1991 Mar-Jun;142(2-3):239-42.

[287] Lazdins JK, Klimkait T, Woods-Cook K, Walker M, Alteri E, Cox D, et al. In vitro effect of transforming growth factor-beta on progression of HIV-1 infection in primary mononuclear phagocytes. J Immunol. 1991 Aug 15;147(4):1201-7.

[288] McKiel V, Gu Z, Wainberg MA, Hiscott J. Inhibition of human immunodeficiency virus type 1 multiplication by transforming growth factor beta 1 and AZT in HIV-1-infected myeloid cells. J Interferon Cytokine Res. 1995 Oct;15(10):849-55.

[289] Poli G, Kinter AL, Justement JS, Bressler P, Kehrl JH, Fauci AS. Retinoic acid mimics transforming growth factor beta in the regulation of human immunodeficiency virus expression in monocytic cells. Proc Natl Acad Sci U S A. 1992 Apr 1;89(7):2689-93.

[290] Poli G, Kinter AL, Justement JS, Bressler P, Kehrl JH, Fauci AS. Transforming growth factor beta suppresses human immunodeficiency virus expression and replication in infected cells of the monocyte/macrophage lineage. J Exp Med. 1991;173(3):589-97.

[291] Perrella O, Carreiri PB, Perrella A, Sbreglia C, Gorga F, Guarnaccia D, et al. Transforming growth factor beta-1 and interferon-alpha in the AIDS dementia complex (ADC): possible relationship with cerebral viral load? Eur Cytokine Netw. 2001 Mar;12(1):51-5.

[292] Pantaleo G, Cohen OJ, Schacker T, Vaccarezza M, Graziosi C, Rizzardi GP, et al. Evolutionary pattern of human immunodeficiency virus (HIV) replication and distribution in lymph nodes following primary infection: implications for antiviral therapy. Nat Med. 1998;4(3):341-5.

[293] Kramer-Hammerle S, Rothenaigner I, Wolff H, Bell JE, Brack-Werner R. Cells of the central nervous system as targets and reservoirs of the human immunodeficiency virus. Virus Res. 2005 Aug;111(2):194-213.

[294] Shattock RJ, Moore JP. Inhibiting sexual transmission of HIV-1 infection. Nat Rev Microbiol. 2003 Oct;1(1):25-34.

[295] John-Stewart G, Mbori-Ngacha D, Ekpini R, Janoff EN, Nkengasong J, Read JS, et al. Breast-feeding and Transmission of HIV-1. Journal of acquired immune deficiency syndromes (1999). 2004 Feb 1;35(2):196-202.

[296] Mattapallil JJ, Douek DC, Hill B, Nishimura Y, Martin M, Roederer M. Massive infection and loss of memory CD4+ T cells in multiple tissues during acute SIV infection. Nature. 2005 Apr 28;434(7037):1093-7.

[297] Fox CH, Kotler D, Tierney A, Wilson CS, Fauci AS. Detection of HIV-1 RNA in the lamina propria of patients with AIDS and gastrointestinal disease. The Journal of infectious diseases. 1989 Mar;159(3):467-71.

[298] Check E. Gut warfare. Nature medicine. 2007 Feb;13(2):116-7.

[299] Schnittman SM, Lane HC, Greenhouse J, Justement JS, Baseler M, Fauci AS. Preferential infection of CD4+ memory T cells by human immunodeficiency virus type 1: evidence for a role in the selective T-cell functional defects observed in infected individuals. Proceedings of the National Academy of Sciences of the United States of America. 1990 Aug;87(16):6058-62.

[300] Cheroutre H, Madakamutil L. Acquired and natural memory T cells join forces at the mucosal front line. Nat Rev Immunol. 2004 Apr;4(4):290-300.

[301] Fletcher PS, Elliott J, Grivel JC, Margolis L, Anton P, McGowan I, et al. Ex vivo culture of human colorectal tissue for the evaluation of candidate microbicides. AIDS (London, England). 2006 Jun 12;20(9):1237-45.

[302] Zeitz M, Schieferdecker HL, Ullrich R, Jahn HU, James SP, Riecken EO. Phenotype and function of lamina propria T lymphocytes. Immunologic research. 1991;10(3-4):199-206.

[303] Lapenta C, Boirivant M, Marini M, Santini SM, Logozzi M, Viora M, et al. Human intestinal lamina propria lymphocytes are naturally permissive to HIV-1 infection. European journal of immunology. 1999 Apr;29(4):1202-8.

[304] Anton PA, Elliott J, Poles MA, McGowan IM, Matud J, Hultin LE, et al. Enhanced levels of functional HIV-1 co-receptors on human mucosal T cells demonstrated using intestinal biopsy tissue. AIDS (London, England). 2000 Aug 18;14(12):1761-5.

[305] Grivel JC, Elliott J, Lisco A, Biancotto A, Condack C, Shattock RJ, et al. HIV-1 pathogenesis differs in rectosigmoid and tonsillar tissues infected ex vivo with CCR5- and CXCR4-tropic HIV-1. AIDS (London, England). 2007 Jun 19;21(10):1263-72.

[306] Wolinsky SM, Wike CM, Korber BT, Hutto C, Parks WP, Rosenblum LL, et al. Selective transmission of human immunodeficiency virus type-1 variants from mothers to infants. Science. 1992 Feb 28;255(5048):1134-7.

[307] Margolis L, Shattock R. Selective transmission of CCR5-utilizing HIV-1: the 'gatekeeper' problem resolved? Nat Rev Microbiol. 2006 Apr;4(4):312-7.

[308] Porter BO, Malek TR. Thymic and intestinal intraepithelial T lymphocyte development are each regulated by the gammac-dependent cytokines IL-2, IL-7, and IL-15. Seminars in immunology. 2000 Oct;12(5):465-74.

[309] Ndolo T, Rheinhardt J, Zaragoza M, Smit-McBride Z, Dandekar S. Alterations in RANTES gene expression and T-cell prevalence in intestinal mucosa during pathogenic or nonpathogenic simian immunodeficiency virus infection. Virology. 1999 Jun 20;259(1):110-8.

[310] Moniuszko M, Edghill-Smith Y, Venzon D, Stevceva L, Nacsa J, Tryniszewska E, et al. Decreased number of CD4+ and CD8+ T cells that express the interleukin-7 receptor in blood and tissues of SIV-infected macaques. Virology. 2006 Dec 5-20;356(1-2):188-97.

[311] Olsson J, Poles M, Spetz AL, Elliott J, Hultin L, Giorgi J, et al. Human immunodeficiency virus type 1 infection is associated with significant mucosal inflammation characterized by increased expression of CCR5, CXCR4, and beta-chemokines. The Journal of infectious diseases. 2000 Dec;182(6):1625-35.

[312] Nilsson J, Kinloch-de-Loes S, Granath A, Sonnerborg A, Goh LE, Andersson J. Early immune activation in gut-associated and peripheral lymphoid tissue during acute HIV infection. AIDS (London, England). 2007 Mar 12;21(5):565-74.

[313] Wang HC, Dann SM, Okhuysen PC, Lewis DE, Chappell CL, Adler DG, et al. High levels of CXCL10 are produced by intestinal epithelial cells in AIDS patients with active cryptosporidiosis but not after reconstitution of immunity. Infection and immunity. 2007 Jan;75(1):481-7.

[314] Dolei A, Biolchini A, Serra C, Curreli S, Gomes E, Dianzani F. Increased replication of T-cell-tropic HIV strains and CXC-chemokine receptor-4 induction in T cells treated with macrophage inflammatory protein (MIP)-1alpha, MIP-1beta and RANTES beta-chemokines. Aids. 1998;12(2):183-90.

[315] Kinter A, Catanzaro A, Monaco J, Ruiz M, Justement J, Moir S, et al. CC-chemokines enhance the replication of T-tropic strains of HIV-1 in CD4(+) T cells: role of signal transduction. Proc Natl Acad Sci U S A. 1998;95(20):11880-5.

[316] Vicenzi E, Alfano M, Ghezzi S, Gatti A, Veglia F, Lazzarin A, et al. Divergent regulation of HIV-1 replication in PBMC of infected individuals by CC chemokines: suppression by RANTES, MIP-1alpha, and MCP-3, and enhancement by MCP-1. J Leukoc Biol. 2000;68(3):405-12.

[317] Aziz S, Fackler OT, Meyerhans A, Muller-Lantzsch N, Zeitz M, Schneider T. Replication of M-tropic HIV-1 in activated human intestinal lamina propria lymphocytes is the main reason for increased virus load in the intestinal mucosa. Journal of acquired immune deficiency syndromes (1999). 2005 Jan 1;38(1):23-30.

[318] Li Q, Duan L, Estes JD, Ma ZM, Rourke T, Wang Y, et al. Peak SIV replication in resting memory CD4+ T cells depletes gut lamina propria CD4+ T cells. Nature. 2005 Apr 28;434(7037):1148-52.

[319] Luster AD. Chemokines--chemotactic cytokines that mediate inflammation. The New England journal of medicine. 1998 Feb 12;338(7):436-45.

[320] Abner SR, Guenthner PC, Guarner J, Hancock KA, Cummins JE, Jr., Fink A, et al. A human colorectal explant culture to evaluate topical microbicides for the prevention of HIV infection. The Journal of infectious diseases. 2005 Nov 1;192(9):1545-56.

[321] Guadalupe M, Reay E, Sankaran S, Prindiville T, Flamm J, McNeil A, et al. Severe CD4+ T-cell depletion in gut lymphoid tissue during primary human immunodeficiency virus type 1 infection and substantial delay in restoration following highly active antiretroviral therapy. J Virol. 2003 Nov;77(21):11708-17.

[322] Moll H. Dendritic cells and host resistance to infection. Cell Microbiol. 2003 Aug;5(8):493-500.

[323] Hlavacek WS, Stilianakis NI, Perelson AS. Influence of follicular dendritic cells on HIV dynamics. Philos Trans R Soc Lond B Biol Sci. 2000 Aug 29;355(1400):1051-8.

[324] Su L, Kaneshima H, Bonyhadi M, Salimi S, Kraft D, Rabin L, et al. HIV-1-induced thymocyte depletion is associated with indirect cytopathogenicity and infection of progenitor cells in vivo. Immunity. 1995 Jan;2(1):25-36.

[325] Gaulton GN, Scobie JV, Rosenzweig M. HIV-1 and the thymus. Aids. 1997 Mar 15;11(4):403-14.

[326] Hazenberg MD, Otto SA, Cohen Stuart JW, Verschuren MC, Borleffs JC, Boucher CA, et al. Increased cell division but not thymic dysfunction rapidly affects the T-cell receptor excision circle content of the naive T cell population in HIV-1 infection. Nat Med. 2000 Sep;6(9):1036-42.

[327] Gibb DM, Newberry A, Klein N, de Rossi A, Grosch-Woerner I, Babiker A. Immune repopulation after HAART in previously untreated HIV-1-infected children. Paediatric European Network for Treatment of AIDS (PENTA) Steering Committee. Lancet. 2000 Apr 15;355(9212):1331-2.

[328] Pido-Lopez J, Burton C, Hardy G, Pires A, Sullivan A, Gazzard B, et al. Thymic output during initial highly active antiretroviral therapy (HAART) and during HAART supplementation with interleukin 2 and/or with HIV type 1 immunogen (Remune). AIDS research and human retroviruses. 2003 Feb;19(2):103-9.

[329] Lapenta C, Santini SM, Proietti E, Rizza P, Logozzi M, Spada M, et al. Type I interferon is a powerful inhibitor of in vivo HIV-1 infection and preserves human CD4(+) T cells from virus-induced depletion in SCID mice transplanted with human cells. Virology. 1999 Oct 10;263(1):78-88.

[330] Haas DW, Lavelle J, Nadler JP, Greenberg SB, Frame P, Mustafa N, et al. A randomized trial of interferon alpha therapy for HIV type 1 infection. AIDS research and human retroviruses. 2000 Feb 10;16(3):183-90.

[331] Lane HC, Kovacs JA, Feinberg J, Herpin B, Davey V, Walker R, et al. Anti-retroviral effects of interferon-alpha in AIDS-associated Kaposi's sarcoma. Lancet. 1988 Nov 26;2(8622):1218-22.

[332] Portales P, Reynes J, Pinet V, Rouzier-Panis R, Baillat V, Clot J, et al. Interferon-alpha restores HIV-induced alteration of natural killer cell perforin expression in vivo. AIDS (London, England). 2003 Mar 7;17(4):495-504.

[333] Uittenbogaart CH, Boscardin WJ, Anisman-Posner DJ, Koka PS, Bristol G, Zack JA. Effect of cytokines on HIV-induced depletion of thymocytes in vivo. AIDS (London, England). 2000 Jul 7;14(10):1317-25.

[334] Kim JJ, Yang JS, Manson KH, Weiner DB. Modulation of antigen-specific cellular immune responses to DNA vaccination in rhesus macaques through the use of IL-2, IFN-gamma, or IL-4 gene adjuvants. Vaccine. 2001 Mar 21;19(17-19):2496-505.

[335] Barouch DH, Craiu A, Kuroda MJ, Schmitz JE, Zheng XX, Santra S, et al. Augmentation of immune responses to HIV-1 and simian immunodeficiency virus DNA vaccines by IL-2/Ig plasmid administration in rhesus monkeys. Proceedings of the National Academy of Sciences of the United States of America. 2000 Apr 11;97(8):4192-7.

[336] Barouch DH, Santra S, Schmitz JE, Kuroda MJ, Fu TM, Wagner W, et al. Control of viremia and prevention of clinical AIDS in rhesus monkeys by cytokine-augmented DNA vaccination. Science. 2000 Oct 20;290(5491):486-92.

[337] Craiu A, Barouch DH, Zheng XX, Kuroda MJ, Schmitz JE, Lifton MA, et al. An IL-2/Ig fusion protein influences CD4+ T lymphocytes in naive and simian immunodeficiency virus-infected Rhesus monkeys. AIDS research and human retroviruses. 2001 Jul 1;17(10):873-86.

[338] Imami N, Hardy GA, Nelson MR, Morris-Jones S, Al-Shahi R, Antonopoulos C, et al. Induction of HIV-1-specific T cell responses by administration of cytokines in late-stage patients receiving highly active anti-retroviral therapy. Clin Exp Immunol. 1999 Oct;118(1):78-86.

[339] Lafeuillade A, Poggi C, Chadapaud S, Hittinger G, Chouraqui M, Pisapia M, et al. Pilot study of a combination of highly active antiretroviral therapy and cytokines to induce HIV-1 remission. J Acquir Immune Defic Syndr. 2001 Jan 1;26(1):44-55.

[340] Nair MP, Schwartz SA. Reversal of human immunodeficiency virus type 1 protein-induced inhibition of natural killer cell activity by alpha interferon and interleukin-2. Clinical and diagnostic laboratory immunology. 2000 Jan;7(1):101-5.

[341] Uittenbogaart CH, Anisman DJ, Jamieson BD, Kitchen S, Schmid I, Zack JA, et al. Differential tropism of HIV-1 isolates for distinct thymocyte subsets in vitro. AIDS (London, England). 1996 Jun;10(7):F9-16.

[342] Khatri VP, Baiocchi RA, Bernstein ZP, Caligiuri MA. Immunotherapy with low-dose interleukin-2: rationale for prevention of immune-deficiency-associated cancer. Cancer J Sci Am. 1997 Dec;3 Suppl 1:S129-36.

[343] Shah MH, Baiocchi RA, Fehniger TA, Khatri VP, Gould M, Poiesz B, et al. Cytokine replacement in patients with HIV-1 non-Hodgkin's lymphoma: the rationale for low-dose interleukin-2 therapy. Cancer J Sci Am. 2000 Feb;6 Suppl 1:S45-51.

[344] Baiocchi RA, Ward JS, Carrodeguas L, Eisenbeis CF, Peng R, Roychowdhury S, et al. GM-CSF and IL-2 induce specific cellular immunity and provide protection against Epstein-Barr virus lymphoproliferative disorder. J Clin Invest. 2001 Sep;108(6):887-94.

[345] Tambussi G, Ghezzi S, Nozza S, Vallanti G, Magenta L, Guffanti M, et al., editors. Efficacy of low-dose intermittent subcutaneous interleukin (IL)--2 in antiviral drug--experienced human immunodeficiency virus--infected persons with detectable virus load: a controlled study of 3 il-2 regimens with antiviral drug therapy. The Journal of infectious diseases; 2001 May 15.

[346] Kovacs JA, Imamichi H, Vogel S, Metcalf JA, Dewar RL, Baseler M, et al. Effects of intermittent interleukin-2 therapy on plasma and tissue human immunodeficiency virus levels and quasi-species expression. J Infect Dis. 2000 Oct;182(4):1063-9.

[347] Kovacs JA, Vogel S, Albert JM, Falloon J, Davey RT, Jr., Walker RE, et al. Controlled trial of interleukin-2 infusions in patients infected with the human immunodeficiency virus. N Engl J Med. 1996 Oct 31;335(18):1350-6.

[348] Armstrong WS, Kazanjian P. Use of cytokines in human immunodeficiency virus-infected patients: colony-stimulating factors, erythropoietin, and interleukin-2. Clin Infect Dis. 2001 Mar 1;32(5):766-73.

[349] Levy YaSSC, editor. Effect of Interleukin-2 on clinical outcomes in patients with CD4+ cell count 50 to 299/mm3: primary results of the SILCAAT study. CROI, 16th Conference on Retroviruses and Opportunistic Infections; 2009 February 8-11; Palais des Congres de Montreal, Montreal, Canada.

[350] Porter B, Lane HC, Kovacs JA, Davey RT, Jr., Rehm C, Lozier J, et al., editors. IL-2 cycling causes transient increase in hsCRP and D-dimer independent of HIV viremia. CROI, 16th Conference on Retroviruses and Opportunistic Infections; 2009 February 8-11; Palais des Congres de Montreal, Montreal, Canada.

[351] Tebas P, Henry WK, Matining R, Weng-Cherng D, Schmitz J, Valdez H, et al. Metabolic and immune activation effects of treatment interruption in chronic HIV-1 infection: implications for cardiovascular risk. PLoS ONE. 2008;3(4):e2021.

[352] Chun TW, Carruth L, Finzi D, Shen X, DiGiuseppe JA, Taylor H, et al. Quantification of latent tissue reservoirs and total body viral load in HIV-1 infection [see comments]. Nature. 1997;387(6629):183-8.

[353] Finzi D, Hermankova M, Pierson T, Carruth LM, Buck C, Chaisson RE, et al. Identification of a reservoir for HIV-1 in patients on highly active antiretroviral therapy [see comments]. Science. 1997;278(5341):1295-300.

[354] Zhu T, Muthui D, Holte S, Nickle D, Feng F, Brodie S, et al. Evidence for human immunodeficiency virus type 1 replication in vivo in CD14(+) monocytes and its potential role as a source of virus in patients on highly active antiretroviral therapy. J Virol. 2002;76:707-16.

[355] Fulcher JA, Hwangbo Y, Zioni R, Nickle D, Lin X, Heath L, et al. Compartmentalization of human immunodeficiency virus type 1 between blood monocytes and CD4+ T cells during infection. J Virol. 2004 Aug;78(15):7883-93.

[356] Boyer JD, Cohen AD, Ugen KE, Edgeworth RL, Bennett M, Shah A, et al. Therapeutic immunization of HIV-infected chimpanzees using HIV-1 plasmid antigens and interleukin-12 expressing plasmids. AIDS (London, England). 2000 Jul 28;14(11):1515-22.

[357] Boyer JD, Cohen AD, Ugen KE, Edgeworth RL, Bennett M, Shah A, et al. Therapeutic immunization of HIV-infected chimpanzees using HIV-1 plasmid antigens and interleuoin-12 expressing plasmiDs. Aids. 2000 Jul 28;14(11):1515-22.

[358] Kohl S, Sigaroudinia M, Charlebois ED, Jacobson MA. Interleukin-12 administered in vivo decreases human NK cell cytotoxicity and antibody-dependent cellular cytotoxicity to human immunodeficiency virus-infected cells. J Infect Dis. 1996 Nov;174(5):1105-8.

[359] Kanai T, Thomas EK, Yasutomi Y, Letvin NL. IL-15 stimulates the expansion of AIDS virus-specific CTL. J Immunol. 1996 Oct 15;157(8):3681-7.

[360] Boullier S, Poquet Y, Debord T, Fournie JJ, Gougeon ML. Regulation by cytokines (IL-12, IL-15, IL-4 and IL-10) of the Vgamma9Vdelta2 T cell response to mycobacterial phosphoantigens in responder and anergic HIV-infected persons. Eur J Immunol. 1999 Jan;29(1):90-9.

[361] Hasan MS, Kallas EG, Thomas EK, Looney J, Campbell M, Evans TG. Effects of interleukin-15 on in vitro human T cell proliferation and activation. J Interferon Cytokine Res. 2000 Feb;20(2):119-23.

[362] Naora H, Gougeon ML. Enhanced survival and potent expansion of the natural killer cell population of HIV-infected individuals by exogenous interleukin-15. Immunol Lett. 1999 Jun 1;68(2-3):359-67.

[363] Lin SJ, Roberts RL, Ank BJ, Nguyen QH, Thomas EK, Stiehm ER. Human immunodeficiency virus (HIV) type-1 GP120-specific cell-mediated cytotoxicity (CMC) and natural killer (NK) activity in HIV-infected (HIV+) subjects: enhancement with interleukin-2(IL-2), IL-12, and IL-15. Clin Immunol Immunopathol. 1997 Feb;82(2):163-73.

[364] Seder RA, Grabstein KH, Berzofsky JA, McDyer JF. Cytokine interactions in human immunodeficiency virus-infected individuals: roles of interleukin (IL)-2, IL-12, and IL-15. J Exp Med. 1995 Oct 1;182(4):1067-77.

[365] Mueller YM, Petrovas C, Bojczuk PM, Dimitriou ID, Beer B, Silvera P, et al. Interleukin-15 increases effector memory CD8+ t cells and NK Cells in simian immunodeficiency virus-infected macaques. Journal of virology. 2005 Apr;79(8):4877-85.

[366] Chong SY, Egan MA, Kutzler MA, Megati S, Masood A, Roopchard V, et al. Comparative ability of plasmid IL-12 and IL-15 to enhance cellular and humoral immune responses elicited by a SIVgag plasmid DNA vaccine and alter disease progression following SHIV(89.6P) challenge in rhesus macaques. Vaccine. 2007 Jun 21;25(26):4967-82.

[367] Hryniewicz A, Price DA, Moniuszko M, Boasso A, Edghill-Spano Y, West SM, et al. Interleukin-15 but not interleukin-7 abrogates vaccine-induced decrease in virus level in simian immunodeficiency virus mac251-infected macaques. J Immunol. 2007 Mar 15;178(6):3492-504.

[368] Wong GH, Goeddel DV. Tumour necrosis factors alpha and beta inhibit virus replication and synergize with interferons. Nature. 1986 Oct 30-Nov 5;323(6091):819-22.

[369] Wong GH, Krowka JF, Stites DP, Goeddel DV. In vitro anti-human immunodeficiency virus activities of tumor necrosis factor-alpha and interferon-gamma. J Immunol. 1988 Jan 1;140(1):120-4.

[370] Fortis C, Biswas P, Soldini L, Veglia F, Careddu AM, Delfanti F, et al. Dual role of TNF-alpha in NK/LAK cell-mediated lysis of chronically HIV-infected U1 cells. Concomitant enhancement of HIV expression and sensitization of cell-mediated lysis. European journal of immunology. 1999 Nov;29(11):3654-62.

[371] Biswas P, Mantelli B, Delfanti F, Cota M, Vallanti G, de Filippi C, et al. Tumor necrosis factor-alpha drives HIV-1 replication in U937 cell clones and upregulates CXCR4. Cytokine. 2001 Jan 7;13(1):55-9.

[372] Brice GT, Mayne AE, Villinger F, Ansari AA. A novel role for tumor necrosis factor-alpha in regulating susceptibility of activated CD4+ T cells from human and nonhuman primates for distinct coreceptor using lentiviruses. Journal of acquired immune deficiency syndromes (1999). 2000 May 1;24(1):10-22.

[373] Lipman M, Breen R. Immune reconstitution inflammatory syndrome in HIV. Current opinion in infectious diseases. 2006 Feb;19(1):20-5.

[374] Carcelain G, Debre P, Autran B. Reconstitution of CD4+ T lymphocytes in HIV-infected individuals following antiretroviral therapy. Current opinion in immunology. 2001 Aug;13(4):483-8.

[375] Meintjes G, Wilkinson KA, Rangaka MX, Skolimowska K, van Veen K, Abrahams M, et al. Type 1 helper T cells and FoxP3-positive T cells in HIV-tuberculosis-associated immune reconstitution inflammatory syndrome. American journal of respiratory and critical care medicine. 2008 Nov 15;178(10):1083-9.

[376] Deayton JR, Sabin CA, Britt WB, Jones IM, Wilson P, Johnson MA, et al. Rapid reconstitution of humoral immunity against cytomegalovirus but not HIV following highly active antiretroviral therapy. AIDS (London, England). 2002 Nov 8;16(16):2129-35.

[377] Wagner AD. [Immune reconstitution inflammatory syndrome (IRIS)]. Zeitschrift fur Rheumatologie. 2008 Jul;67(4):284, 6-9.

[378] Dhasmana DJ, Dheda K, Ravn P, Wilkinson RJ, Meintjes G. Immune reconstitution inflammatory syndrome in HIV-infected patients receiving antiretroviral therapy : pathogenesis, clinical manifestations and management. Drugs. 2008;68(2):191-208.

[379] Pires A, Nelson M, Pozniak AL, Fisher M, Gazzard B, Gotch F, et al. Mycobacterial immune reconstitution inflammatory syndrome in HIV-1 infection after antiretroviral therapy is associated with deregulated specific T-cell responses: beneficial effect of IL-2 and GM-CSF immunotherapy. Journal of immune based therapies and vaccines. 2005 Sep 25;3:7.

CHAPTER 3

Defensins and HIV Infection

Theresa L. Chang and Mary Klotman*

Department of Medicine, Division of Infectious Diseases, Mount Sinai School of Medicine, New York, NY.

Abstract: The innate immune system provides the first line of defense against a wide variety of microorganisms before the development of an adaptive immune response. Epithelial cells at mucosal surfaces and recruited leukocytes are often the first to contact microbial pathogens and mount an innate immune response including the production of Antimicrobial Peptides (AMPs) such as defensins and cathelicidins and pro-inflammatory cytokines through pattern recognition receptors (e.g. Toll-like receptors, TLRs). Defensins exhibit a broad spectrum of action against microorganisms including Gram-positive and Gram-negative bacteria, fungi and viruses. In addition to their microbicidal effects they act as immunomodulators involved in inflammation, tissue repair and angiogenesis. However, increasing evidence suggests that the innate immunity including production of AMPs can act as a double-edged sword by providing protection against invading pathogens but at the same time causing potentially harmful inflammation. This review focuses on the role of defensins as innate effectors and immunodulators in HIV infection, the multiple and complex mechanisms by which defensins inhibit or enhance HIV infection in vitro as well as recent clinical evidence supporting an association between defensins and HIV transmission.

AN OVERVIEW OF CLASSIFICATION AND STRUCTURE OF MAMMALIAN DEFENSINS:

Defensins are cationic peptides with β-sheet structures stabilized by three disulfide bonds between the cysteine residues [1, 2]. In humans, defensins are classified into two subfamilies: α and β defensins, differing in their disulfide bond paring. The linkages of Cys residues in a-defensins are $Cys^1–Cys^6$, $Cys^2–Cys^4$, $Cys^3–Cys^5$, whereas in b-defensins the linkages are $Cys^1–Cys^5$, $Cys^2–Cys^4$, $Cys^3–Cys^6$ (Table **1**, reviewed in [2-4]. Despite variation in sequences and disulfide bond linkages, both families have similar structures [5-8]. The α-defensins are synthesized as a prepropeptide, consisting of an amino (N)-terminal signal sequence, an anionic propiece, and a carboxyl (C) terminal mature peptide with approximate 30 amino acids in length [2]. Neutrophil α-defensins (HNPs 1-4) are mainly synthesized in promyelocytes, neutrophil precursor cells in the bone marrow, and the mature peptide is stored in primary granules of neutrophils [2]. Unlike leukocyte α-defensins such as HNPs, human α-defensin-5 (HD5) is released as a propeptide that is processed extracellularly [9, 10]. An additional class of mammalian defensins is the θ-defensin originally found in rhesus monkeys [11]. It has a circular structure with the Cys residues linking Cys^1-Cys^6, Cys^2-Cys^5, Cys^3-Cys^4 [11]. The q-defensins are formed by the fusion of two truncated α-defensin nonapeptides that are connected by fusion of the N- and C-termini [11-13].

Defensin structure appears to be important for its chemotactic and antiviral activities but not antibacterial activities. For examples, disulfide bonds are not required for antibacterial functions of HNP1, human β-defensin-3 (HBD3), and cryptdin-4, a mouse Paneth cells α defensin [14-16]. However, properly folded HBD3 is important for its chemotactic activity [15]. Similarly, HNPs 1-3 or θ-defensins after treatment with the reducing agents dithiothreitol and iodoacetamide loose their direct effect of on the virion [17, 18] and HD5 and HD6 linear analogs loose their HIV enhancing effect [19]. Mutagenesis studies of cryptdin-4 indicates that the disulfide bonds may play a role in protection from proteolysis by matrix metalloproteinase-7 [14].

CELL SOURCES AND TISSUE DISTRIBUTION

Human defensins are mainly produced by leukocytes and epithelial cells. HNPs 1-3 were first isolated from neutrophilic granulocytes (polymorphonucleated neutrophilic leukocytes; PMN), and account for 30-50% of

---

__Address Correspondence to this Author Mary E. Klotman at:__ Department of Medicine, Division of Infectious Diseases, Box 1090, One Gustave L. Levy Place, New York, NY, 10029, USA. Tel: (212) 241-6471, Fax: (212)-534-3240. E-mail: mary.klotman@mssm.edu

Massimo Alfano (Ed)

total protein in azurophil granules of neutrophils [20]. They share high similarity in sequence with only a single amino acid difference [21]. No gene encoding HNP2 was found and thus it is proposed to be a proteolytic product of HNP1 or HNP3. HNP4 comprises less than 2% of defensins in neutrophils and has a relatively distinct sequence but similar structure to HNPs1-3 [2, 22]. While neutrophils produce the highest amount of HNPs, these peptides can be found in other immune cells including natural killer cells, B cells, $\gamma\delta$ T cells, monocytes/macrophages and immature dendritic cells [23, 24]. In addition, cells can absorb and internalize HNPs intracellularly [25-27], underlining the complexity in defining true HNP producing cells and the questions regarding the function of the up-taken defensins. HNPs have been detected in placenta, spleen, thymus, intestinal mucosa, saliva, and cervical mucus plugs [24, 28-30] . Elevation of HNPs has been reported in the vaginal mucosa in women with *N. gonorrhoeae* (GC)*, T. vaginalis, or C. trachomatis* (CT) [31-33], suggesting their role in mucosal immunity against infections *in vivo* [32, 34].

Although leukocyte α defensins are conserved evolutionarily and have been isolated from many species including human, rabbits, rats, guinea pigs and hamsters, mice lack α-defensin expression by neutrophils [2]. Mice express many enteric a-defensins known as cryptdins in intestinal Paneth cells [1, 2]. Similarly, HD5 and HD6 are produced predominantly by intestinal Paneth cells [2]. Interestingly, endogenous cryptdins do not protect mice against salmonellosis, whereas transgenic mice with an HD5 minigene that contains 2 exons and 1.4 kilobases of 5'-flanking sequence are markedly resistant to oral challenge with virulent *Salmonella typhimurium* [35]. In rhesus macaques, an animal model used for studying HIV pathogenesis, six Paneth cell defensins have been identified and their coding sequences are distinct from HD5 and HD6 [36]. HD5 is also found in other tissues such as the salivary glands, the female genital tract and the inflamed large bowel [29, 37-39]. In addition, increased levels of HD5 have been observed in urethral secretions of men with *Neisseria gonorrhoeae* and urethritis associated with *Chlamydia trachomatis* infection [10] and in cervicovaginal secretions from women with bacterial vaginosis [40].

Six human β-defensins (HBD1, -2, -3, -4, -5,-6) have been identified and characterized [4, 41, 42], although an additional 28 human β-defensins [43] have been identified by gene-based searches. HBDs are expressed by epithelial cells and non-epithelial cells including monocytes, macrophages and monocyte-derived dendritic cells (DCs) [2, 4, 44]. While HBD1 is often constitutively expressed, expression of HBD2 and HBD3 can be induced by viruses, bacteria, microbial products and pro-inflammatory cytokines, such as tumour-necrosis factor (TNF) and interleukin-1 (IL-1) [2, 45-48]. HBD1, HBD2 and HBD3 have been detected in various epithelial tissues [29, 49, 50]. Both human α- and β-defensins have been found in breast milk [51, 52], suggesting a role for defensins in protecting infants from infection. Constitutive expression of HBD4 seems to be restricted to testis and gastric antrum, although HBD4 expression can be induced in human respiratory epithelial cells after exposure to phorbol 12-myristate 13-acetate (PMA) or bacteria infection *in vitro* [53]. HBD5 and HBD6 are specifically expressed in human epididymis [41].

Old World monkeys including rhesus macaques, orangutans and a lesser ape species express intact θ-defensins [54]. In contrast, primates including human, chimpanzees and gorillas contain pseudogenes of θ-defensin mRNAs with a conserved stop codon upstream of the signal sequence that prevents translation [54]. Three θ-defensins have been found in leukocytes of rhesus macaques: rhesus θ-defensin-1 (RTD1), RTD2 and RTD3 [11-13]. Retrocyclin, an artificially made circular peptide based on the sequence of the mature peptide that would be encoded by the human θ-defensin pseudogene, has been shown to display antiviral activity *in vitro* [55].

Regulation

HNPs are primarily synthesized in promyelocytes and early myelocytes, the bone-marrow precursors of neutrophils [56]. HNP1 and HNP3 are transcriptionally regulated in promyelocytic cells by the binding of CCAAT/enhancer-binidng protein (C/EBP a) to C/EBP/c-Myb sites in the HNP promoter [57]. In response to bacterial infection, high concentrations of HNPs (mg/ml) are present in neutrophils phagosomes as the result of the fusion of granules and phagocytic vacuoles of neutrophils [2, 58]. HNPs can also be released by chemokines, FCg receptor cross-linking and PMA [25, 59-61]. Pathogen-associated molecular patterns (PAMPs) from the outer membrane protein A of *Klebsiella pneumoniae* and flagellin of *Escherichia coli*, which signal via toll-like receptors 2 and 5, respectively, trigger the release of HNPs 1-3 by CD3$^+$CD56$^+$

natural killer T cells [60]. Direct interaction of *Mycobacterium bovis* BCG with eosinophils induces the production and release of HNPs 1-3 in a TLR2 dependent manner [62].

HD5, the most abundant AMP in the small intestine, is constitutively expressed by Paneth cells but can be found in the colon of patients with inflammatory bowel disease [35, 63, 64]. A NOD2 mutation in patients with ileal Crohn's disease (CD), a chronic mucosal inflammation, has been associated with a pronounced reduction in HD5 production [65]. A reduced expression Wnt signaling transcription factor Tcf-4 protein has been correlated with a decrease in HD5 and HD6 expression in the small intestine of patients with ileal CD, although this association is independent of the NOD2 genotype [66]. HD5 is induced in the genital mucosa in patients with bacterial vaginosis, *Neisseria gonorrhoeae* and *Chlamydia trachomatis* infections [10, 40], although the mechanism of induction remains to be defined.

The mechanisms of induction of HBD1, HBD2 and HBD3 have been shown to be distinct from each other [42]. HBD2 can be induced by TLR2, TLR3, TLR4, TLR7, NOD1 and NOD2 signaling in various epithelial cells and keratinocytes [67-71]. Stimulation of TLR3 has been shown to induce HBD1 and HBD2 expression in uterine epithelial cells [72]. Induction of HBD2 and HBD3 but not HBD1 in bronchial epithelial cells in response to human rhinovirus infection is mediated by nuclear factor-κB (NF-κB) activation but not of IL-1 [45]. As TLR3 activation also induces HBD2 and HBD3, it is possible that intracellular double-stranded RNA generated during replication of rhinovirus may be involved in the regulation of HBDs [45, 46]. Similarly, HBD2 and HBD3 are induced in normal human oral epithelial cells [73]. In oral epithelium, TLR2 and NOD1/2 ligands synergistically activate NF-κB and induce HBD2 gene expression [74]. Cytokines such as IL-1 and IL-17 also play important roles in the regulation of HBD2 expression. Induction of HBD2 by IL-17A is mediated by the PI3K and MAPK pathways to activate NF-κB in airway epithelial cells, whereas regulation of HBD2 by the activation of NF-κB is not dependent on PI3K pathway in bronchial epithelial cell, [75-77], indicating that specific pathways involved in regulation of HBDs are cell type dependent.

Functions

Defensins are originally thought to kill mammalian target cells and microorganisms though a common mechanism by permeabilization of target membranes, which involves electrostatic interactions between positively charged defensins and negatively charged membrane lipids (reviewed in [78]). Recent studies revealed that defensins have differential antibacterial activity and specificity. The varying degree of antibacterial activity of HBD3 against different bacteria is in part attributed to its lipid-specificity [79]. For example, HD6, distinct from other α-defensins including HNPs1-4 and HD5, does not exhibit anti-bacterial activity [80]. Additionally, HNPs and HBDs have differential effects on cytokine production in bronchial epithelial cells [81]. Thus, the functions of defensins appear to be specific to the defensin and target.

Defensins have a wide range of functions in modulating innate and adaptive immunity [4] as well as a number of other defensin specific biological functions [82-87]. Many of these effects could directly or indirectly influence HIV. Both HNPs and HBDs exhibit chemotactic activity for T cells, monocytes and immature DCs and can induce production of cytokines and chemokines [4, 88, 89]. HNP1 also regulates the release of IL-1β and enhances phagocytosis [90, 91]. HBDs1-3 recruit memory T cells and immature DCs through binding to CCR6, the receptor for the CC-chemokine ligand 20 (CCL20; also known as MIP3α) [92, 93]. HBD2 has multiple activities on mast cells, including induction of cell migration, degranulation and prostaglandin D_2 production [94]. Murine β-defensin-2 can recruit bone-marrow-derived immature DCs through CCR6 and can induce DC maturation through TLR4 [95]. HBD3 activates antigen-presenting cells such as monocytes and DCs through TLRs 1 and 2 [96]. HBD3 actives antigen presenting cells (DCs and monocytes) via TLR1/2 [96], suggesting a role for defensins in HIV transmission. Defensins are frequently induced by pro-inflammatory cytokines or TLR activation [2, 97]. Conversely, defensins can induce cytokines and chemokines. HNPs upregulate the expression of CC-chemokines and IL-8 in macrophages and epithelial cells, respectively [98, 99]. HBD2, known to be inducible in response to bacterial infection and pro-inflammatory cytokines [2, 4] can up-regulate IL-6, IL-8, IL-10, MCP-1, IL-1β, MIP-1β and RANTES in PBMCs [100]. HD5 can induce IL-8 [101] that enhances HIV infection in cervical tissues [102].

Defensins can bind to other host proteins to modulate immune or metabolic functions [82]. HNPs bind to low-density lipoprotein receptor-related proteins and interact with protein kinase Cα and β leading to decreased smooth muscle contraction in response to phenylephrine [103]. HNPs also interact with adrenocorticotrophic hormone (ACTH) receptors and heparan sulfate-containing proteoglycan (HSPGs) to modulate other biological activities [104, 105]. HNP1 has been shown to inhibit the activity of conventional PKC isoforms in a cell-free system [106]. This PKC inhibitory activity appears to be important for HNP1-mediated inhibition of HIV replication in primary CD4$^+$ T cells [107]. As defensins display various biological functions, the roles of defensins in HIV-associated metabolic disorders or cancers in addition to HIV transmission and pathogenesis remain to be investigated.

EFFECT OF DEFENSINS ON HIV INFECTION: MECHANISM(S) OF ACTION

Recent studies indicate that, specific defensins can inhibit or enhance HIV infection. With respect to anti-HIV activities of defensins, these peptides have at least two mechanisms of antiviral activity. One aspect of antiviral activity involves direct interaction with viral envelopes with possibly disruption of the envelope, similar to their antibacterial activity. This interaction, even in the absence of disruption, could interfere with viral entry. The other antiviral pathway involves indirect effects through interactions with potential target cells. These defensin-cell interactions are complex and at least in part mediated by interacting with cell surface glycoproteins and/or interfering with cell-signaling pathways that are required for viral replication. A recent report demonstrates that HD5 and HD6, induced in cervicovaginal epithelial cells in response to *Neisseria gonorrhoeae* infection, enhances HIV infectivity [19]. Interestingly, the enhancing effect of HD5 and HD6 is more pronounced with R5 virus compared with X4 virus, which may have clinical relevance relative to the selective transmission of R5 viruses. The enhancing effects, as discussed below may be through similar interactions with viral envelope and cell membranes. The influence of specific defensins on HIV replication is summarized in Table **1**.

Inhibition of HIV replication by synthetic guinea-pig, rabbit and rat α-defensins was first reported in 1993 [108], when it was shown that these peptides could inhibit HIV-1 infection *in vitro* following viral entry into transformed CD4$^+$ T cells in the presence of serum [108]. It has subsequently been appreciated that HNPs1-3 block HIV infection through multiple mechanisms [26, 109-111].

Table 1: Effects of defensins on HIV infection and their mechanisms of action.

Defensin	Effect	Mechanisms of action	Refs
NP1	Inhibitory	Inactivates virion	34,114
HNPs1-2	Inhibitory	Induce CC-chemokine production by macrophages	102
HNPs1-3	Inhibitory	Bind to gp120 and CD4	117
HNP2	Inhibitory	Binds to gp120 and CD4, blocks fusion Down-regulates CD4 in the absence of serum	112
HNP1	Inhibitory	Blocks viral nuclear import and transcription	114
HNP4	Inhibitory	Blocks HIV infection in a lectin-independent manner	115,117
HD5, HD6	Enhancement	Enhance viral entry	27
Cryptidin-3	Enhancement	Not available	120
HBD1	None		81,121
HBD2	Inhibitory	Blocks early reverse transcription product formation	121
HBD2, HBD3	Inhibitory	Downregulate CXCR4 expression Bind to HIV virions	81
Retrocyclin	Inhibitory	Blocks viral entry, Binds to gp120 and CD4	26,63, 117,122,
Retrocyclin1	Inhibitory	Blocks viral fusion	124
RTD 1-3	Inhibitory	Binds to gp120 and CD4	117
Guinea-ping, rabbit, rat α-defensins	Inhibitory	Block infection after viral entry	111

HIV, human immunodeficiency virus; HNP, human neutrophil peptide; HBD, human β-defensin; HD5, human defensin 5; RTD, rhesus θ-defensin.

HNPs1 -3 all have similar activities against HIV primary isolates [112], in contrast to their differential chemotactic activities on monocytes, where HNP3 has no effect [113]. They can inhibit HIV-1 replication by a direct interaction with the virus as well by affecting multiple steps of the HIV life cycle [26, 107, 109, 111, 114]. In the absence of serum, HNP1 can directly inactivate the virus prior to infection of a cell [107]. The influence of conditions including serum and salt on defensin activity has been well described [17, 73, 107] and clearly influence this direct virus interaction. Some defensins (e.g. HNPs but not HD5 or HD6) at high concentrations are known to cause cytotoxicity in the absence of serum, which is associated with changes in cell membrane permeability, similar to their anti-bacterial activity. This cytotoxicity is abolished by the presence of serum [115, 116]. This type of membrane effect may partially account for the antiviral effect [26] which is also lost in the presence of serum. While most defensins display potent direct antibacterial activities in conditions of low salt [78], neither a low concentration of salt nor the absence of serum are required for the chemotactic effects of defensins [89, 92].

In the presence of serum and at non-cytotoxic concentrations (low dose), HNP1 acts on primary CD4$^+$ T cells and blocks HIV-1 infection at the steps of nuclear import and transcription by interfering with PKC signaling [107]. The post-entry inhibitory effect of HIV infection occurs in primary CD4$^+$ T cells and macrophages but not in several transformed T-cell lines [107, 111]. In the presence of serum, HNP1 does not affect expression of cell-surface CD4 and HIV-co-receptors on primary CD4+ T cells [107], whereas HNP2 down-regulates CD4 expression in the absence of serum [109]. HNPs block HIV-mediated cell-cell fusion and the early steps of HIV infection by interacting with HIVgp120 and CD4 through their lectin-like properties [109]. In macrophages, HNPs 1 and 2 upregulate the expression of CC-chemokines, which could contribute to inhibition of HIV through competition for receptors [99] . CC-chemokines can also induce the release of HNPs from neutrophils by degranulation [61]. Both effects could play a role *in vivo* in an innate immune response to HIV; at the mucosal surface, HNPs might work to directly inactivate the virions in the absence of serum; however, in the presence of serum, their inhibitory effect would largely be on the infected cell.

HNPs are positively charged, so direct binding to HIV virions through charge interactions may account for some of their direct inhibition of HIV virions as well as account for sensitivity to serum through competing interactions with serum proteins. Acting as lectins, HNPs1-3 bind to HIV envelope glycoprotein gp120 and to its receptor, CD4 with high affinity [114]. Binding to gp120 is strongly attenuated by serum. Interestingly, in contrast to HNPs1-3, HNP4 acts in a lectin-independent manner and does not bind to CD4 or HIV gp120 [112, 114]. However, HNP4 inhibits HIV replication more effectively than HNPs-13 [112].

Other α-defensins, including HD5 and HD6, mouse Paneth cell cryptdin-3 and cryptdin-4, and rhesus macaque myeloid α-defensin-3 (RMAD3) and RMAD4 have been tested for their ability to block HIV infection [19, 117]. While HD5 does not exhibit any effect on X4 HIV-1$_{LAI}$ infection of transformed CD4+ T cell lines [117], HD5 and HD6 significantly enhances infectivity of HIV-1R5 strains [19]. At high concentrations associated with cytotoxicity, RMAD4 blocks HIV replication, whereas similar to human Paneth cell defensins, cryptdin-3 enhances viral replication.

Similar to HNP1 [107], HBD2 and HBD3 have dual anti-HIV activities through direct interactions with the virus and by altering the target cell. The binding of defensins to cellular membranes and HIV virions has been demonstrated by electron microscopy, although membrane disruption is not apparent [73]. HBD2 does not affect viral fusion but inhibits the formation of early reverse transcribed HIV DNA products [118]. There are conflicting reports on the downregulation of expression of HIV co-receptors by β-defensins. Sun *et al.* [118] reported that HBD1 and HBD2 did not modulate cell-surface HIV co-receptor expression by primary CD4+ T cells, whereas Quinones-Mateu *et al.* [73] showed HBD2- and HBD3-mediated downregulation of surface CXCR4 but not CCR5 expression on peripheral blood mononuclear cells (PBMCs) at high salt conditions and in the absence of serum. Interestingly, HBD2 is constitutively expressed in the healthy adult oral mucosa but the level seems to be diminished in HIV-infected individuals [118].

Retrocyclins, and RTD1, -2 and -3 act as lectins and can inhibit entry of X4 and R5 viruses, including primary isolates [18, 55, 114, 119]. Unlike α- and β-defensins, retrocyclin does not appear to directly inactivate the HIV virion [55]. Retrocyclin does however bind to HIV gp120 as well as CD4 with high affinity, which is consistent with inhibition of viral entry [55, 119]. This high-binding affinity to glycosylated gp120 and CD4 is mediated through interactions with their O-linked and N-linked sugars [120] and is strongly reduced in the presence of serum [114]. RTD1 binds directly to the C-terminal heptad repeat of HIV envelope gp41, blocking formation of the six helix bundle required for fusion [121]. Studies on retrocyclin-1 analogues indicate that modification of this peptide can enhance its potency against HIV *in vitro* [122], suggesting a therapeutic potential.

ROLE OF DEFENSINS IN HIV PATHOGENESIS AND TRANSMISSION

Reported *in vivo* levels of defensins vary most likely due to the individuals studied and the analytic methods used. In addition, defensins have been found to interact with other cellular proteins in plasma [105, 123, 124], which may affect the quantitation of defensins by ELISA. In healthy donors, the plasma concentrations of HNPs1-3 range from ~150-500 ng/ml [125]. The levels of defensins in the plasma or at the mucosal surface are frequently elevated in patients with infections or diseases [83, 126]. For example, defensin levels in plasma from patients with sepsis reach 900-170,000 ng/ml [127]. Using liquid chromatography-tandem mass spectrometry, the levels of HNPs in the saliva from healthy donors range from 1 to 10 ug/ml, whereas the level of HBDs 1-2 range from undetectable to 33 ng/ml [128]. The level of HNPs in cervicovaginal fluid from healthy women ranges from 250 ng/ml to 5 µg/ml [31, 129].

HNPs1-3

The role of HNPs in HIV pathogenesis was first suggested by the association made between HNPs 1-3 and soluble anti-HIV activity of CD8$^+$ T cells (CAF) isolated from patients infected with HIV but remaining free of AIDS for a prolonged period (long-term nonprogressors, LTNPs) [110]. These peptides were detected in the media of stimulated CD8$^+$ T cells from normal healthy controls and LTNPs but not from HIV progressors. Subsequent studies on the cell source of defensins revealed that HNPs were probably produced by co-cultured monocytes and residual granulocytes of allogenic normal donor irradiated PBMCs that were used as feeder cells, but they were not produced by the CD8$^+$ T cells themselves [26, 27], suggesting uptake might differ between the groups studied. Using similar co-culture systems, levels of HNPs1-3 were measured in CD8$^+$ T-cell supernatants and cervical-vaginal mononuclear cells (CVMCs) derived from HIV-exposed seronegative individuals, HIV-infected patients, and normal controls [130]. Higher levels of HNPs were found in CD8+ T cells from HIV-exposed seronegative individuals and HIV patients compared to normal controls.

An association between production of HNPs1-3 in breast milk and transmission of HIV has also been reported [131]. In a case-controlled study of HIV-positive women, levels of HNPs in breast milk correlated with HIV RNA copy number in breast milk, which was a strong predictor of transmission. However, after adjusting for breast milk HIV copy number, higher levels of HNPs in breast milk were associated with a decreased incidence of intrapartum or postnatal HIV transmission. Bosire and colleagues performed similar studies to determine the correlation between HNPs in breast milk and transmission risk in a cohort of 260 HIV-1-infected pregnant women in Nairobi followed for 12 months postpartum with their infants [132]. Analysis of breast milk from these women at one month postpartum demonstrated that women with detectable HNPs1-3 had significantly higher mean breast milk HIV-1 RNA levels than women with undetectable α-defensins. Increased α-defensin concentrations in breast milk were also associated with subclinical mastitis and increased CC-chemokines in breast milk. Interestingly, in contrast to the report by Kuhn *et al.* [131], the level of defensins was not associated with vertical transmission, indicating a complex interplay between innate effectors, inflammation and HIV transmission.

There is a correlation between the abundance of several anti-HIV proteins, including HNPs1-3 and cell-associated HIV replication in lymphoid follicles compared with extrafollicular lymphoid tissue [133]. Expression of these antiviral proteins is significantly lower in the follicular region, where HIV replication is concentrated, compared with the extrafollicular regions in lymph nodes from HIV-positive individuals.

Cationic peptides including defensins are associated with anti-HIV activity of vaginal fluid from healthy women [134]. While it is well established that sexual transmitted infections (STIs) significantly increase the likelihood of HIV transmission [135-139] and that levels of defensins including HNPs, HBDs and HD5 in genital fluid, are elevated in patients with STIs [10, 31-33], the role of defensins in HIV transmission seems to be quite complex. A study involving a cohort of HIV uninfected sex workers in Kenya demonstrated an association between an increase in HNPs and LL-37 levels in the IgA-depleted cervicovaginal secretions from women with bacterial STIs and increased in HIV acquisition compared to women without STIs. In this case, the high levels of HNPs and LL-37 did not appear to be protective although it is hard to determine if they provide some level of protection in the permissive environment presented by active inflammation associated with an STI [129]. This study underscores the complex role of defensins in HIV transmission at the vaginal mucosa and the urgent need to define the role of innate effectors in HIV acquisition.

HBDs

Polymorphisms in the *DEFB1* gene (coding for HBD1) have been associated with susceptibility to and severity of pulmonary diseases [140-144]. Interestingly, single-nucleotide polymorphisms (SNPs) in the 5' untranslated region of *DEFB1* influence transmission rates to children and this is most likely due to the influence of these genetic variants on expression of HBD1 and ultimately on plasma and/or breast milk levels viral loads [145-148]. Although HBD1 has no effect on HIV infection in vitro [73, 118], the presence of SNPs may modulate the overall immune response by down-or up regulation of HBD1.

The role of defensins in protection against HIV infection has been studied in HIV-exposed seronegative (ESN) individuals. ESN expressed significantly greater mRNA copy number of HBD2 and 3 in oral mucosa compared to healthy controls, while there was no difference in mRNA copy number of HBDs1-3 in vaginal/endocervical mucosa between ESN and controls [149]. In addition, homozygosity for the A692G polymorphism is significantly more frequent in ESN than in seropositive individuals [149]. Sequence analysis of θ-defensin pseudogenes (DEFT) in ESN female sex-workers from Thailand revealed that all subjects had premature stop codons [150]. Therefore, restoration of endogenous θ-defensin production does not account for the resistance to HIV-1 infection in these women.

CONCLUSION

Innate immunity is the first line of defense against pathogens. Leukocytes and mucosal epithelial cells are the main cells that produce defensins and play a major role in innate immune response. Defensins display versatile functions in modulating various immunological and biological aspects. Aberrant defensin expression has been associated with many human diseases [151], although studies on the role of defensins in HIV pathogenesis and transmission in humans have just begun to reveal the complex functions of defensins in modulating HIV infection. While the innate immune system including defensins is evolutionarily conserved among multicellular organisms, it is challenging to find a suitable animal model to study the role of defensins in HIV pathogenesis and transmission due to the complex diversity of defensins in mammals as well as apparent differences in mechanisms of action. Future studies focusing on the development of a better animal model for studying innate immunity in HIV transmission and pathogenesis as well as careful assessments of immune responses (soluble factors and immune cells) in patients with reduced or elevated levels of defensins will shed light on the development of novel therapeutics for HIV prevention.

REFERENCES

[1]   Selsted ME, Ouellette AJ. Mammalian defensins in the antimicrobial immune response. Nat Immunol. 2005;6(6):551-557.
[2]   Ganz T. Defensins: antimicrobial peptides of innate immunity. Nat Rev Immunol. 2003;3(9):710-720.
[3]   Yang D, Biragyn A, Kwak LW, Oppenheim JJ. Mammalian defensins in immunity: more than just microbicidal. Trends Immunol. 2002;23(6):291-296.
[4]   Yang D, Biragyn A, Hoover DM, Lubkowski J, Oppenheim JJ. Multiple roles of antimicrobial defensins, cathelicidins, and eosinophil-derived neurotoxin in host defense. Annu Rev Immunol. 2004;22:181-215.
[5]   Szyk A, Wu Z, Tucker K, Yang D, Lu W, Lubkowski J. Crystal structures of human alpha-defensins HNP4, HD5, and HD6. Protein Sci. 2006;15(12):2749-2760.

[6]   Pardi A, Zhang XL, Selsted ME, Skalicky JJ, Yip PF. NMR studies of defensin antimicrobial peptides. 2. Three-dimensional structures of rabbit NP-2 and human HNP-1. Biochemistry. 1992;31(46):11357-11364.

[7]   Hill CP, Yee J, Selsted ME, Eisenberg D. Crystal structure of defensin HNP-3, an amphiphilic dimer: mechanisms of membrane permeabilization. Science. 1991;251(5000):1481-1485.

[8]   Hoover DM, Chertov O, Lubkowski J. The structure of human beta-defensin-1: new insights into structural properties of beta-defensins. J Biol Chem. 2001;276(42):39021-39026.

[9]   Ghosh D, Porter E, Shen B, Lee SK, Wilk D, Drazba J, *et al.* Paneth cell trypsin is the processing enzyme for human defensin-5. Nat Immunol. 2002;3(6):583-590.

[10]   Porter E, Yang H, Yavagal S, Preza GC, Murillo O, Lima H, *et al.* Distinct defensin profiles in Neisseria gonorrhoeae and Chlamydia trachomatis urethritis reveal novel epithelial cell-neutrophil interactions. Infect Immun. 2005;73(8):4823-4833.

[11]   Tang YQ, Yuan J, Osapay G, Osapay K, Tran D, Miller CJ, *et al.* A cyclic antimicrobial peptide produced in primate leukocytes by the ligation of two truncated alpha-defensins. Science. 1999;286(5439):498-502.

[12]   Leonova L, Kokryakov VN, Aleshina G, Hong T, Nguyen T, Zhao C, *et al.* Circular minidefensins and posttranslational generation of molecular diversity. J Leukoc Biol. 2001;70(3):461-464.

[13]   Tran D, Tran PA, Tang YQ, Yuan J, Cole T, Selsted ME. Homodimeric theta-defensins from rhesus macaque leukocytes: isolation, synthesis, antimicrobial activities, and bacterial binding properties of the cyclic peptides. J Biol Chem. 2002;277(5):3079-3084.

[14]   Maemoto A, Qu X, Rosengren KJ, Tanabe H, Henschen-Edman A, Craik DJ, *et al.* Functional analysis of the alpha-defensin disulfide array in mouse cryptdin-4. J Biol Chem. 2004;279(42):44188-44196.

[15]   Wu Z, Hoover DM, Yang D, Boulegue C, Santamaria F, Oppenheim JJ, *et al.* Engineering disulfide bridges to dissect antimicrobial and chemotactic activities of human beta-defensin 3. Proc Natl Acad Sci USA. 2003;100(15):8880-8885.

[16]   Mandal M, Nagaraj R. Antibacterial activities and conformations of synthetic alpha-defensin HNP-1 and analogs with one, two and three disulfide bridges. J Pept Res. 2002;59(3):95-104.

[17]   Daher KA, Selsted ME, Lehrer RI. Direct inactivation of viruses by human granulocyte defensins. J Virol. 1986;60(3):1068-1074.

[18]   Wang W, Cole AM, Hong T, Waring AJ, Lehrer RI. Retrocyclin, an antiretroviral theta-defensin, is a lectin. J Immunol. 2003;170(9):4708-4716.

[19]   Klotman ME, Rapista A, Teleshova N, Micsenyi A, Jarvis GA, Lu W, *et al.* Neisseria gonorrhoeae-Induced Human Defensins 5 and 6 Increase HIV Infectivity: Role in Enhanced Transmission. J Immunol. 2008;180(9):6176-6185.

[20]   Ganz T, Selsted ME, Szklarek D, Harwig SS, Daher K, Bainton DF, *et al.* Defensins. Natural peptide antibiotics of human neutrophils. J Clin Invest. 1985;76(4):1427-1435.

[21]   Selsted ME, Harwig SS, Ganz T, Schilling JW, Lehrer RI. Primary structures of three human neutrophil defensins. J Clin Invest. 1985;76(4):1436-1439.

[22]   Wilde CG, Griffith JE, Marra MN, Snable JL, Scott RW. Purification and characterization of human neutrophil peptide 4, a novel member of the defensin family. J Biol Chem. 1989;264(19):11200-11203.

[23]   Rodriguez-Garcia M, Oliva H, Climent N, Garcia F, Gatell JM, Gallart T. Human immature monocyte-derived dendritic cells produce and secrete alpha-defensins 1-3. J Leukoc Biol. 2007;82(5):1143-1146.

[24]   Agerberth B, Charo J, Werr J, Olsson B, Idali F, Lindbom L, *et al.* The human antimicrobial and chemotactic peptides LL-37 and alpha-defensins are expressed by specific lymphocyte and monocyte populations. Blood. 2000;96(9):3086-3093.

[25]   Ganz T. Extracellular release of antimicrobial defensins by human polymorphonuclear leukocytes. Infect Immun. 1987;55(3):568-571.

[26]   Mackewicz CE, Yuan J, Tran P, Diaz L, Mack E, Selsted ME, *et al.* alpha-Defensins can have anti-HIV activity but are not CD8 cell anti-HIV factors. AIDS. 2003;17(14):F23-32.

[27]   Zaharatos GJ, He T, Lopez P, Yu W, Yu J, Zhang L. alpha-Defensins Released Into Stimulated CD8+ T-Cell Supernatants Are Likely Derived From Residual Granulocytes Within the Irradiated Allogeneic Peripheral Blood Mononuclear Cells Used as Feeders. J Acquir Immune Defic Syndr. 2004;36(5):993-1005.

[28]   Hein M, Valore EV, Helmig RB, Uldbjerg N, Ganz T. Antimicrobial factors in the cervical mucus plug. Am J Obstet Gynecol. 2002;187(1):137-144.

[29]   Fellermann K, Stange EF. Defensins -- innate immunity at the epithelial frontier. Eur J Gastroenterol Hepatol. 2001;13(7):771-776.

[30]   Cunliffe RN. Alpha-defensins in the gastrointestinal tract. Mol Immunol. 2003;40(7):463-467.

[31] Simhan HN, Anderson BL, Krohn MA, Heine RP, Martinez de Tejada B, Landers DV, *et al.* Host immune consequences of asymptomatic Trichomonas vaginalis infection in pregnancy. Am J Obstet Gynecol. 2007;196(1):59 e51-55.

[32] Wiesenfeld HC, Heine RP, Krohn MA, Hillier SL, Amortegui AA, Nicolazzo M, *et al.* Association between elevated neutrophil defensin levels and endometritis. J Infect Dis. 2002;186(6):792-797.

[33] Valore EV, Wiley DJ, Ganz T. Reversible deficiency of antimicrobial polypeptides in bacterial vaginosis. Infect Immun. 2006;74(10):5693-5702.

[34] Heine RP, Wiesenfeld H, Mortimer L, Greig PC. Amniotic fluid defensins: potential markers of subclinical intrauterine infection. Clin Infect Dis. 1998;27(3):513-518.

[35] Salzman NH, Underwood MA, Bevins CL. Paneth cells, defensins, and the commensal microbiota: a hypothesis on intimate interplay at the intestinal mucosa. Semin Immunol. 2007;19(2):70-83.

[36] Tanabe H, Yuan J, Zaragoza MM, Dandekar S, Henschen-Edman A, Selsted ME, *et al.* Paneth cell alpha-defensins from rhesus macaque small intestine. Infect Immun. 2004;72(3):1470-1478.

[37] Fahlgren A, Hammarstrom S, Danielsson A, Hammarstrom ML. Increased expression of antimicrobial peptides and lysozyme in colonic epithelial cells of patients with ulcerative colitis. Clin Exp Immunol. 2003;131(1):90-101.

[38] Svinarich DM, Wolf NA, Gomez R, Gonik B, Romero R. Detection of human defensin 5 in reproductive tissues. Am J Obstet Gynecol. 1997;176(2):470-475.

[39] Quayle AJ, Porter EM, Nussbaum AA, Wang YM, Brabec C, Yip KP, *et al.* Gene expression, immunolocalization, and secretion of human defensin-5 in human female reproductive tract. Am J Pathol. 1998;152(5):1247-1258.

[40] Fan SR, Liu XP, Liao QP. Human defensins and cytokines in vaginal lavage fluid of women with bacterial vaginosis. Int J Gynaecol Obstet. 2008.

[41] Yamaguchi Y, Nagase T, Makita R, Fukuhara S, Tomita T, Tominaga T, *et al.* Identification of multiple novel epididymis-specific beta-defensin isoforms in humans and mice. J Immunol. 2002;169(5):2516-2523.

[42] Pazgier M, Hoover DM, Yang D, Lu W, Lubkowski J. Human beta-defensins. Cell Mol Life Sci. 2006;63(11):1294-1313.

[43] Schutte BC, Mitros JP, Bartlett JA, Walters JD, Jia HP, Welsh MJ, *et al.* Discovery of five conserved beta - defensin gene clusters using a computational search strategy. Proc Natl Acad Sci USA. 2002;99(4):2129-2133.

[44] Duits LA, Ravensbergen B, Rademaker M, Hiemstra PS, Nibbering PH. Expression of beta-defensin 1 and 2 mRNA by human monocytes, macrophages and dendritic cells. Immunology. 2002;106(4):517-525.

[45] Proud D, Sanders SP, Wiehler S. Human rhinovirus infection induces airway epithelial cell production of human beta-defensin 2 both in vitro and in vivo. J Immunol. 2004;172(7):4637-4645.

[46] Duits LA, Nibbering PH, van Strijen E, Vos JB, Mannesse-Lazeroms SP, van Sterkenburg MA, *et al.* Rhinovirus increases human beta-defensin-2 and -3 mRNA expression in cultured bronchial epithelial cells. FEMS Immunol Med Microbiol. 2003;38(1):59-64.

[47] Yang D, Chertov O, Oppenheim JJ. Participation of mammalian defensins and cathelicidins in anti-microbial immunity: receptors and activities of human defensins and cathelicidin (LL-37). J Leukoc Biol. 2001;69(5):691-697.

[48] Sorensen OE, Thapa DR, Rosenthal A, Liu L, Roberts AA, Ganz T. Differential regulation of beta-defensin expression in human skin by microbial stimuli. J Immunol. 2005;174(8):4870-4879.

[49] Harder J, Bartels J, Christophers E, Schroder JM. Isolation and characterization of human beta -defensin-3, a novel human inducible peptide antibiotic. J Biol Chem. 2001;276(8):5707-5713.

[50] Garcia JR, Jaumann F, Schulz S, Krause A, Rodriguez-Jimenez J, Forssmann U, *et al.* Identification of a novel, multifunctional beta-defensin (human beta-defensin 3) with specific antimicrobial activity. Its interaction with plasma membranes of Xenopus oocytes and the induction of macrophage chemoattraction. Cell Tissue Res. 2001;306(2):257-264.

[51] Armogida SA, Yannaras NM, Melton AL, Srivastava MD. Identification and quantification of innate immune system mediators in human breast milk. Allergy Asthma Proc. 2004;25(5):297-304.

[52] Jia HP, Starner T, Ackermann M, Kirby P, Tack BF, McCray PB, Jr. Abundant human beta-defensin-1 expression in milk and mammary gland epithelium. J Pediatr. 2001;138(1):109-112.

[53] Garcia JR, Krause A, Schulz S, Rodriguez-Jimenez FJ, Kluver E, Adermann K, *et al.* Human beta-defensin 4: a novel inducible peptide with a specific salt-sensitive spectrum of antimicrobial activity. FASEB J. 2001;15(10):1819-1821.

[54] Nguyen TX, Cole AM, Lehrer RI. Evolution of primate theta-defensins: a serpentine path to a sweet tooth. Peptides. 2003;24(11):1647-1654.

[55] Cole AM, Hong T, Boo LM, Nguyen T, Zhao C, Bristol G, *et al.* Retrocyclin: a primate peptide that protects cells from infection by T- and M-tropic strains of HIV-1. Proc Natl Acad Sci USA. 2002;99(4):1813-1818.

[56] Cowland JB, Borregaard N. The individual regulation of granule protein mRNA levels during neutrophil maturation explains the heterogeneity of neutrophil granules. J Leukoc Biol. 1999;66(6):989-995.

[57] Tsutsumi-Ishii Y, Hasebe T, Nagaoka I. Role of CCAAT/enhancer-binding protein site in transcription of human neutrophil peptide-1 and -3 defensin genes. J Immunol. 2000;164(6):3264-3273.

[58] Joiner KA, Ganz T, Albert J, Rotrosen D. The opsonizing ligand on Salmonella typhimurium influences incorporation of specific, but not azurophil, granule constituents into neutrophil phagosomes. J Cell Biol. 1989;109(6 Pt 1):2771-2782.

[59] Tanaka S, Edberg JC, Chatham W, Fassina G, Kimberly RP. Fc gamma RIIIb allele-sensitive release of alpha-defensins: anti-neutrophil cytoplasmic antibody-induced release of chemotaxins. J Immunol. 2003;171(11):6090-6096.

[60] Chalifour A, Jeannin P, Gauchat JF, Blaecke A, Malissard M, N'Guyen T, et al. Direct bacterial protein PAMP recognition by human NK cells involves TLRs and triggers alpha-defensin production. Blood. 2004;104(6):1778-1783.

[61] Jan MS, Huang YH, Shieh B, Teng RH, Yan YP, Lee YT, et al. CC Chemokines Induce Neutrophils to Chemotaxis, Degranulation, and alpha-Defensin Release. J Acquir Immune Defic Syndr. 2006;41(1):6-16.

[62] Driss V, Legrand F, Hermann E, Loiseau S, Guerardel Y, Kremer L, et al. TLR2-dependent eosinophil interactions with mycobacteria : role of {alpha}-defensins. Blood. 2009 Apr 2;113(14):3235-44.

[63] Cunliffe RN, Rose FR, Keyte J, Abberley L, Chan WC, Mahida YR. Human defensin 5 is stored in precursor form in normal Paneth cells and is expressed by some villous epithelial cells and by metaplastic Paneth cells in the colon in inflammatory bowel disease. Gut. 2001;48(2):176-185.

[64] George MD, Wehkamp J, Kays RJ, Leutenegger CM, Sabir S, Grishina I, et al. In vivo gene expression profiling of human intestinal epithelial cells: analysis by laser microdissection of formalin fixed tissues. BMC Genomics. 2008;9:209.

[65] Wehkamp J, Harder J, Weichenthal M, Schwab M, Schaffeler E, Schlee M, et al. NOD2 (CARD15) mutations in Crohn's disease are associated with diminished mucosal alpha-defensin expression. Gut. 2004;53(11):1658-1664.

[66] Wehkamp J, Wang G, Kubler I, Nuding S, Gregorieff A, Schnabel A, et al. The Paneth cell alpha-defensin deficiency of ileal Crohn's disease is linked to Wnt/Tcf-4. J Immunol. 2007;179(5):3109-3118.

[67] Hertz CJ, Wu Q, Porter EM, Zhang YJ, Weismuller KH, Godowski PJ, et al. Activation of Toll-like receptor 2 on human tracheobronchial epithelial cells induces the antimicrobial peptide human beta defensin-2. J Immunol. 2003;171(12):6820-6826.

[68] Vora P, Youdim A, Thomas LS, Fukata M, Tesfay SY, Lukasek K, et al. Beta-defensin-2 expression is regulated by TLR signaling in intestinal epithelial cells. J Immunol. 2004;173(9):5398-5405.

[69] Uehara A, Fujimoto Y, Fukase K, Takada H. Various human epithelial cells express functional Toll-like receptors, NOD1 and NOD2 to produce anti-microbial peptides, but not proinflammatory cytokines. Mol Immunol. 2007;44(12):3100-3111.

[70] Nagy I, Pivarcsi A, Koreck A, Szell M, Urban E, Kemeny L. Distinct strains of Propionibacterium acnes induce selective human beta-defensin-2 and interleukin-8 expression in human keratinocytes through toll-like receptors. J Invest Dermatol. 2005;124(5):931-938.

[71] Pivarcsi A, Nagy I, Koreck A, Kis K, Kenderessy-Szabo A, Szell M, et al. Microbial compounds induce the expression of pro-inflammatory cytokines, chemokines and human beta-defensin-2 in vaginal epithelial cells. Microbes Infect. 2005;7:1117-1127.

[72] Schaefer TM, Fahey JV, Wright JA, Wira CR. Innate immunity in the human female reproductive tract: antiviral response of uterine epithelial cells to the TLR3 agonist poly(I:C). J Immunol. 2005;174(2):992-1002.

[73] Quinones-Mateu ME, Lederman MM, Feng Z, Chakraborty B, Weber J, Rangel HR, et al. Human epithelial beta-defensins 2 and 3 inhibit HIV-1 replication. AIDS. 2003;17(16):F39-48.

[74] Uehara A, Takada H. Synergism between TLRs and NOD1/2 in oral epithelial cells. J Dent Res. 2008;87(7):682-686.

[75] Huang F, Kao CY, Wachi S, Thai P, Ryu J, Wu R. Requirement for both JAK-mediated PI3K signaling and ACT1/TRAF6/TAK1-dependent NF-kappaB activation by IL-17A in enhancing cytokine expression in human airway epithelial cells. J Immunol. 2007;179(10):6504-6513.

[76] Jang BC, Lim KJ, Suh MH, Park JG, Suh SI. Dexamethasone suppresses interleukin-1beta-induced human beta-defensin 2 mRNA expression: involvement of p38 MAPK, JNK, MKP-1, and NF-kappaB transcriptional factor in A549 cells. FEMS Immunol Med Microbiol. 2007;51(1):171-184.

[77] Kao CY, Kim C, Huang F, Wu R. Requirements for two proximal NF-kappaB binding sites and IkappaB-zeta in IL-17A-induced human beta-defensin 2 expression by conducting airway epithelium. J Biol Chem. 2008;283(22):15309-15318.

[78]   Lehrer RI, Lichtenstein AK, Ganz T. Defensins: antimicrobial and cytotoxic peptides of mammalian cells. Annu Rev Immunol. 1993;11:105-128.

[79]   Bohling A, Hagge SO, Roes S, Podschun R, Sahly H, Harder J, *et al.* Lipid-specific membrane activity of human beta-defensin-3. Biochemistry. 2006;45(17):5663-5670.

[80]   Ericksen B, Wu Z, Lu W, Lehrer RI. Antibacterial activity and specificity of the six human {alpha}-defensins. Antimicrob Agents Chemother. 2005;49(1):269-275.

[81]   Sakamoto N, Mukae H, Fujii T, Ishii H, Yoshioka S, Kakugawa T, *et al.* Differential effects of alpha- and beta-defensin on cytokine production by cultured human bronchial epithelial cells. Am J Physiol Lung Cell Mol Physiol. 2005;288(3):L508-513.

[82]   Rehaume LM, Hancock RE. Neutrophil-derived defensins as modulators of innate immune function. Crit Rev Immunol. 2008;28(3):185-200.

[83]   Coffelt SB, Scandurro AB. Tumors sound the alarmin(s). Cancer Res. 2008;68(16):6482-6485.

[84]   Liu HY, Collins QF, Moukdar F, Zhuo D, Han J, Hong T, *et al.* Suppression of hepatic glucose production by human neutrophil alpha-defensins through a signaling pathway distinct from insulin. J Biol Chem. 2008;283(18):12056-12063.

[85]   Joseph G, Tarnow L, Astrup AS, Hansen TK, Parving HH, Flyvbjerg A, *et al.* Plasma alpha-defensin is associated with cardiovascular morbidity and mortality in type 1 diabetic patients. J Clin Endocrinol Metab. 2008;93(4):1470-1475.

[86]   Saraheimo M, Forsblom C, Pettersson-Fernholm K, Flyvbjerg A, Groop PH, Frystyk J. Increased levels of alpha-defensin (-1, -2 and -3) in type 1 diabetic patients with nephropathy. Nephrol Dial Transplant. 2008;23(3):914-918.

[87]   Kruse T, Kristensen HH. Using antimicrobial host defense peptides as anti-infective and immunomodulatory agents. Expert Rev Anti Infect Ther. 2008;6(6):887-895.

[88]   Yang D, Chen Q, Chertov O, Oppenheim JJ. Human neutrophil defensins selectively chemoattract naive T and immature dendritic cells. J Leukoc Biol. 2000;68(1):9-14.

[89]   Chertov O, Michiel DF, Xu L, Wang JM, Tani K, Murphy WJ, *et al.* Identification of defensin-1, defensin-2, and CAP37/azurocidin as T-cell chemoattractant proteins released from interleukin-8-stimulated neutrophils. J Biol Chem. 1996;271(6):2935-2940.

[90]   Tecle T, White MR, Gantz D, Crouch EC, Hartshorn KL. Human neutrophil defensins increase neutrophil uptake of influenza A virus and bacteria and modify virus-induced respiratory burst responses. J Immunol. 2007;178(12):8046-8052.

[91]   Shi J, Aono S, Lu W, Ouellette AJ, Hu X, Ji Y, *et al.* A novel role for defensins in intestinal homeostasis: regulation of IL-1beta secretion. J Immunol. 2007;179(2):1245-1253.

[92]   Yang D, Chertov O, Bykovskaia SN, Chen Q, Buffo MJ, Shogan J, *et al.* Beta-defensins: linking innate and adaptive immunity through dendritic and T cell CCR6. Science. 1999;286(5439):525-528.

[93]   Zlotnik A, Yoshie O. Chemokines: a new classification system and their role in immunity. Immunity. 2000;12(2):121-127.

[94]   Niyonsaba F, Hirata M, Ogawa H, Nagaoka I. Epithelial cell-derived antibacterial peptides human beta-defensins and cathelicidin: multifunctional activities on mast cells. Curr Drug Targets Inflamm Allergy. 2003;2(3):224-231.

[95]   Biragyn A, Ruffini PA, Leifer CA, Klyushnenkova E, Shakhov A, Chertov O, *et al.* Toll-like receptor 4-dependent activation of dendritic cells by beta-defensin 2. Science. 2002;298(5595):1025-1029.

[96]   Funderburg N, Lederman MM, Feng Z, Drage MG, Jadlowsky J, Harding CV, *et al.* Human -defensin-3 activates professional antigen-presenting cells via Toll-like receptors 1 and 2. Proc Natl Acad Sci USA. 2007;104(47):18631-18635.

[97]   Klotman ME, Chang TL. Defensins in innate antiviral immunity. Nat Rev Immunol. 2006;6(6):447-456.

[98]   Van Wetering S, Mannesse-Lazeroms SP, Van Sterkenburg MA, Daha MR, Dijkman JH, Hiemstra PS. Effect of defensins on interleukin-8 synthesis in airway epithelial cells. Am J Physiol. 1997;272(5 Pt 1):L888-896.

[99]   Guo CJ, Tan N, Song L, Douglas SD, Ho WZ. Alpha-defensins inhibit HIV infection of macrophages through upregulation of CC-chemokines. Aids. 2004;18(8):1217-1218.

[100]   Boniotto M, Jordan WJ, Eskdale J, Tossi A, Antcheva N, Crovella S, *et al.* Human beta-defensin 2 induces a vigorous cytokine response in peripheral blood mononuclear cells. Antimicrob Agents Chemother. 2006;50(4):1433-1441.

[101]   Liu CY, Lin HC, Yu CT, Lin SM, Lee KY, Chen HC, *et al.* The concentration-dependent chemokine release and pro-apoptotic effects of neutrophil-derived alpha-defensin-1 on human bronchial and alveolar epithelial cells. Life Sci. 2007;80(8):749-758.

[102]   Narimatsu R, Wolday D, Patterson BK. IL-8 increases transmission of HIV type 1 in cervical explant tissue. AIDS Res Hum Retroviruses. 2005;21(3):228-233.

[103] Nassar T, Akkawi S, Bar-Shavit R, Haj-Yehia A, Bdeir K, Al-Mehdi AB, *et al.* Human alpha-defensin regulates smooth muscle cell contraction: a role for low-density lipoprotein receptor-related protein/alpha 2-macroglobulin receptor. Blood. 2002;100(12):4026-4032.

[104] Higazi AA, Nassar T, Ganz T, Rader DJ, Udassin R, Bdeir K, *et al.* The alpha-defensins stimulate proteoglycan-dependent catabolism of low-density lipoprotein by vascular cells: a new class of inflammatory apolipoprotein and a possible contributor to atherogenesis. Blood. 2000;96(4):1393-1398.

[105] Higazi AA, Ganz T, Kariko K, Cines DB. Defensin modulates tissue-type plasminogen activator and plasminogen binding to fibrin and endothelial cells. J Biol Chem. 1996;271(30):17650-17655.

[106] Charp PA, Rice WG, Raynor RL, Reimund E, Kinkade JM, Jr., Ganz T, *et al.* Inhibition of protein kinase C by defensins, antibiotic peptides from human neutrophils. Biochem Pharmacol. 1988;37(5):951-956.

[107] Chang TL, Vargas J, Jr., DelPortillo A, Klotman ME. Dual role of alpha-defensin-1 in anti-HIV-1 innate immunity. J Clin Invest. 2005;115(3):765-773.

[108] Nakashima H, Yamamoto N, Masuda M, Fujii N. Defensins inhibit HIV replication in vitro. Aids. 1993;7(8):1129.

[109] Furci L, Sironi F, Tolazzi M, Vassena L, Lusso P. Alpha-defensins block the early steps of HIV-1 infection: interference with the binding of gp120 to CD4. Blood. 2007;109(7):2928-2935.

[110] Zhang L, Yu W, He T, Yu J, Caffrey RE, Dalmasso EA, *et al.* Contribution of human alpha-defensin 1, 2, and 3 to the anti-HIV-1 activity of CD8 antiviral factor. Science. 2002;298(5595):995-1000.

[111] Chang TL, Francois F, Mosoian A, Klotman ME. CAF-mediated human immunodeficiency virus (HIV) type 1 transcriptional inhibition is distinct from alpha-defensin-1 HIV inhibition. J Virol. 2003;77(12):6777-6784.

[112] Wu Z, Cocchi F, Gentles D, Ericksen B, Lubkowski J, Devico A, *et al.* Human neutrophil alpha-defensin 4 inhibits HIV-1 infection in vitro. FEBS Lett. 2005;579(1):162-166.

[113] Territo MC, Ganz T, Selsted ME, Lehrer R. Monocyte-chemotactic activity of defensins from human neutrophils. J Clin Invest. 1989;84(6):2017-2020.

[114] Wang W, Owen SM, Rudolph DL, Cole AM, Hong T, Waring AJ, *et al.* Activity of alpha- and theta-defensins against primary isolates of HIV-1. J Immunol. 2004;173(1):515-520.

[115] Okrent DG, Lichtenstein AK, Ganz T. Direct cytotoxicity of polymorphonuclear leukocyte granule proteins to human lung-derived cells and endothelial cells. Am Rev Respir Dis. 1990;141(1):179-185.

[116] Van Wetering S, Mannesse-Lazeroms SP, Dijkman JH, Hiemstra PS. Effect of neutrophil serine proteinases and defensins on lung epithelial cells: modulation of cytotoxicity and IL-8 production. J Leukoc Biol. 1997;62(2):217-226.

[117] Tanabe H, Ouellette AJ, Cocco MJ, Robinson WE, Jr. Differential effects on human immunodeficiency virus type 1 replication by alpha-defensins with comparable bactericidal activities. J Virol. 2004;78(21):11622-11631.

[118] Sun L, Finnegan CM, Kish-Catalone T, Blumenthal R, Garzino-Demo P, La Terra Maggiore GM, *et al.* Human {beta}-Defensins Suppress Human Immunodeficiency Virus Infection: Potential Role in Mucosal Protection. J Virol. 2005;79(22):14318-14329.

[119] Munk C, Wei G, Yang OO, Waring AJ, Wang W, Hong T, *et al.* The theta-defensin, retrocyclin, inhibits HIV-1 entry. AIDS Res Hum Retroviruses. 2003;19(10):875-881.

[120] Wang SZ, Smith PK, Lovejoy M, Bowden JJ, Alpers JH, Forsyth KD. The apoptosis of neutrophils is accelerated in respiratory syncytial virus (RSV)-induced bronchiolitis. Clin Exp Immunol. 1998;114(1):49-54.

[121] Gallo SA, Wang W, Rawat SS, Jung G, Waring AJ, Cole AM, *et al.* Theta-defensins prevent HIV-1 Env-mediated fusion by binding gp41 and blocking 6-helix bundle formation. J Biol Chem. 2006;281(27):18787-18792.

[122] Owen SM, Rudolph DL, Wang W, Cole AM, Waring AJ, Lal RB, *et al.* RC-101, a retrocyclin-1 analogue with enhanced activity against primary HIV type 1 isolates. AIDS Res Hum Retroviruses. 2004;20(11):1157-1165.

[123] Panyutich AV, Szold O, Poon PH, Tseng Y, Ganz T. Identification of defensin binding to C1 complement. FEBS Lett. 1994;356(2-3):169-173.

[124] Panyutich A, Ganz T. Activated alpha 2-macroglobulin is a principal defensin-binding protein. Am J Respir Cell Mol Biol. 1991;5(2):101-106.

[125] Mukae H, Iiboshi H, Nakazato M, Hiratsuka T, Tokojima M, Abe K, *et al.* Raised plasma concentrations of alpha-defensins in patients with idiopathic pulmonary fibrosis. Thorax. 2002;57(7):623-628.

[126] Ihi T, Nakazato M, Mukae H, Matsukura S. Elevated concentrations of human neutrophil peptides in plasma, blood, and body fluids from patients with infections. Clin Infect Dis. 1997;25(5):1134-1140.

[127] Panyutich AV, Panyutich EA, Krapivin VA, Baturevich EA, Ganz T. Plasma defensin concentrations are elevated in patients with septicemia or bacterial meningitis. J Lab Clin Med. 1993;122(2):202-207.

[128] Gardner MS, Rowland MD, Siu AY, Bundy JL, Wagener DK, Stephenson JL. Comprehensive defensin assay for saliva. Anal Chem. 2009;81(2):557-566.

[129] Levinson P, Kaul R, Kimani J, Ngugi E, Moses S, Macdonald KS, *et al.* Levels of innate immune factors in genital fluids: association of alpha defensins and LL-37 with genital infections and increased HIV acquisition. AIDS. 2008.

[130] Trabattoni D, Caputo SL, Maffeis G, Vichi F, Biasin M, Pierotti P, *et al.* Human alpha Defensin in HIV-Exposed But Uninfected Individuals. J Acquir Immune Defic Syndr. 2004;35(5):455-463.

[131] Kuhn L, Trabattoni D, Kankasa C, Semrau K, Kasonde P, Lissoni F, *et al.* Alpha-defensins in the prevention of HIV transmission among breastfed infants. J Acquir Immune Defic Syndr. 2005;39(2):138-142.

[132] Bosire R, John-Stewart GC, Mabuka JM, Wariua G, Gichuhi C, Wamalwa D, *et al.* Breast milk alpha-defensins are associated with HIV type 1 RNA and CC chemokines in breast milk but not vertical HIV type 1 transmission. AIDS Res Hum Retroviruses. 2007;23(2):198-203.

[133] Folkvord JM, Armon C, Connick E. Lymphoid follicles are sites of heightened human immunodeficiency virus type 1 (HIV-1) replication and reduced antiretroviral effector mechanisms. AIDS Res Hum Retroviruses. 2005;21(5):363-370.

[134] Venkataraman N, Cole AL, Svoboda P, Pohl J, Cole AM. Cationic polypeptides are required for anti-HIV-1 activity of human vaginal fluid. J Immunol. 2005;175(11):7560-7567.

[135] Galvin SR, Cohen MS. The role of sexually transmitted diseases in HIV transmission. Nat Rev Microbiol. 2004;2(1):33-42.

[136] Plummer FA. Heterosexual transmission of human immunodeficiency virus type 1 (HIV): interactions of conventional sexually transmitted diseases, hormonal contraception and HIV-1. AIDS Res Hum Retroviruses. 1998;14 Suppl 1:S5-10.

[137] Cohen MS, Hoffman IF, Royce RA, Kazembe P, Dyer JR, Daly CC, *et al.* Reduction of concentration of HIV-1 in semen after treatment of urethritis: implications for prevention of sexual transmission of HIV-1. AIDSCAP Malawi Research Group. Lancet. 1997;349(9069):1868-1873.

[138] Chesson HW, Pinkerton SD. Sexually transmitted diseases and the increased risk for HIV transmission: implications for cost-effectiveness analyses of sexually transmitted disease prevention interventions. J Acquir Immune Defic Syndr. 2000;24(1):48-56.

[139] Mabey D. Interactions between HIV infection and other sexually transmitted diseases. Trop Med Int Health. 2000;5(7):A32-36.

[140] Matsushita I, Hasegawa K, Nakata K, Yasuda K, Tokunaga K, Keicho N. Genetic variants of human beta-defensin-1 and chronic obstructive pulmonary disease. Biochem Biophys Res Commun. 2002;291(1):17-22.

[141] Salvatore F, Scudiero O, Castaldo G. Genotype-phenotype correlation in cystic fibrosis: the role of modifier genes. Am J Med Genet. 2002;111(1):88-95.

[142] Vankeerberghen A, Scudiero O, De Boeck K, Macek M, Jr., Pignatti PF, Van Hul N, *et al.* Distribution of human beta-defensin polymorphisms in various control and cystic fibrosis populations. Genomics. 2005;85(5):574-581.

[143] Levy H, Raby BA, Lake S, Tantisira KG, Kwiatkowski D, Lazarus R, *et al.* Association of defensin beta-1 gene polymorphisms with asthma. J Allergy Clin Immunol. 2005;115(2):252-258.

[144] Dork T, Stuhrmann M. Polymorphisms of the human beta-defensin-1 gene. Mol Cell Probes. 1998;12(3):171-173.

[145] Braida L, Boniotto M, Pontillo A, Tovo PA, Amoroso A, Crovella S. A single-nucleotide polymorphism in the human beta-defensin 1 gene is associated with HIV-1 infection in Italian children. AIDS. 2004;18(11):1598-1600.

[146] Milanese M, Segat L, Pontillo A, Arraes LC, de Lima Filho JL, Crovella S. DEFB1 gene polymorphisms and increased risk of HIV-1 infection in Brazilian children. Aids. 2006;20(12):1673-1675.

[147] Ricci E, Malacrida S, Zanchetta M, Montagna M, Giaquinto C, Rossi AD. Role of beta-Defensin-1 Polymorphisms in Mother-to-Child Transmission of Human Immunodeficiency Virus Type 1. J Acquir Immune Defic Syndr. 2009;51(1):13-9.

[148] Milanese M, Segat L, Crovella S. Transcriptional effect of DEFB1 gene 5' untranslated region polymorphisms. Cancer Res. 2007;67(12):5997; author reply 5997.

[149] Zapata W, Rodriguez B, Weber J, Estrada H, Quinones-Mateu ME, Zimermman PA, *et al.* Increased levels of human beta-defensins mRNA in sexually HIV-1 exposed but uninfected individuals. Curr HIV Res. 2008;6(6):531-538.

[150] Yang C, Boone L, Nguyen TX, Rudolph D, Limpakarnjanarat K, Mastro TD, *et al.* theta-Defensin pseudogenes in HIV-1-exposed, persistently seronegative female sex-workers from Thailand. Infect Genet Evol. 2005;5(1):11-15.

[151] de Leeuw E, Lu W. Human defensins: turning defense into offense? Infect Disord Drug Targets. 2007;7(1):67-70.

CHAPTER 4

Extracellular HMGB1: an Ambiguous Messenger During HIV-1 Infection

Joël Gozlan[1,2,*], Chloe Borde[1] and Vincent Marechal[1]

[1]*Centre de Recherche des Cordeliers, Université Pierre et Marie Curie – Paris 6, UMRS 872, Paris, F-75006 France; Université Paris Descartes, UMRS 872, Paris, F-75006 France; INSERM, U872, Paris, F-75006 France;* [2]*Laboratoire de Virologie, Hôpital Saint-Antoine, 184 rue du Faubourg Saint-Antoine, 75012, Paris, France.*

Abstract: High Mobility Group Box 1 (HMGB1) protein is an abundant nuclear protein that is released outside the cell, upon immune activation or primary cell necrosis. In the extra-cellular space, HMGB1 acts as a potent soluble factor that coordinates cellular events that are crucial for the amplification of inflammation, establishment of early immune responses and tissue repair. HMGB1 is therefore considered as the leading member of a subgroup of the Damage Associated Pattern Molecules named "Alarmins".

Its critical position between innate and adaptive immunity targets HMGB1 is an important soluble factor that may interfere with HIV-1 infection. Indeed, recent works from our laboratory and others brought evidences for significant - although ambiguous - impact of HMGB1 on HIV-1 infection and/or expression.

This review will summarize the current understanding of this exciting molecule, before focusing on the main data available in the literature regarding its relationship with HIV-1. Its potential role during AIDS pathogenesis will be discussed.

HMGB1: AN OVERVIEW

HMGB1, previously named HMG1 or amphoterin, belongs to the High Mobility Group (HMG) proteins, a category of nuclear DNA-binding proteins that are widely expressed in most mammalian cells. HMGs were named according to their electrophoretic mobility in polyacrylamide gels. HMGB1 is especially abundant in mammalian cells nuclei (more than one million molecules per cell). Since its discovery HMGB1 has been mostly analyzed for its various functions in the nucleus. However, recent studies uncovered a quite unexpected albeit presumably essential activity for HMGB1. In addition to its nuclear activity, HMGB1 was indeed demonstrated to act outside of the cells where it behaves as a potent intercellular mediator. Extracellular forms of HMGB1 may provide either from an active secretion in immuno-competent cells such as activated macrophages or natural killer cells, or from a passive release in cells whose plasma membrane has been damaged, such as necrotic cells.

Under this form, HMGB1 may coordinate various cell responses linking septic or aseptic stress signals to innate immunity and tissue repair. Due to this property, HMGB1 is now considered as the main prototype of the "damage-associated pattern molecules" (DAMPs) called "alarmins".

The B box also contains the cytokine activity of HMGB1. The first 20 amino acids of the B box induce TNF release from macrophages, whereas residues 106-123 are sufficient to induce IL6 secretion from dendritic cells [31, 90, 91]. The domain involved in the binding of HMGB1 to RAGE is located between amino acid residues 150 and 183 [9, 35].

HMGB1 STRUCTURE AND NUCLEAR FUNCTIONS

HMGB1 gene is highly conserved, with a 99% homology between humans and rodents. It encodes for a 215 amino-acids protein in human that is organized into two DNA-binding domains (named A- and B-boxes) followed by an acidic tail that confers a globally negative charge at the C-terminus of the protein (Fig. **1**). Two nuclear localization signals (NLS1 and NLS2) control the nuclear translocation of HMGB1 [1]. They

---

*****Address correspondence to this Author Dr. Joël Gozlan at:** [1]Centre de Recherche des Cordeliers, Université Pierre et Marie Curie – Paris 6, UMRS 872, Paris, F-75006 France; Université Paris Descartes, UMRS 872, Paris, F-75006 France; INSERM, U872, Paris, F-75006 France; E-mail: joel.gozlan@sat.aphp.fr

both contain a cluster of lysine residues whose acetylation is thought to modulate the intra-cellular dynamics of HMGB1 [2].

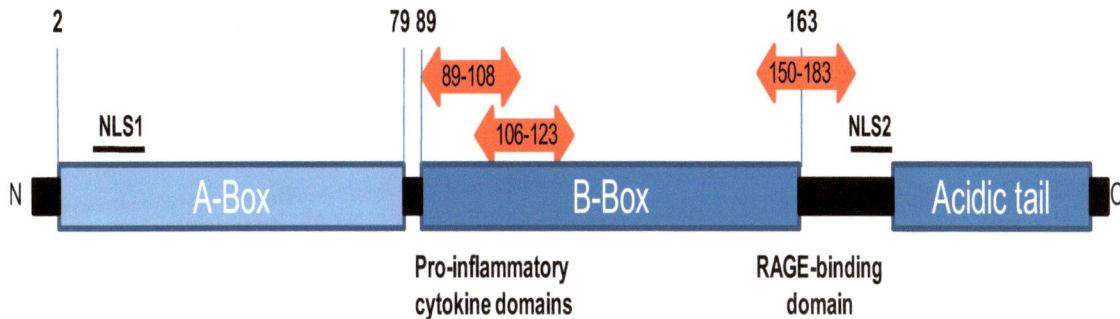

Figure 1: Structural and functional regions of HMGB1. HMGB1 is composed of 3 domains: two positively charged domains (A and B-boxes) involved in DNA binding and a carboxy-terminal acidic tail. Two NLS (nuclear localization signal) have been identified.

Biochemical investigations demonstrated that HMGB1 exhibited a moderated affinity for B-form double-stranded DNA with no sequence specificity, but had a higher affinity for sharply bent structures such as cruciform, cis-platinated and hemicatenated DNA [3-5]. Both the A- and B- boxes exhibit a triple helix conformation and bind to the minor groove of the double-stranded DNA. In turn, HMGB1 promotes the bending of the DNA to which it binds, a property that may help other proteins to gain access and to bind DNA. Its ability to interact with histones and various DNA binding factors progressively led to the notion that HMGB1 could act as a general architectural protein with multiple roles in transcription, replication, recombination and DNA repair. Surprisingly, although HMGB1 inactivation is lethal in knockout mice, it does not impair cell growth [6].

EXTRA-CELLULAR HMGB1: ORIGINS AND MECHANISMS OF RELEASE FROM CELL

HMGB1 biological properties cannot be limited to its nuclear functions, as recently illustrated by a series of surprising observations. H. Rauvala and co-workers were the first ones to describe extracellular activities for HMGB1. In a series of remarkable publications, they showed that a cellular, membrane-bound protein called amphoterin (another name for HMGB1) was highly expressed in embryonic rat neurons, and could promote neurite outgrowth even in a purified form. Later, this activity was proved to require the binding of amphoterin to RAGE, the receptor for advanced glycation end-products [7-9].

The potential of HMGB1 as a soluble factor was eventually recognized in 1999 when Kevin Tracey's group established that HMGB1 was a central pro-inflammatory cytokine involved in the most severe forms of sepsis [10]. Notably, the authors demonstrated that HMGB1 could be actively secreted by activated macrophages in response to bacterial lipopolysaccharide (LPS) and took part to the late phase of sepsis, at the contrary to TNF-alpha or IL-1ß that are known to act in the earliest phases of the disease. This discovery immediately pointed out the therapeutic potential of strategies that would modulate HMGB1 pro-inflammatory activities in sepsis and in the numerous inflammatory conditions where it has been involved later.

Two different mechanisms may lead to the release of HMGB1 into the extracellular environment (Fig. **2**). The first relies on an active secretion by immuno-competent cells, such as mononuclear phagocytes, dendritic cells or natural killer cells, following exposure to exogenous bacterial products such as LPS or classical pro-inflammatory cytokines such as TNF-α, IL-1β or IFN-γ [11-13]. Similarly to IL-1β, HMGB1 lacks leader sequence and its extracellular release may result from an unusual secretory pathway. Notably, HMGB1 secretion would rely on the acetylation of several clusters of lysine that are distributed throughout HMGB1 sequence [2,13]. HMGB1 is highly mobile within the nucleus [14], but it can also shuffle between the nucleus and the cytoplasm. HMGB1 acetylation takes place in the nucleus upon cell stimulation, and prevents HMGB1 re-entry into the nucleus, which may be a prerequisite for addressing HMGB1 to the secretory pathway. The cytosolic HMGB1 would then travel to still un-characterized secretory vesicles that eventually deliver the protein out the cells. The mechanisms controlling HMGB1 acetylation are not yet fully characterized, but they likely involve the inhibition of nuclear deacetylases. Other post-translational modifications have been shown to promote intracytoplasmic sequestration into the cytoplasm and subsequent secretion, such as phosphorylation [15].

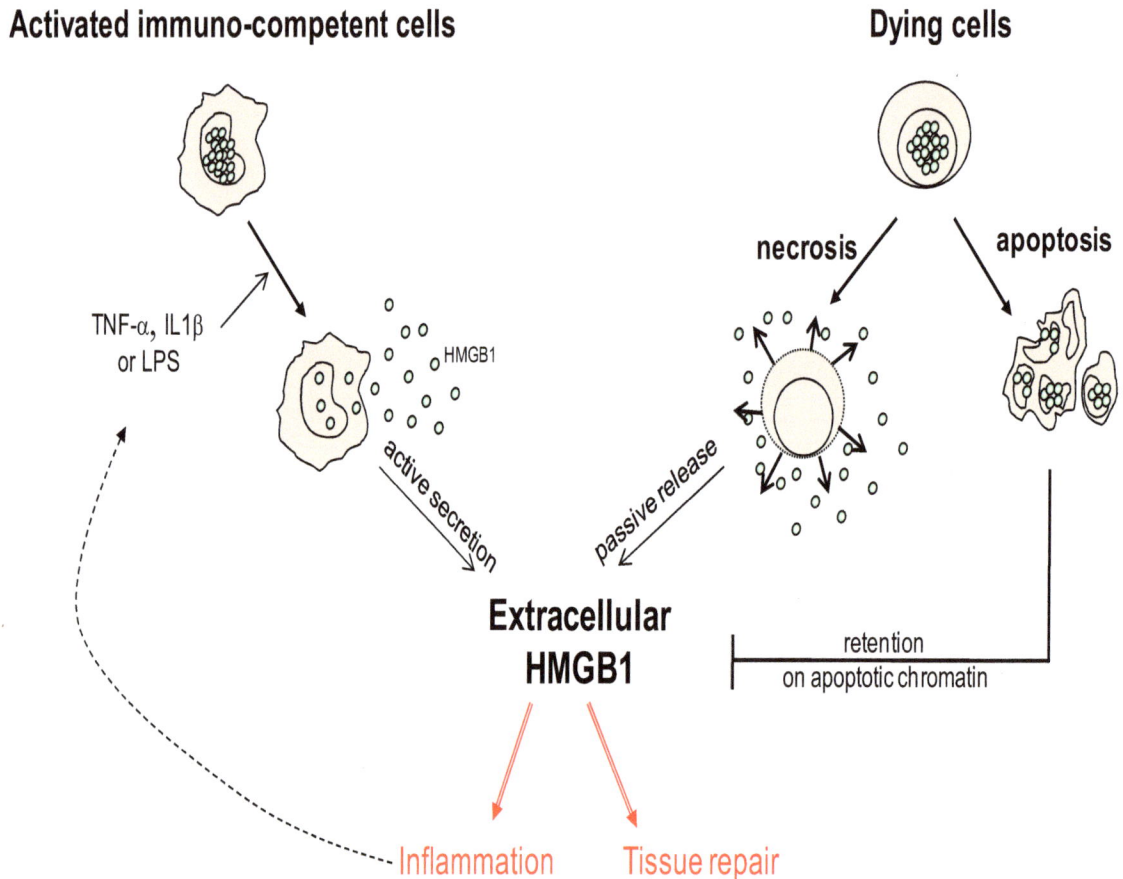

Figure 2: Release of HMGB1 into the extracellular environment. The two recognized sources of HMGB1 release are activated immuno-competent cells (left) and necrotic cells dying through a necrosis process (right), although some forms of apoptosis can also lead to HMGB1 release.

An important contribution to the understanding of the origin and possible functions of extracellular HMGB1 was provided by Bianchi's laboratory, demonstrating a close link between HMGB1 release and cell death signalisation [16]. Indeed, it was established for the first time that HMGB1 can passively diffuse out of the cells when the plasma membranes are damaged, a process that is observed during primary necrosis. This extracellular form of HMGB1 could promote the secretion of TNF-α from monocytes as well, providing strong evidence that HMGB1 may initiate necrosis-induced inflammation. Conversely, HMGB1 did not diffuse out of apoptotic cells, even during secondary necrosis (also called post-apoptotic necrosis), which was in agreement with the general observation that apoptosis does not promote inflammation most of the time. In this situation HMGB1 was found in a close association with the chromatin, possibly in response to the general histone hypoacetylation that is observed during apoptosis. Importantly, HMGB1 itself does not appear hypoacetylated during apoptosis [16]. This model is widely recognized, but recent works have suggested that some forms of apoptosis could still be compatible with HMGB1 release [17]. The immune tolerance observed during apoptosis may rely in this case on the caspase-induced production of reactive oxygen species (ROS) by mitochondria. ROS indeed mediated the oxidation of cystein residues of HMGB1 that has been shown to inactivate its immunostimulatory activity [18].

HMGB1 AS A MAJOR "ALARMIN"

Signaling cellular stress or infection to the immune system is a critical obligation for multicellular organisms. Due to their microbial origin, a subset of these warning signals has been recognized as a coherent functional group called "pathogen-associated molecular pattern" or PAMPs. These molecules alert the immune system following their recognition by toll-like receptors (TLRs) expressed at the surface of immuno-competent cells belonging to both innate and adaptive immunity, therefore triggering inflammatory and immune responses to the microbial invaders.

Another subset of non-microbial "danger signals" has been more recently recognized. The term "alarmins" has been proposed at the last EMBO Workshop on Innate Danger Signals and HMGB1 for these molecules [19]. Indeed, cell and tissue damages are not only caused by pathogens but also by physical stress (wounding, cold or heat etc…), radiations, chemicals, nutrients or oxygen starvation. These traumas trigger a non-septic immune/inflammatory response and the alarmins would be the endo-genous molecules that initiate this process. Exogenous PAMPS and endo-genous "alarmins" are therefore consi-dered as two subgroups of a larger set of molecules, the Damage Associated Molecular Patterns (DAMPs) [19].

Alarmins share several characteristics [19,20]:

a   They are from cellular origin.

b   They are rapidly released by cell dying through non-programmed cell processes, but they are usually not released during apoptosis.

c   They should be secreted by living immuno-competent cells following activation.

d   They activate cells from the innate immunity so they can initiate the adaptive response.

e   Finally, they promote the healing and reconstruction of the damages tissues.

Among other putative candidates, HMGB1 fully meets these criteria and it is now considered as the leading member of this new group of molecules.

HMGB1: RECEPTORS AND BIOLOGICAL ACTIVITIES

Several potential receptors for HMGB1 have been described. Among them, the receptor for Advanced Glycation End-products (RAGE) is certainly one of the most relevant. RAGE is a trans-membrane protein that belongs to the immunoglobulin superfamily. RAGE acts as a receptor for multiple ligands including HMGB1, the amyloid peptide, some members of S100/calgranulin peptides and above all advanced glycation end products (AGEs). AGEs are a group of heterogeneous complex molecules produced by the non-enzymatic glycation between aldoses and free amino groups on proteins [21], DNA [22] or lipids [23]. RAGE is expressed at high level in lung type-1 pneumocytes, but its expression is found at low levels in almost all cell types. Increased levels of RAGE expression has been observed in patients suffering from diabetes, Alzheimer's disease and atherosclerosis [24]. Engagement of RAGE by its ligands results in the activation of several intracellular signaling pathways, including the mitogen activated protein (MAP) kinases ERK and p38 [25], that eventually lead to NF-kB activation [26]. Although it is not clear whether different ligands promote different cell responses, these pathways have been frequently associated with the production of pro-inflammatory cytokines, cell migration, survival and proliferation.

Accumulating evidences lead to the notion that HMGB1 could also be recognized by at least two Toll-Like receptors (TLRs). Park *et al.* first demonstrated that TLR-2 and TLR-4 could be engaged by HMGB1 [27], an event that would be especially important for leucocytes activation. Importantly, interaction of HMGB1 with TLR-2 and TLR-4 also mediates NF-kB activation (even through different pathways), which promotes inflammatory responses similar to those triggered by bacterial components (Fig. **3**).

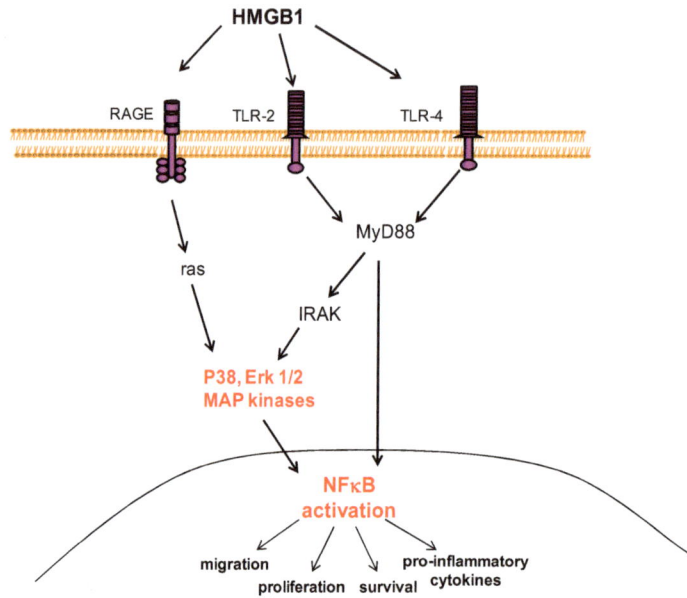

Figure 3. HMGB1 signal transduction pathways. HMGB1 binds to the receptor for advanced glycation end products (RAGE) and two members of the toll like receptors (TLRs). These interactions induce the NFkB nuclear translocation via the ras/MAP kinase or the MyD88/IRAK/MAP kinase pathways, respectively.

MAIN BIOLOGICAL EFFECTS OF EXTRACELLULAR HMGB1

The large pattern of cells expressing these receptors explains at least in part the pleiotropic actions of extracellular HMGB1 (Fig. **4**).

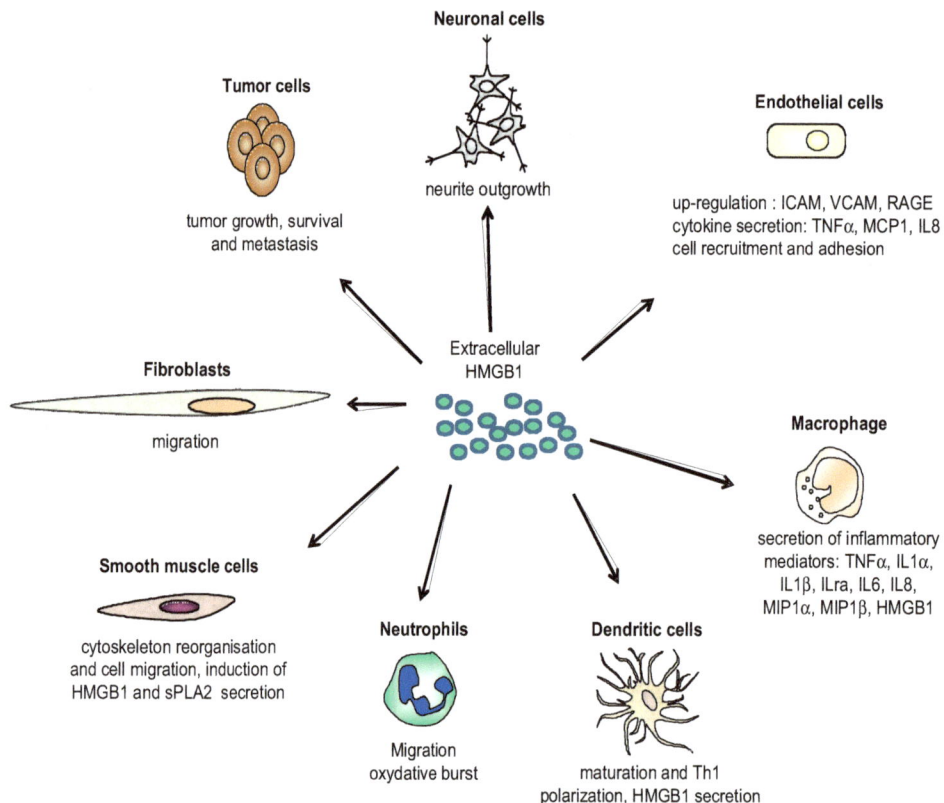

Figure 4: Biological effects of extracellular HMGB1. The major and pleiotropic activities of extracellular HMGB1.

HMGB1: An Active "Go-Between" Linking Innate and Adaptive Immunity

Considering the contribution of HMGB1 to inflammation, a considerable amount of work has been done to define its effect on immune cells. Independently from the mechanism responsible for its release (active secretion or passive diffusion outside a necrotic cells), HMGB1 has been shown to participate to the recruitment of inflammatory cells to the site of the "danger". Then, it takes part to an active cross-talk between natural killers cells (NKs), dendritic cells (DCs) and macrophages. HMGB1-mediated recruitment of leukocytes through the endothelial barrier is linked at least in part to its ability to activate endothelial cells (ECs). The increased expression of various adhesion molecules, at the surface of activated ECs, will in turn stimulates the adhesion of leukocytes, including neutrophils [28-30].

In addition, HMGB1 enhances DCs maturation [31,32] and acts in synergy with IL-1, IL-2 and IL-18 to promote interactions between NKs, DCs and monocytes [33,34].

HMGB1: Chemoattraction and Tissue Repair

The role of HMGB1 as a chemoattractant is not restricted to the cells of the immune system. Other cell types, including the mesoangioblasts, heart myocytes, smooth muscle cells, fibroblats, monocytes and endothelial cells have been shown to migrate in response to HMGB1 [35-37] (S. Barnay, unpublished results). These observations suggested that HMGB1 might contribute to tissue repair and/or remodeling processes, concomitantly or following its participation in damage signaling and immune activation.

In agreement with this model, an increased regeneration has been observed *in vivo* in various pathological tissues treated by HMGB1, including infarcted heart [36] and the skin of diabetic mice [38]. However, HMGB1 chemoattractant properties may have some drawbacks, since HMGB1/RAGE interactions have also been implicated in cell growth and tumor metastasis [39-42].

To be or not to be … A Cytokine?

When K. Tracey and colleagues discovered HMGB1 contribution to severe sepsis, it seemed quite obvious that it was a new and important pro-inflammatory cytokine. Experiments conducted *in vitro* and in animal models of sepsis [10,43] lead to the exciting proposal that HMGB1 was secreted by activated macrophages and, in turn, could act as a secondary activator of immunocompetent cells. Therefore, HMGB1 activation was considered as a central part of a classical pro-inflammatory response involving TNF, IL-1 and IL-6. Moreover, the delayed pattern of HMGB1 secretion (several hours after the initiation of sepsis) compared to the rapid accumulation of TNF and IL-1 opened very promising therapeutic possibilities, using either antibodies against HMGB1, recombinant inhibitory HMGB1 box A or chemical inhibitors of HMGB1 secretion [10,44].

This model was also strengthened by the accumulation of HMGB1 in the sera of patients with sepsis, the highest concentrations of HMGB1 being correlated with the severity of sepsis. Recent data using highly purified forms of the protein however challenged the hypothesis of HMGB1 being a pro-inflammatory cytokine "by its own".

Investigating the secretion of pro-inflammatory mediators by smooth muscle cells exposed to HMGB1, our laboratory provided evidences that highly purified forms of HMGB1 had barely no pro-inflammatory activity in this model, whereas it could cooperate very efficiently with IL-1ß to promote the secretion of soluble phospholipase A2 (sPLA2) [45]. In the same respect, Rouhiainen and coll. confirmed that the pro-inflammatory activity (i.e. its ability to induce TNF-α secretion and nitric oxide release from mononuclear cells) of recombinant HMGB1 was mainly due to its natural ability to bind to phosphatidylserine [46]. In fact, there are now accumulating evidences that HMGB1 exerts its pro-inflammatory activity mainly by forming non-covalent complexes with pro-inflammatory molecules such as LPS or CpG-DNA [47-49].

In the case of CpG DNA, it has been suggested that HMGB1 ability to form complexes and to interact with RAGE may promote the subsequent interaction of CpG DNA to its final receptor, TLR-9.

Altogether, these results may arise questions about some conclusions drawn from experiments conducted with HMGB1 purified from E.coli under native conditions, since this protein can contain minute amounts of LPS, phosphatidylserine, but also significant amounts bacterial nucleic acids as shown by our group (S. Thierry and V. Maréchal, unpublished, Fig. **5**). Importantly, these contaminants do not appear to induce artefacts nor cooperate with HMGB1 in cell migration assays.

CONTRIBUTION OF HMGB1 TO HUMAN DISEASES

Besides its crucial implication in acute conditions such as severe sepsis, HMGB1 has been implicated in the pathogenesis of several chronic inflammatory diseases or in pathologies where chronic local inflammation is important, such as atherosclerosis. Some examples are presented below.

Rheumatoid Arthritis

HMGB1 has been implicated in the development of rheumatoid arthritis. In animal models, HMGB1 is highly expressed in synovial tissue and fluid as well, and the symptoms are reduced by the administration of antibodies against

HMGB1 or by recombinant box-A [50]. Reversely, intra-articular injection of HMGB1 in healthy animals induces arthritis [51] whereas high levels of HMGB1 have been found *in vivo*, in the synovial fluid of patients with rheumatoid arthritis [52].

Cancer

HMGB1 is over-expressed in many tumor cells but the link between HMGB1 and cancer development is complex and still partially understood. This may be due at least in part to the ability of HMGB1 to modulate gene expression. In colon carcinomas for example, HMGB1 overexpression has been associated with a pronounced activation of NF-kB responsive genes, including c-IAP2, a protein that prevents apoptosis. In the same study, the authors were also able to correlate HMGB1 over expression to the reduced activity of two pro-apoptotic proteins, namely the caspase-3 and -9 [53].

As indicated before, numerous studies demonstrated that interaction between HMGB1 and RAGE promoted the growth, spread and metastasis of tumors from diverse origins, including colon and prostate [42,54]. Importantly, blockade of this interaction by soluble or mutated RAGE reversed tumor aggressiveness [55].

On the opposite, the adjuvant action of HMGB1 may be beneficial to the anti-tumoral immune response. Indeed, the release of HMGB1 by dying tumor cells after radiotherapy or chemotherapy can promote an efficient tumor antigen-specific immune responses, a process that involve HMGB1 recognition by TLR-4 at the surface of dendritic cells [56]. In the same respect, HMGB1 released by dying tumor cells may contribute to brain tumor regression, a process that is dependent of TLR-2 [57].

Atherosclerosis

Local chronic inflammation plays a key role in atherogenesis. Recent data demonstrated the expression of HMGB1 in activated vascular smooth muscle cells in human atherosclerotic lesions. HMGB1 stimulates in turn the production of both C-reactive protein and matrix metalloproteinase through its interaction with RAGE, thus contributing to the progression and vulnerability of the atherosclerotic plaque [58]. An intimate interplay between smooth muscle cells and HMGB1 has been described. On the first hand, smooth muscle cells actively secrete HMGB1 after cholesterol loading. On the other hand, SMCs proliferate, migrate, produce soluble phospholipase A2 and secrete more HMGB1 when exposed to HMGB1 [45,59].

HMGB1 AND HIV-1

Extracellular HMGB1: Putative Mechanisms of Interference with HIV-1 Infection.

HMGB1 may influence HIV infection at three levels at least. First, HMGB1 pro-inflammatory activity, alone or in combination with other factors, may elicit the production of numerous soluble factors – including TNF-α – that are known to modulate HIV-1 infection and/or replication [60]. Second, HMGB1 may play an important function during the early phase of HIV-1 infection, as a growing set of evidences indicates that it could link innate to adaptive immunity. Third, HMGB1 may act directly on the multiple HIV-1 target cells that have been shown to express RAGE, TLR-2 or TLR-4, such as the monocytes/macrophages, the CD4 T cells and the dendritic cells [61-63]. This is especially relevant for the control of HIV-1 expression since most if not all the signaling pathways induced by soluble HMGB1 converge to NF-kB, a well-known regulator of HIV-1 transcription [60,64].

HMGB1, Natural Killer Cells and Dendritic Cells: When Innate Immunity Talks to the Adaptive Response

The sexual route is the main way of HIV-1 acquisition. During infection of the sexual mucosa, the first target cells encountered by the virus in the genital epithelium and sub-epithelium are the CCR5 expressing dendritic cells (DCs) and their subtypes the Langherans cells (LCs). These cells are professional antigen presenting cells (APCs) that can play an opposite (and not mutually exclusive) role during HIV infection.

On the first hand, they contribute to HIV-1 transmission to its main target, the CD4 T cells, since they migrate after their activation to the lymphoid tissues where they can find significant amounts of these major target cells. This is mainly due to the ability of HIV-1 to bind to the C-type lectins expressed at the surface of these cells, such as DC-SIGN for the DCs and langerin for the LCs even if a recent study suggests the lectin langerin might also protect LCs from infection [65].

One the other hand, these cells are also important to initiate specific immunity against the HIV-1. Migration of dendritic cells to the lymphoid compartment induces their maturation, allowing the priming of a specific immune response against the virus through the presentation of viral antigen to naïve T cells. Maturation of DCs is also known to be essential for the subsequent orientation of CD4 T cell to a Th1 phenotype [66]. Therefore, DCs are located at the cross road between innate and specific immunity. Their fate has been recently linked to their interaction with another key actor of the innate immunity, the Natural Killer cells (NKs). Importantly, the reciprocal activation of these two cell types involves HMGB1. During DC-NK interaction, NKs trigger the polarized secretion of IL-18 at the synaptic space by immature DCs, whereas DC-activated NKs secrete in turn hyper-acetylated HMGB1 [33]. Many works demonstrated that HMGB1 can induce maturation of DCs [31,32,67] and it is now believed that this protein is a key actor of the DC-NK cross talk. Indeed HMGB1 secreted by NK matures DCs and triggers these cells to secrete the pro-inflammatory cytokines IL-1β and IL-12. Moreover, secreted HMGB1 at the NK-DC synapse also appears to induce the resistance displayed by matured DC to NK cells cytotoxicity [33].

A recent work investigated how this NK-DC cross-talk may impact the fate of infected DCs in the context of HIV-1 infection [68]. HIV-1 infected DCs retain their susceptibility to NK-induced maturation and this cross talk still involves the secretion of HMGB1 by both cell types. As for uninfected DCs, maturation of HIV-1 infected DCs by HMGB1 involves RAGE expression on these cells [67,68]. However, this cross-talk is not fully functional when DCs are infected by HIV-1, since infected DCs do not properly secrete IL-12 and IL-18 after their maturation via NKs interactions. These cytokines are important in the subsequent polarization of autologous CD4 T cell to a Th1 phenotype [66] and no increase in IFN-γ secreting T cells was indeed observed when naïve CD4+CD45RO-T cells were co-cultured with autologous NKs and infected DCs [68]. The effective contribution of HIV to this defect is demonstrated by the restoration of the Th1 polarization upon addition of the reverse transcriptase inhibitor AZT to the co-cultures.

Another consequence of the cross talk between activated NKs and infected DCs is an increased viral expression in DCs, as demonstrated by the percentage of positive p24 antigen expressing DCs, the p24 release in the co-cultures supernatants and the amount of viral DNA within the cells. Importantly, this increase in HIV expression in dependent on HMGB1 since it is alleviated by specific anti-HMGB1 antibodies or by glycyrrhizin, another direct inhibitor of HMGB1 [68].

This last result opens another very exciting field of work on HMGB1 and HIV-1 that is its impact on viral expression. Whereas an early work did demonstrate that intracellular expression of HMGB1 could inhibit

HIV-1 LTR-directed transcription in a cell-specific manner [69], recent studies focused on the putative impact of extracellular HMGB1 on HIV-1 expression.

HMGB1 and HIV-1 Expression

Soluble factors such as cytokines or chemokines have long been shown to modulate viral expression [70]. Both HIV infection itself and other conditions that are frequent in HIV infected patients (cellular stress, immune stimulation, co-infections) may deeply alter the balanced production of these factors. The various and sometimes controversial properties of extracellular HMGB1 lead our laboratory and others to investigate the potential impact of HMGB1 on HIV-1 expression. Two key moments in HIV-1 life cycle may be influenced by extracellular HMGB1: i) the early stages of HIV-1 infection and ii) the expression of the integrated provirus.

HMGB1 Induces HIV-1 Expression from Latently Infected Cells

To investigate the effect of soluble HMGB1 on latently infected cells, we used two different sources of HMGB1 protein [71]. A native form of HMGB1 was obtained from necrotic HeLa cells, whereas a highly purified recombinant protein was produced in *Escherichia coli*. As shown before (Fig. **5**), many precautions were taken to exclude contaminant from bacterial origin, including LPS and nucleic acids.

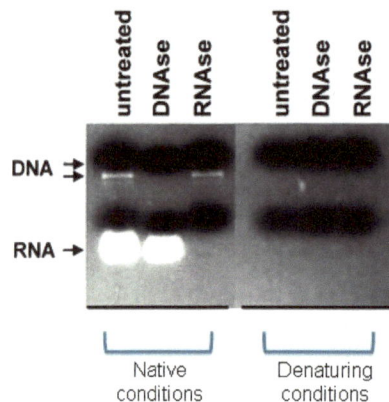

Figure 5: HMGB1 co-purifies with DNA and RNA in E.coli. Recombinant human HMGB1 was purified from *E. coli* under native or denaturing conditions. Following purification, 10µg of recombinant protein was subjected to DNA or RNA extraction. As illustrated, native HMGB1 was associated with large amounts of nucleic acids from bacterial origin.

Several models of viral persistence were used for this study, including two well characterized cell lines, ACH-2 and U1 cells. These cells have been widely used in other laboratories to investigate post-integration latency in T lymphocytes and monocytic cells respectively, since they both exhibit a low level of basal retroviral expression that can be increased by chemical or biological agents. A strong dose-dependant increase in viral expression was observed in both cell lines when they were exposed to HMGB1 concentrations ranging from 100 ng/ml to 10 µg/ml. Nowak and colleagues did also report that HMGB1 reactivated HIV-1 in U1 but, surprisingly, not in ACH-2 cells [72]. This discrepancy could be largely explained by the high basal level of HIV-1 expression in the ACH-2 clone used in their study compared to U1 cells.

Then, we delineated the mechanisms of HMGB1-mediated increase of viral expression in great details, confirming that (1) HIV-1 reactivation was transcriptional, (2) it did not required de novo protein synthesis and (3) it relied on the interaction between HMGB1 and RAGE. Finally, intracellular signaling was proved to be mediated by MAP kinases p38 and ERK activation that finally resulted in the binding of NFkB to the nucleosome nuc-1, a region of the 5' LTR that plays a pivotal role in HIV-1 expression. We prolonged these results in the highly relevant context of the HIV-1 persistency in infected patients, aviraemic under highly active antiretroviral therapy (HAART). We randomly choose six HIV-1-infected volunteers, efficiently controlled by HAART for more than 4 years (viral load below 50 copies/ml, median CD4 cell count: 723 c/µl [minimum 419-maximum 961]) and collected their PBMCs for *ex vivo* reactivation experiments. Long-term

HIV-1 cultures were performed from 2×10^6 CD8 depleted PBMC in the presence or in the absence of recombinant human HMGB1 (Fig. **6**). One culture from one patient could not be analyzed since it displayed a moderate HIV-1 production without any induction. For the other five patients, HMGB1 was at least as efficient as phyto-hemagglutinine A (PHA) in reactivating HIV-1 since it induced virus outgrowth for 4 out of 5 PBMC cultures, with a viral production similar (patients 5 and 6) or even higher (patients 2 and 3) than observed for PHA-treated cells. In this experiment, HMGB1 did also reactivate HIV-1 in the absence of IL-2, confirming its strong ability to reactivate the virus from these controlled patients. Although this was not formerly proved *in vivo*, this work strongly suggests that HMGB1 could positively influence HIV1 reactivation from latently infected cells when necrosis or immune activation occurs (Fig. **7**). This may be especially relevant during AIDS, where cell injury is frequent in organs targeted by opportunistic diseases. Interestingly, recent data confirmed that virus-induced cell toxicity might indeed induce HMGB1 release [73,74]. Furthermore, HIV itself could participate to cell injury since both necrosis and apoptosis were observed during HIV-mediated cell killing [75,76].

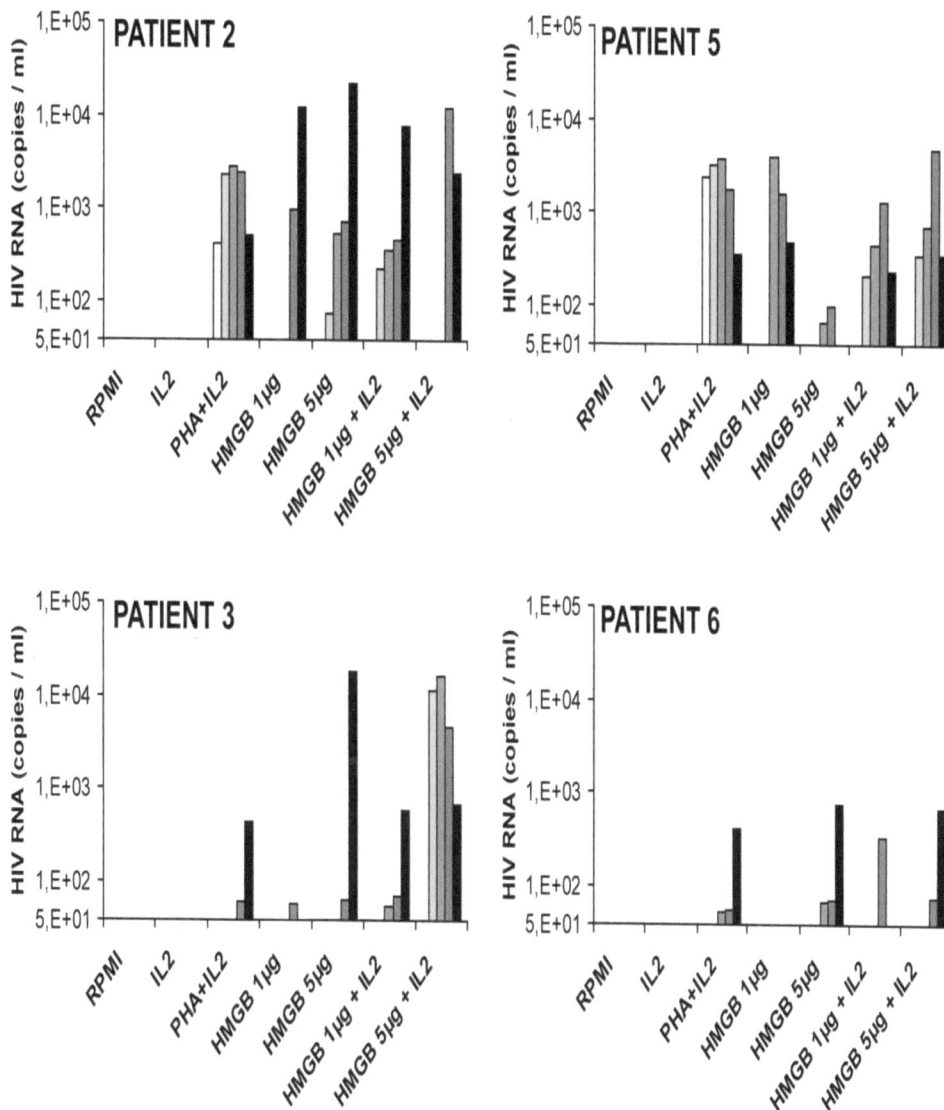

Figure 6: Ex vivo HIV-1 recovery induced by HMGB1. CD8 depleted PBMC, obtained from aviraemic patients controlled by HAART, were cultured for 35 days in the presence of IL-2, PHA and/or HMGB1 at various concentrations. HIV-1 outgrowth was evaluated by quantification of viral RNA in the cell culture supernatants. Adapted from [71].

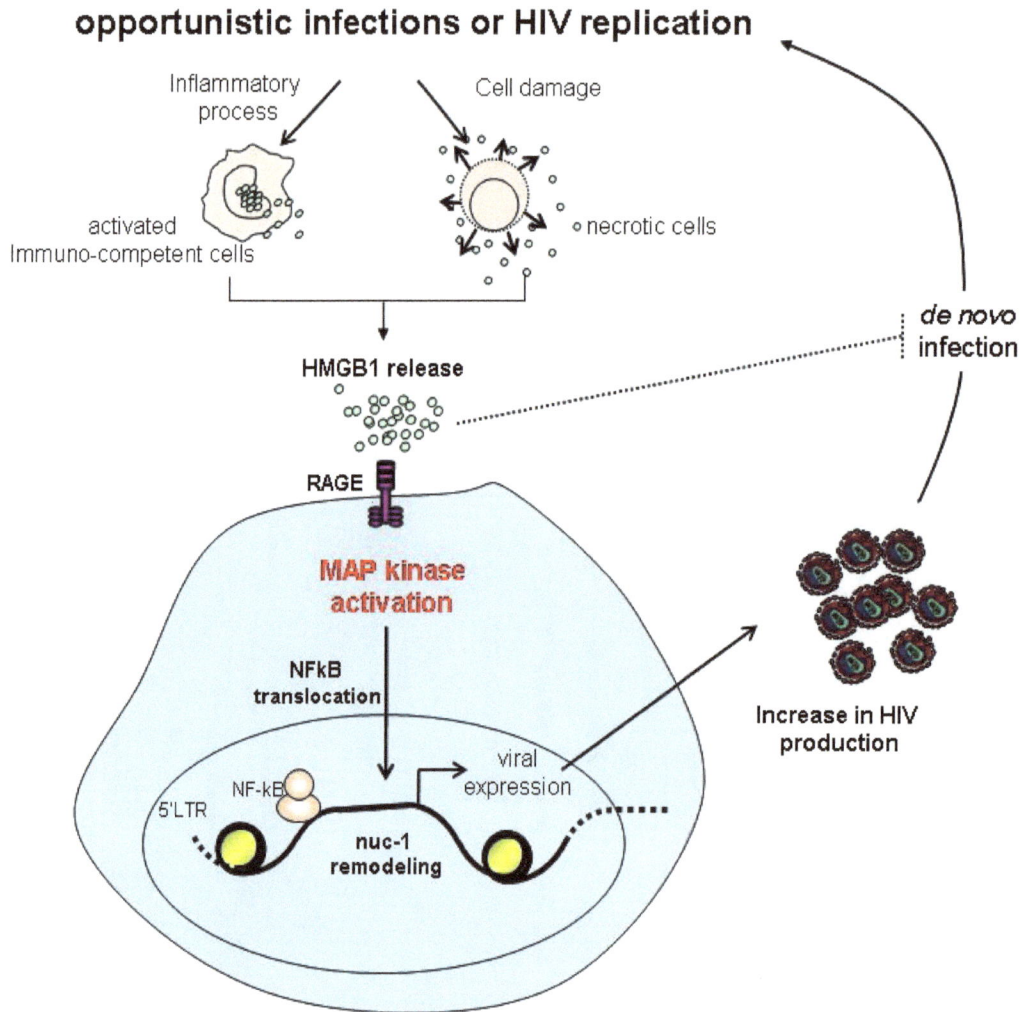

Figure 7: Potential impact of HMGB1 on HIV viral cycle. Extracellular HMGB1, released through cell damage or immune activation, inhibits HIV-1 de novo infection but increases HIV-1 production by persistently infected cells.

Two independent works demonstrated that HMGB1 might influence very differently the process of *de novo* infection [72,77]. In both instances, necrotic and recombinant HMGB1 were shown to decrease viral expression when primary monocyte-derived macrophages (MDM) were infected by the R5-tropic isolate BaL. The mechanism of this inhibition still remains controversial.

Nowak *et al.* explained this result by the ability of HMGB1 to induce the secretion of RANTES, MIP-1α and MIP-1β, a series of chemokines that bind to the CCR5 co-receptor and therefore inhibit HIV infection.

However, Cassetta and colleagues did not observe any increase of these chemokines in their study. Rather, the authors suggested that HMGB1 might interfere with viral entry by decreasing CCR5 expression at the surface of MDM.

This result is quite reminiscent of a recent work from our lab, which also demonstrated a decrease in HIV-1 co-receptors expression at the surface of dendritic cells when the cells were incubated in the presence of AGEs, another ligand of RAGE (N. Nasreddine, manuscript submitted for publication).

Cassetta and colleagues also observed a restriction in the replication of X4-tropic strains in some U937 monocytic clones. In that case, the reduced infection was not explained by a reduction of the surface expression of the CXCR4 co-receptor.

Whatever the mechanisms involved, the dual impact of HMGB1 on HIV replication in monocytic cells is strikingly reminiscent of what has already been reported for other soluble factors such as TNF-α [78]or IFN-γ [79].

HMGB1 Concentration *In Vivo*

Various techniques have been used to quantify extra-cellular HMGB1 in peripheral blood or other biological specimens. The western blotting was initially used [11, 80] before an easier and more sensitive commercial ELISA test became available [81,82]. This new assay allowed more extensive studies on the levels of HMGB1 during various conditions, even if some concerns have been raised regarding the possible interference of factors that may mask HMGB1 in the serum, such as antibodies [82]. This may notably explain some observed discrepancies between the severity of sepsis and the concentration of HMGB1 in serum [83].

To investigate this question, our team has recently developed an original and very sensitive gel shift assay to quantify HMGB1 [84]. This assay is based on the ability of HMGB1 to bind with extremely high affinity to a particular form of double-stranded DNA, the hemicatenated DNA loops [5,85]. The protocol was then modified to introduce an additional step where HMGB1 is chemically dissociated from other molecules, such as antibodies. Some unpublished work from our lab suggested that the ELISA would often underestimate the effective amount of HMGB1 in serum (S.Barnay, manuscript submitted for publication). Whatever the method used, HMGB1 concentrations are usually undetectable or very low (below 1 ng/ml) in serum or plasma collected from healthy controls, even if frequent occurrence of detectable HMGB1 can be scarcely observed in individuals without any apparent condition [84,86]. On the contrary, increased concentrations of HMGB1 have been detected in the serum of patients with severe sepsis [10,83]. The range of HMGB1 levels in this setting appears to be large (from 1 to 160 ng/ml) and may depend on the method used. However, HMGB1 concentrations globally correlate in this setting with clinical outcome, the highest levels being observed most often in non-survivors. Importantly, much higher concentrations (up to 10 µg/ml) can be measured *in vivo*, when samples are collected from local inflammatory sites. This has been notably observed in bronchoalveolar lavages from patients suffering from acute lung injury [87], synovial fluid of individuals with rheumatoid arthritis [52] and in cervico-vaginal swabs from women with genital herpes (C. Borde, unpublished data).In the context of HIV-1 infection, HMGB1 levels have been measured in plasma samples from healthy volunteers and from untreated HIV infected patients at various stages of their disease [88]. Three patient categories have been defined: group A (n = 14), with preserved immunological status (CD4 cell count above 600/µl) and a low viral load (below 2000 c/ml); group B (n = 13), with deteriorated immunological status (CD4 cell count below 400/µl) and a high viral load (above 20000 c/ml); group C (n = 16), with a deteriorated immunological status, a high viral load and an opportunistic disease at the moment of sampling. Despite the limited size of the different groups, the authors found that HIV infected patients globally displayed increased concentrations of HMGB1 in plasma (median 5.3 ng/ml, range 0.5-87.5) compared with uninfected controls (median 1.4 ng/ml, range 0.0-4.4; p<0.001). Furthermore, infected patients with opportunistic infections have higher levels (median 8.4 ng/ml, range 1.1-71.8) compared with asymptomatic HIV infected patients with preserved (median 4.7 ng/ml, range 1.7-87.5; p<0.05) or deteriorated (median 3.8 ng/ml, range 0.5-83.5; p<0.05) immune status.

Even if the biological origin of HMGB1 in these patients was not documented, these data suggested that HMGB1 might indeed significantly contribute to AIDS pathogenesis. It is still possible however that HMGB1 levels only mirror AIDS progression and/or opportunistic infections.

CONCLUSIONS AND PERSPECTIVES

This review underlined the many aspects that might link HMGB1 to HIV-1 infection in a direct or indirect manner. In this complex pathology, HMGB1 could bring to the infected organism both the armor and the sword.

Its active participation to the cross-talk between innate and adaptive immunity may be critical to the organism to bring up an appropriate response to the early phases of acute infection. The impairment of this cross-talk during HIV-1 infection might be one important key among many others to explain why infected individuals do not build a strong and efficient immune response against HIV *in vivo* [68]. The ability of HMGB1 to inhibit HIV-1 acute infection of macrophages, probably through a restriction of the entry of R5-tropic - and possibly X4-tropic isolates - may also be an unexpected and positive effect of the protein. The real impact of HMGB1 on HIV entry still remains to be investigated *in vivo*, and on a larger spectrum of target cells. Nonetheless the recent demonstration of the clinical efficacy of new CCR5 inhibitors in patients evading classical HAART [89] indicates that blocking viral entry remains a key step, even during an established infection.

Conversely, HMGB1 may exhibit an opposite and deleterious effect on infected cells since it has been shown to activate latent infection. This has been demonstrated in chronically infected cell lines but also in mononuclear cells from patients efficiently controlled by HAART. Wheter HMGB1 modulates HIV infection and transcription by itself, or in conjunction with still unknown cellular (or exogenous) molecules, remains to be clarified regarding to the recent notion that pure HMGB1 may not induce pro-inflammatory cytokines.

In any cases, HMGB1 might overall be an important actor in the known deleterious consequences brought by opportunistic or co-infections status on AIDS progression.

ACKNOWLEDGMENTS

We thank S. Barnay, C. Gaillard, S. Thierry and P.M. Girard for their help in some studies summarized in this paper.

This research program was supported by Sidaction, ANRS and by the University Pierre et Marie Curie (Bonus Qualité Recherche).

C. Borde is recipient of fellowships from the Ministère de l'Education Nationale, de la Recherche et des Technologies and from the INSERM network "herpesviruses and cancer".

REFERENCES

[1]   Cokol M, Nair R, Rost B. Finding nuclear localization signals. EMBO Rep 2000 Nov;1(5):411-5.
[2]   Bonaldi T, Talamo F, Scaffidi P, Ferrera D, Porto A, Bachi A, *et al*. Monocytic cells hyperacetylate chromatin protein HMGB1 to redirect it towards secretion. EMBO J 2003 Oct 15;22(20):5551-60.
[3]   Bianchi ME, Beltrame M, Paonessa G. Specific recognition of cruciform DNA by nuclear protein HMG1. Science 1989 Feb 24;243(4894 Pt 1):1056-9.
[4]   Ohndorf UM, Rould MA, He Q, Pabo CO, Lippard SJ. Basis for recognition of cisplatin-modified DNA by high-mobility-group proteins. Nature 1999 Jun 17;399(6737):708-12.
[5]   Gaillard C, Strauss F. High affinity binding of proteins HMG1 and HMG2 to semicatenated DNA loops. BMC Mol Biol 2000;1:1.
[6]   Calogero S, Grassi F, Aguzzi A, Voigtlander T, Ferrier P, Ferrari S, *et al*. The lack of chromosomal protein Hmg1 does not disrupt cell growth but causes lethal hypoglycaemia in newborn mice. Nat Genet 1999 Jul;22(3):276-80.
[7]   Rauvala H, Pihlaskari R. Isolation and some characteristics of an adhesive factor of brain that enhances neurite outgrowth in central neurons. J Biol Chem 1987 Dec 5;262(34):16625-35.
[8]   Merenmies J, Pihlaskari R, Laitinen J, Wartiovaara J, Rauvala H. 30-kDa heparin-binding protein of brain (amphoterin) involved in neurite outgrowth. Amino acid sequence and localization in the filopodia of the advancing plasma membrane. J Biol Chem 1991 Sep 5;266(25):16722-9.
[9]   Hori O, Brett J, Slattery T, Cao R, Zhang J, Chen JX, *et al*. The receptor for advanced glycation end products (RAGE) is a cellular binding site for amphoterin. Mediation of neurite outgrowth and co-expression of rage and amphoterin in the developing nervous system. J Biol Chem 1995 Oct 27;270(43):25752-61.
[10] Wang H, Bloom O, Zhang M, Vishnubhakat JM, Ombrellino M, Che J, *et al*. HMG-1 as a late mediator of endotoxin lethality in mice. Science 1999 Jul 9;285(5425):248-51.
[11] Wang H, Vishnubhakat JM, Bloom O, Zhang M, Ombrellino M, Sama A, *et al*. Proinflammatory cytokines (tumor necrosis factor and interleukin 1) stimulate release of high mobility group protein-1 by pituicytes. Surgery 1999 Aug;126(2):389-92.

[12]   Rendon-Mitchell B, Ochani M, Li J, Han J, Wang H, Yang H, *et al*. IFN-gamma induces high mobility group box 1 protein release partly through a TNF-dependent mechanism. J Immunol 2003 Apr 1;170(7):3890-7.

[13]   Gardella S, Andrei C, Ferrera D, Lotti LV, Torrisi MR, Bianchi ME, *et al*. The nuclear protein HMGB1 is secreted by monocytes via a non-classical, vesicle-mediated secretory pathway. EMBO Rep 2002 Oct;3(10):995-1001.

[14]   Pallier C, Scaffidi P, Chopineau-Proust S, Agresti A, Nordmann P, Bianchi ME, *et al*. Association of chromatin proteins high mobility group box (HMGB) 1 and HMGB2 with mitotic chromosomes. Mol Biol Cell 2003 Aug;14(8):3414-26.

[15]   Youn JH, Shin JS. Nucleocytoplasmic shuttling of HMGB1 is regulated by phosphorylation that redirects it toward secretion. J Immunol 2006 Dec 1;177(11):7889-97.

[16]   Scaffidi P, Misteli T, Bianchi ME. Release of chromatin protein HMGB1 by necrotic cells triggers inflammation. Nature 2002 Jul 11;418(6894):191-5.

[17]   Bell CW, Jiang W, Reich CF, 3rd, Pisetsky DS. The extracellular release of HMGB1 during apoptotic cell death. Am J Physiol Cell Physiol 2006 Dec;291(6):C1318-25.

[18]   Kazama H, Ricci JE, Herndon JM, Hoppe G, Green DR, Ferguson TA. Induction of immunological tolerance by apoptotic cells requires caspase-dependent oxidation of high-mobility group box-1 protein. Immunity 2008 Jul;29(1):21-32.

[19]   Bianchi ME. DAMPs, PAMPs and alarmins: all we need to know about danger. J Leukoc Biol 2007 Jan;81(1):1-5.

[20]   Harris HE, Raucci A. Alarmin(g) news about danger: workshop on innate danger signals and HMGB1. EMBO Rep 2006 Aug;7(8):774-8.

[21]   Dunn JA, Patrick JS, Thorpe SR, Baynes JW. Oxidation of glycated proteins: age-dependent accumulation of N epsilon-(carboxymethyl)lysine in lens proteins. Biochemistry 1989 Nov 28;28(24):9464-8.

[22]   Lee AT, Cerami A. *In vitro* and *in vivo* reactions of nucleic acids with reducing sugars. Mutat Res 1990 May;238(3):185-91.

[23]   Bucala R, Makita Z, Koschinsky T, Cerami A, Vlassara H. Lipid advanced glycosylation: pathway for lipid oxidation *in vivo*. Proc Natl Acad Sci USA 1993 Jul 15;90(14):6434-8.

[24]   Rong LL, Gooch C, Szabolcs M, Herold KC, Lalla E, Hays AP, *et al*. RAGE: a journey from the complications of diabetes to disorders of the nervous system - striking a fine balance between injury and repair. Restor Neurol Neurosci 2005;23(5-6):355-65.

[25]   Park JS, Arcaroli J, Yum HK, Yang H, Wang H, Yang KY, *et al*. Activation of gene expression in human neutrophils by high mobility group box 1 protein. Am J Physiol Cell Physiol 2003 Apr;284(4):C870-9.

[26]   Bierhaus A, Humpert PM, Morcos M, Wendt T, Chavakis T, Arnold B, *et al*. Understanding RAGE, the receptor for advanced glycation end products. J Mol Med 2005 Nov;83(11):876-86.

[27]   Park JS, Svetkauskaite D, He Q, Kim JY, Strassheim D, Ishizaka A, *et al*. Involvement of toll-like receptors 2 and 4 in cellular activation by high mobility group box 1 protein. J Biol Chem 2004 Feb 27;279(9):7370-7.

[28]   Fiuza C, Bustin M, Talwar S, Tropea M, Gerstenberger E, Shelhamer JH, *et al*. Inflammation-promoting activity of HMGB1 on human microvascular endothelial cells. Blood 2003 Apr 1;101(7):2652-60.

[29]   Chavakis T, Bierhaus A, Al-Fakhri N, Schneider D, Witte S, Linn T, *et al*. The pattern recognition receptor (RAGE) is a counterreceptor for leukocyte integrins: a novel pathway for inflammatory cell recruitment. J Exp Med 2003 Nov 17;198(10):1507-15.

[30]   Orlova VV, Choi EY, Xie C, Chavakis E, Bierhaus A, Ihanus E, *et al*. A novel pathway of HMGB1-mediated inflammatory cell recruitment that requires Mac-1-integrin. EMBO J 2007 Feb 21;26(4):1129-39.

[31]   Messmer D, Yang H, Telusma G, Knoll F, Li J, Messmer B, *et al*. High mobility group box protein 1: an endogenous signal for dendritic cell maturation and Th1 polarization. J Immunol 2004 Jul 1;173(1):307-13.

[32]   Rovere-Querini P, Capobianco A, Scaffidi P, Valentinis B, Catalanotti F, Giazzon M, *et al*. HMGB1 is an endogenous immune adjuvant released by necrotic cells. EMBO Rep 2004 Aug;5(8):825-30.

[33]   Semino C, Angelini G, Poggi A, Rubartelli A. NK/iDC interaction results in IL-18 secretion by DCs at the synaptic cleft followed by NK cell activation and release of the DC maturation factor HMGB1. Blood 2005 Jul 15;106(2):609-16.

[34]   DeMarco RA, Fink MP, Lotze MT. Monocytes promote natural killer cell interferon gamma production in response to the endogenous danger signal HMGB1. Mol Immunol 2005 Feb;42(4):433-44.

[35]   Palumbo R, Sampaolesi M, De Marchis F, Tonlorenzi R, Colombetti S, Mondino A, *et al*. Extracellular HMGB1, a signal of tissue damage, induces mesoangioblast migration and proliferation. J Cell Biol 2004 Feb 2;164(3):441-9.

[36]   Limana F, Germani A, Zacheo A, Kajstura J, Di Carlo A, Borsellino G, *et al*. Exogenous high-mobility group box 1 protein induces myocardial regeneration after infarction via enhanced cardiac C-kit+ cell proliferation and differentiation. Circ Res 2005 Oct 14;97(8):e73-83.

[37] Mitola S, Belleri M, Urbinati C, Coltrini D, Sparatore B, Pedrazzi M, *et al.* Cutting edge: extracellular high mobility group box-1 protein is a proangiogenic cytokine. J Immunol 2006 Jan 1;176(1):12-5.

[38] Straino S, Di Carlo A, Mangoni A, De Mori R, Guerra L, Maurelli R, *et al.* High-mobility group box 1 protein in human and murine skin: involvement in wound healing. J Invest Dermatol 2008 Jun;128(6):1545-53.

[39] Huttunen HJ, Fages C, Kuja-Panula J, Ridley AJ, Rauvala H. Receptor for advanced glycation end products-binding COOH-terminal motif of amphoterin inhibits invasive migration and metastasis. Cancer Res 2002 Aug 15;62(16):4805-11.

[40] Kuniyasu H, Oue N, Wakikawa A, Shigeishi H, Matsutani N, Kuraoka K, *et al.* Expression of receptors for advanced glycation end-products (RAGE) is closely associated with the invasive and metastatic activity of gastric cancer. J Pathol 2002 Feb;196(2):163-70.

[41] Kuniyasu H, Chihara Y, Takahashi T. Co-expression of receptor for advanced glycation end products and the ligand amphoterin associates closely with metastasis of colorectal cancer. Oncol Rep 2003 Mar-Apr;10(2):445-8.

[42] Kuniyasu H, Yano S, Sasaki T, Sasahira T, Sone S, Ohmori H. Colon cancer cell-derived high mobility group 1/amphoterin induces growth inhibition and apoptosis in macrophages. Am J Pathol 2005 Mar;166(3):751-60.

[43] Wang H, Yang H, Tracey KJ. Extracellular role of HMGB1 in inflammation and sepsis. J Intern Med 2004 Mar;255(3):320-31.

[44] Yang H, Ochani M, Li J, Qiang X, Tanovic M, Harris HE, *et al.* Reversing established sepsis with antagonists of endogenous high-mobility group box 1. Proc Natl Acad Sci USA 2004 Jan 6;101(1):296-301.

[45] Jaulmes A, Thierry S, Janvier B, Raymondjean M, Marechal V. Activation of sPLA2-IIA and PGE2 production by high mobility group protein B1 in vascular smooth muscle cells sensitized by IL-1beta. FASEB J 2006 Aug;20(10):1727-9.

[46] Rouhiainen A, Tumova S, Valmu L, Kalkkinen N, Rauvala H. Pivotal advance: analysis of proinflammatory activity of highly purified eukaryotic recombinant HMGB1 (amphoterin). J Leukoc Biol 2007 Jan;81(1):49-58.

[47] Tian J, Avalos AM, Mao SY, Chen B, Senthil K, Wu H, *et al.* Toll-like receptor 9-dependent activation by DNA-containing immune complexes is mediated by HMGB1 and RAGE. Nat Immunol 2007 May;8(5):487-96.

[48] Ivanov S, Dragoi AM, Wang X, Dallacosta C, Louten J, Musco G, *et al.* A novel role for HMGB1 in TLR9-mediated inflammatory responses to CpG-DNA. Blood 2007 Sep 15;110(6):1970-81.

[49] Youn JH, Oh YJ, Kim ES, Choi JE, Shin JS. High mobility group box 1 protein binding to lipopolysaccharide facilitates transfer of lipopolysaccharide to CD14 and enhances lipopolysaccharide-mediated TNF-alpha production in human monocytes. J Immunol 2008 Apr 1;180(7):5067-74.

[50] Kokkola R, Li J, Sundberg E, Aveberger AC, Palmblad K, Yang H, *et al.* Successful treatment of collagen-induced arthritis in mice and rats by targeting extracellular high mobility group box chromosomal protein 1 activity. Arthritis Rheum 2003 Jul;48(7):2052-8.

[51] Pullerits R, Jonsson IM, Verdrengh M, Bokarewa M, Andersson U, Erlandsson-Harris H, *et al.* High mobility group box chromosomal protein 1, a DNA binding cytokine, induces arthritis. Arthritis Rheum 2003 Jun;48(6):1693-700.

[52] Taniguchi N, Kawahara K, Yone K, Hashiguchi T, Yamakuchi M, Goto M, *et al.* High mobility group box chromosomal protein 1 plays a role in the pathogenesis of rheumatoid arthritis as a novel cytokine. Arthritis Rheum 2003 Apr;48(4):971-81.

[53] Volp K, Brezniceanu ML, Bosser S, Brableltz T, Kirchner T, Gottel D, *et al.* Increased expression of high mobility group box 1 (HMGB1) is associated with an elevated level of the antiapoptotic c-IAP2 protein in human colon carcinomas. Gut 2006 Feb;55(2):234-42.

[54] Kuniyasu H, Chihara Y, Kondo H, Ohmori H, Ukai R. Amphoterin induction in prostatic stromal cells by androgen deprivation is associated with metastatic prostate cancer. Oncol Rep 2003 Nov-Dec;10(6):1863-8.

[55] Taguchi A, Blood DC, del Toro G, Canet A, Lee DC, Qu W, *et al.* Blockade of RAGE-amphoterin signalling suppresses tumour growth and metastases. Nature 2000 May 18;405(6784):354-60.

[56] Apetoh L, Ghiringhelli F, Tesniere A, Obeid M, Ortiz C, Criollo A, *et al.* Toll-like receptor 4-dependent contribution of the immune system to anticancer chemotherapy and radiotherapy. Nat Med 2007 Sep;13(9):1050-9.

[57] Curtin JF, Liu N, Candolfi M, Xiong W, Assi H, Yagiz K, *et al.* HMGB1 mediates endogenous TLR2 activation and brain tumor regression. PLoS Med 2009 Jan 13;6(1):e10.

[58] Inoue K, Kawahara K, Biswas KK, Ando K, Mitsudo K, Nobuyoshi M, *et al.* HMGB1 expression by activated vascular smooth muscle cells in advanced human atherosclerosis plaques. Cardiovasc Pathol 2007 May-Jun;16(3):136-43.

[59] Porto A, Palumbo R, Pieroni M, Aprigliano G, Chiesa R, Sanvito F, *et al.* Smooth muscle cells in human atherosclerotic plaques secrete and proliferate in response to high mobility group box 1 protein. FASEB J 2006 Dec;20(14):2565-6.

[60] Decrion AZ, Dichamp I, Varin A, Herbein G. HIV and inflammation. Curr HIV Res2005 Jul;3(3):243-59.

[61] Xu D, Komai-Koma M, Liew FY. Expression and function of Toll-like receptor on T cells. Cell Immunol 2005 Feb;233(2):85-9.

[62] Hemmi H, Akira S. TLR signalling and the function of dendritic cells. Chem Immunol Allergy 2005;86:120-35.

[63] Kaisho T, Akira S. Toll-like receptors as adjuvant receptors. Biochim Biophys Acta 2002 Feb 13;1589(1):1-13.

[64] Akira S, Yamamoto M, Takeda K. Role of adapters in Toll-like receptor signalling. Biochem Soc Trans 2003 Jun;31(Pt 3):637-42.

[65] de Witte L, Nabatov A, Pion M, Fluitsma D, de Jong MA, de Gruijl T, *et al*. Langerin is a natural barrier to HIV-1 transmission by Langerhans cells. Nat Med 2007 Mar;13(3):367-71.

[66] Mailliard RB, Son YI, Redlinger R, Coates PT, Giermasz A, Morel PA, *et al*. Dendritic cells mediate NK cell help for Th1 and CTL responses: two-signal requirement for the induction of NK cell helper function. J Immunol 2003 Sep 1;171(5):2366-73.

[67] Dumitriu IE, Baruah P, Bianchi ME, Manfredi AA, Rovere-Querini P. Requirement of HMGB1 and RAGE for the maturation of human plasmacytoid dendritic cells. Eur J Immunol 2005 Jul;35(7):2184-90.

[68] Saidi H, Melki MT, Gougeon ML. HMGB1-dependent triggering of HIV-1 replication and persistence in dendritic cells as a consequence of NK-DC cross-talk. PLoS ONE 2008;3(10):e3601.

[69] Naghavi MH, Nowak P, Andersson J, Sonnerborg A, Yang H, Tracey KJ, *et al*. Intracellular high mobility group B1 protein (HMGB1) represses HIV-1 LTR-directed transcription in a promoter- and cell-specific manner. Virology 2003 Sep 15;314(1):179-89.

[70] Alfano M, Poli G. Role of cytokines and chemokines in the regulation of innate immunity and HIV infection. Mol Immunol 2005 Feb;42(2):161-82.

[71] Thierry S, Gozlan J, Jaulmes A, Boniface R, Nasreddine N, Strauss F, *et al*. High-mobility group box 1 protein induces HIV-1 expression from persistently infected cells. AIDS 2007 Jan 30;21(3):283-92.

[72] Nowak P, Barqasho B, Treutiger CJ, Harris HE, Tracey KJ, Andersson J, *et al*. HMGB1 activates replication of latent HIV-1 in a monocytic cell-line, but inhibits HIV-1 replication in primary macrophages. Cytokine 2006 Apr;34(1-2):17-23.

[73] Chu JJ, Ng ML. The mechanism of cell death during West Nile virus infection is dependent on initial infectious dose. J Gen Virol 2003 Dec;84(Pt 12):3305-14.

[74] Wang H, Ward MF, Fan XG, Sama AE, Li W. Potential role of high mobility group box 1 in viral infectious diseases. Viral Immunol 2006 Spring;19(1):3-9.

[75] Plymale DR, Tang DS, Comardelle AM, Fermin CD, Lewis DE, Garry RF. Both necrosis and apoptosis contribute to HIV-1-induced killing of CD4 cells. AIDS 1999 Oct 1;13(14):1827-39.

[76] Lenardo MJ, Angleman SB, Bounkeua V, Dimas J, Duvall MG, Graubard MB, *et al*. Cytopathic killing of peripheral blood CD4(+) T lymphocytes by human immunodeficiency virus type 1 appears necrotic rather than apoptotic and does not require env. J Virol 2002 May;76(10):5082-93.

[77] Cassetta L, Fortunato O, Adduce L, Rizzi C, Hering J, Rovere-Querini P, *et al*. Extracellular high mobility group box-1 inhibits R5 and X4 HIV-1 strains replication in mononuclear phagocytes without induction of chemokines and cytokines. AIDS 2009 Feb 3.

[78] Lane BR, Markovitz DM, Woodford NL, Rochford R, Strieter RM, Coffey MJ. TNF-alpha inhibits HIV-1 replication in peripheral blood monocytes and alveolar macrophages by inducing the production of RANTES and decreasing C-C chemokine receptor 5 (CCR5) expression. J Immunol 1999 Oct 1;163(7):3653-61.

[79] Biswas P, Poli G, Kinter AL, Justement JS, Stanley SK, Maury WJ, *et al*. Interferon gamma induces the expression of human immunodeficiency virus in persistently infected promonocytic cells (U1) and redirects the production of virions to intracytoplasmic vacuoles in phorbol myristate acetate-differentiated U1 cells. J Exp Med 1992 Sep 1;176(3):739-50.

[80] Sunden-Cullberg J, Norrby-Teglund A, Rouhiainen A, Rauvala H, Herman G, Tracey KJ, *et al*. Persistent elevation of high mobility group box-1 protein (HMGB1) in patients with severe sepsis and septic shock. Crit Care Med 2005 Mar;33(3):564-73.

[81] Yamada S, Inoue K, Yakabe K, Imaizumi H, Maruyama I. High mobility group protein 1 (HMGB1) quantified by ELISA with a monoclonal antibody that does not cross-react with HMGB2. Clin Chem 2003 Sep;49(9):1535-7.

[82] Urbonaviciute V, Furnrohr BG, Weber C, Haslbeck M, Wilhelm S, Herrmann M, *et al*. Factors masking HMGB1 in human serum and plasma. J Leukoc Biol 2007 Jan;81(1):67-74.

[83] Gibot S, Massin F, Cravoisy A, Barraud D, Nace L, Levy B, *et al*. High-mobility group box 1 protein plasma concentrations during septic shock. Intensive Care Med 2007 Aug;33(8):1347-53.

[84]   Gaillard C, Borde C, Gozlan J, Marechal V, Strauss F. A high-sensitivity method for detection and measurement of HMGB1 protein concentration by high-affinity binding to DNA hemicatenanes. PLoS ONE 2008;3(8):e2855.

[85]   Gaillard C, Strauss F. DNA loops and semicatenated DNA junctions. BMC Biochem 2000;1:1.

[86]   Angus DC, Yang L, Kong L, Kellum JA, Delude RL, Tracey KJ, *et al.* Circulating high-mobility group box 1 (HMGB1) concentrations are elevated in both uncomplicated pneumonia and pneumonia with severe sepsis. Crit Care Med 2007 Apr;35(4):1061-7.

[87]   Ueno H, Matsuda T, Hashimoto S, Amaya F, Kitamura Y, Tanaka M, *et al.* Contributions of high mobility group box protein in experimental and clinical acute lung injury. Am J Respir Crit Care Med 2004 Dec 15;170(12):1310-6.

[88]   Nowak P, Barqasho B, Sonnerborg A. Elevated plasma levels of high mobility group box protein 1 in patients with HIV-1 infection. AIDS 2007 Apr 23;21(7):869-71.

[89]   Gulick RM, Lalezari J, Goodrich J, Clumeck N, DeJesus E, Horban A, *et al.* Maraviroc for previously treated patients with R5 HIV-1 infection. N Engl J Med 2008 Oct 2;359(14):1429-41.

[90]   Li J, Kokkola R, Tabibzadeh S, Yang R, Ochani M, Qiang X, *et al.* Structural basis for the proinflammatory cytokine activity of high mobility group box 1. Mol Med 2003 Jan-Feb;9(1-2):37-45.

[91]   Telusma G, Datta S, Mihajlov I, Ma W, Li J, Yang H, *et al.* Dendritic cell activating peptides induce distinct cytokine profiles. Int Immunol 2006 Nov;18(11):1563-73.

CHAPTER 5

The uPA/uPAR System and suPAR in HIV Infection

Sisse R. Ostrowski[1], Eva Haastrup[1], Anne Langkilde[2], Henrik Ullum[1] and Jesper Eugen-Olsen[2,*]

[1]Department of Clinical Immunology, Copenhagen University Hospital, Rigshospitalet and [2]Clinical Research Centre 136, Copenhagen University Hospital, Hvidovre Hospital, Denmark.

Abstract: The urokinase Plasminogen Activator Receptor (uPAR) is linked to the surface of immune cells and involved in multiple immune functions including cell adhesion, chemotaxis, migration, angiogenesis, fibrinolysis, proliferation, differentiation and signal transduction. uPAR binds and activates urokinase resulting in extracellular matrix degradation and remodeling. Also, uPAR can bind the extracellular matrix protein vitronectin promoting cell adhesion and migration.

uPAR can be cleaved from the cell surface resulting in soluble uPAR (suPAR). suPAR levels are increased by various infectious diseases associated with systemic inflammation such as HIV infection. Several studies have shown that those with the highest suPAR levels have increased disease progression and high risk of mortality.

Furthermore, uPA was demonstrated to exert antiretroviral activity by inhibiting late steps in HIV replication cycle in various cell lines, through mechanisms dependent on cell adhesion. Future research will determine whether the emerging role of the uPA/uPAR/suPAR-system in HIV infection can be implemented in HIV drug development and in the use of suPAR measurements for initiating antiretroviral therapy and for monitoring treatment efficacy.

INTRODUCTION

Urokinase-type plasminogen activator (uPA) and uPA receptor (uPAR) are central components of the plasminogen activation system. Plasminogen is converted to plasmin by uPA and the conversion is enhanced when uPA is bound to its cell surface receptor, uPAR. Most physiological with tissue remodelling processes depend on activation of plasminogen to the proteolytically active enzyme plasmin, i.e., fibrinolysis, cell migration, wound healing, ovulation, trophoblast invasion, postlactational mammary gland involution, angiogenesis, activation of growth factors, cytokines and other proteolytic enzymes. In addition, tumour growth, invasion and metastasis also depend on the plasminogen activator (PA)-system [1-6]. However, uPAR not only functions as a protease receptor but also modulates cell adhesion, migration, chemotaxis, proliferation and differentiation through intracellular signalling [7-10]. Thus, through proteolytic and non-proteolytic functions, the PA-system, and uPA and uPAR in particular, are also involved in the inflammatory response and in innate as well as adaptive immunity.

In 2000 it was demonstrated that high blood levels of soluble uPAR (suPAR) independently predicted mortality in antiretroviral-untreated HIV-1 infected patients [11]. Later studies confirmed the negative predictive value of high circulating suPAR levels in HIV-1 [12-15] and HIV-2 infection [13]. In addition to HIV-1 infection, the blood level of suPAR is increased in several diseases categorized by systemic inflammation and immune activation: Sepsis [16-19], Streptococcus pneumoniae bacteraemia [20,21], endotoxemia [17,22,23], systemic inflammatory response syndrome (SIRS) [24], certain CNS infections [25], pulmonary [13] and extra-pulmonary [26] tuberculosis, hepatitis B virus (HBV) infection [27], malaria [28-30], uremia [31], rheumatoid arthritis and primary Sjögrens syndrome [32], multiple sclerosis and stroke [25] and several malignant diseases [33]. In many of these diseases, a high blood level of suPAR has negative prognostic value and may serve as a marker to monitor disease progression and treatment response: Streptococcus pneumoniae bacteraemia [20], SIRS [24], pulmonary tuberculosis [13], malaria [28,29], rheumatoid arthritis [32] and certain malignant diseases [34].

*****Address Correspondence to this Author Dr. Jesper Eugen-Olsen at:** Clinical Research Centre 136, Copenhagen University Hospital, Hvidovre Hospital, Denmark E-mail: jeo@virogates.com

Massimo Alfano (Ed)

In 2001, it was demonstrated that uPA exerts antiretroviral activity by inhibiting late steps in HIV replication cycle in various cell lines [35], a finding later confirmed by independent groups [36-38].

Given the strong prognostic value of suPAR and the molecular association between uPA and HIV-1 infection, the uPA/uPAR system and suPAR have been intensively investigated within the past 10 years.

In this chapter, the actors in the plasminogen activation system will briefly be introduced – with focus on uPA, uPAR and suPAR and their link to inflammation. The association between HIV-1 infection and uPA, uPAR and suPAR will be discussed in detail with reference to HIV-1 pathogenesis and highly active antiretroviral therapy (HAART). Finally, future perspectives will be discussed.

Biology of uPA, uPAR and suPAR

uPA is secreted as an inactive single-chain proenzyme, pro-uPA [2]. Secreted pro-uPA binds to uPAR and is converted, faster than soluble pro-uPA, to active uPA through proteolytic cleavage by plasmin [4,5]. A positive feedback mechanism (referred to as reciprocal proenzyme activation) exists between pro-uPA and plasmin generation (and hence cell-associated proteolysis) since plasmin cleaves uPAR-bound pro-uPA which then converts neighbouring membrane-associated plasminogen to plasmin, tethering the proteolytic activity of plasmin to the membrane and hereby in close proximity to uPAR-bound pro-uPA [4,5]. Other serine proteases can also activate pro-uPA although their physiological significance remains unknown [1,2,4,5,39] (Fig. 1).

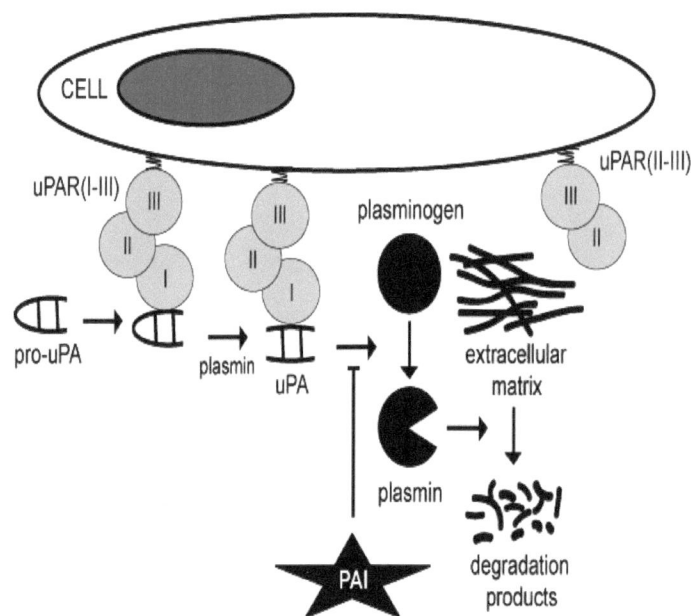

Figure 1: The urokinase PA-system. The cascade is initiated by conversion of pro-uPA to active uPA by plasmin. uPA then converts plasminogen to plasmin, which degrades ECM components. The reaction is enhanced by binding of uPA to uPAR and by binding of plasminogen to its cellular receptor(s). The reaction is inhibited by plasminogen activator inhibitor (PAI)-1 and 2. The truncated receptor uPAR(II-III) can neither bind uPA nor pro-uPAuPA comprises two polypeptide chains that are held together by disulfide bridges. The carboxy-terminal B-chain contains the serine protease domain. The amino-terminal A-chain (ATF) contains the EGF-like domain and the kringle domain [2]. The serine protease domain is responsible for the catalytic activity whereas the EGF-like and kringle domains are responsible for the binding of pro-uPA/uPA to uPAR and for interaction with cell surfaces, respectively [3-5]. The enzymatic activity of uPA is about 250-fold higher than that of pro-uPA [5].

Although uPA has restricted substrate specificity, it can activate latent forms of hepatocyte growth factor, macrophage-stimulating protein, pro-TGF-β, pro-IL-1, pro-IL-6 and MMPs [3,5,8]. Furthermore, uPA can convert the precursor chemokine HCC-1 (amino-acid residues 1-74) into a potent truncated form (amino-acid residues 9-74) which is a strong CCR5 agonist [40]. Finally, uPA catalyzes cleavage of PAI-1 and intra-domain cleavage of uPAR with subsequent release of uPAR(I).

Due to the excessive background level of protease inhibitors, the most abundant circulating form of uPA is pro-uPA and complexes between uPA and PAI-1, as pro-uPA activation rapidly leads to complex formation between uPA and PAI-1 [41]. The activity of uPA is regulated by uPAR, plasmin, PAIs and by endocytosis.

uPAR is the cellular receptor for uPA [42]. It is a 55-60 kDa single-chain highly glycosylated protein consisting of three homologous domains (uPAR(I), uPAR(II) and uPAR(III)) [43,44]. uPAR contains no intracellular domain as the carboxy-terminal (uPAR(III)) is attached to the cell membrane by a GPI-anchor [45].

The amino-terminal uPAR(I) contains the binding site for uPA [44], but high affinity binding requires interaction with uPAR(II) and uPAR(III) as the intact receptor (and uPAR(I-II)) binds uPA with 102 to 103-fold higher affinity than uPAR(I) alone [46]. uPAR(I) can also bind vitronectin, and again, the intact molecule is required for high affinity binding [47]. uPA and vitronectin can bind simultaneously to uPAR(I-III), and uPAR(I-III) binds more readily to vitronectin when it is pre-bound to either pro-uPA, uPA, ATF or the uPA/PAI-1 complex [47-51].

uPAR is expressed by most APCs (monocytes, macrophages, DCs) [52,53], neutrophils, eosinophils [52], activated T cells and NK cells [52,54-56], megakaryocytes [57], ECs [58-61], tubular epithelial cells [17], smooth muscle cells [60], keratinocytes, fibroblasts and many malignant cells [33,52]. It is absent on the cell surface of erythrocytes, platelets (though observed on platelets in [62]) and B cells [52,57] and only expressed in low levels by naive/resting T cells [54-56]. In the hematopoietic system, uPAR-expression follows a differentiation-dependent pattern in the myelomonocytic and megakaryocytic cell lineages but an activation-dependent pattern in monocytes, neutrophils and T cells [52,63].

uPA, plasmin, chymotrypsin and other proteases can cleave uPAR(I-III) in the linker region between uPAR(I) and uPAR(II), with subsequent release of uPAR(I) [8,41,42,44,64]. uPA-catalyzed cleavage of membrane-bound uPAR(I-III) is favoured compared to cleavage of suPAR(I-III) whereas plasmin-catalyzed cleavage of membrane-bound and soluble uPAR(I-III) is comparable [65]. The intra-domain cleavage of uPAR(I-III) leaves the two-domain receptor uPAR(II-III) on the cell surface without ligand binding capacity [42,47,64]. Thus, uPAR is present on the surface of cells as three-domain uPAR(I-III) or as a cleaved receptor, uPAR(II-III) [64] (Fig. **2**).

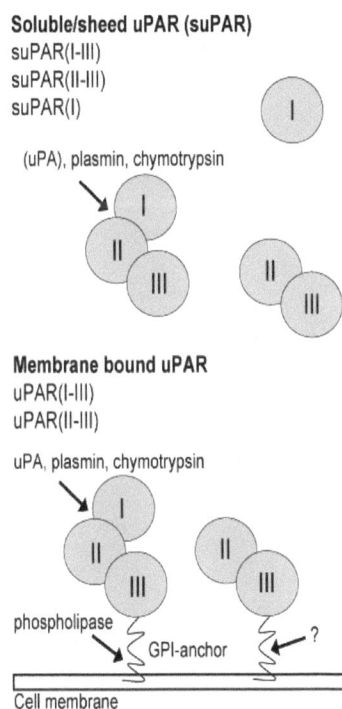

Figure 2: The urokinase receptor. Domains and cleavage sites are shown. uPAR can be shed from the cell membrane by phospholipase C and D-catalyzed cleavage. uPA, plasmin, chymotrypsin and other proteases can cleave uPAR in the linker region between uPAR(I) and uPAR(II) with subsequent release of uPAR(I).

uPAR(I-III) is shed from the cell membrane by neutrophil derived Cathepsin G, phospholipase C and D-catalyzed cleavage of the GPI-anchor [45,66] and by yet unknown mechanisms resulting in shedding of GPI-uPAR (suPAR(I-III) with an intact GPI-anchor) [42,66]. However, in contrast to previous findings, a recent study has found uPAR cleavage to be PLD independent [67], which might highlight the importance of neutrophil derived cathepsin D cleavage or yet undefined proteases responsible for uPAR cleavage. In addition, a soluble form of uPAR(I-III) resulting from alternative splicing of mRNA has also been reported [68]. It is not known whether and/or how uPAR(II-III) is shed from the cell surface, but suPAR is present in various human body fluids (blood, pleural-, pericardial-, peritoneal- and cystic-fluids, urine) and in cell-culture supernatant as suPAR(I-III), suPAR(II-III) and suPAR(I) [16,69-72]. In addition, complexes between suPAR(I-III) and uPA, PAI, vitronectin, uPA/PAI, uPA/vitronectin and uPA/PAI/vitronectin are also present in body fluids [4,5,42].

PAI-1 can inhibit both soluble uPA and uPAR-bound uPA through assembly of a PAI-1/uPAR/uPA complex. The complex is internalized through interactions between uPAR and LRP [4,42], which is followed by degradation of uPA and PAI-1 and recycling of uPAR [73].

Cleavage of cell-bound uPAR(I-III) also regulates the function of uPAR as uPAR(II-III) is unable to bind pro-uPA [65], uPA/PAI-1 complexes and vitronectin [47,65]. Consequently, uPAR(II-III) cannot promote plasminogen activation or be internalized and uPAR(II-III) is probably unable to mediate cell adhesion through integrin binding [74-76]. However, cleavage of cell-bound uPAR(I-III) exposes a potent chemotactic epitope that may function as a cell-bound or soluble chemokine (if shed from cell surface).

uPA AND uPAR FUNCTION

Localized Proteolysis

The primary function of uPAR was initially thought to be cell-associated proteolysis through localization of uPA and hence the plasminogen activation cascade to the cell surface. By polarizing uPA at focal areas of the cell membrane, uPAR participates in cell-associated proteolysis during physiological processes with tissue remodelling and during tumour growth, invasion and metastasis [2,42,63]. Although the primary initiator of the cell-associated PA-system is unknown, pro-uPA itself, tPA, other proteases or autoactivation (specific orientation effects that favour the interaction between cell-bound uPA and cell-bound plasminogen) may initiate the cell-associated cascade [39,42]. However, acceleration of the positive feed back mechanism between plasmin-catalyzed activation of pro-uPA and uPA-catalyzed activation of plasminogen requires not only the binding of pro-uPA to uPAR but also binding of plasminogen to components on the cell surface. The acceleration is therefore most likely due to an effect on both reactions [39,42].

In addition to localized proteolysis, uPAR can also modulate cell adhesion and migration, chemotaxis, proliferation and differentiation through intracellular signalling [5-10].

Signal Transduction

Although uPAR lacks a cytoplasmatic domain, binding of uPA (or pro-uPA or ATF) activates several signal transduction pathways involved in adhesion, migration, chemotaxis, cytoskeleton dynamics, proliferation and differentiation [7,77]. Initiation of intracellular signalling may either be induced by a conformational change, by proteolytic cleavage of uPAR or through interaction with molecules containing cytoplasmic domains (transmembrane adaptor molecules) such as integrins, caveolin and a G-protein coupled receptor [7,75,77,78].

Adhesion and Migration

To migrate, cells must adhere to the ECM and activate the integrin-dependent signalling pathway that induces cytoskeleton reorganization and cell-shape changes. During cell migration, cell-ECM adhesion at the leading edge provides guidance and mechanical force whereas dissociation of the adhesion molecule/ligand complexes allows retraction of the trailing edge [5,79].

uPAR mediates the initial binding of cells to a matrix substrate either by direct binding to vitronectin [80] or by integrin interaction/activation [78,79]. uPAR has high lateral mobility in the cell membrane and during cell migration it usually becomes concentrated at focal adhesion sites (cell-cell or cell-ECM contact sites) and at the leading edge, co-localizing with various transmembrane adaptor molecules [7,74,78,79]. The co-localization often occurs in cell surface areas termed lipid rafts which are membrane components enriched in cholesterol, glycosphingolipids, gangliosides and GPI-anchored molecules [7,81].

The cell-associated proteolysis, which occurs upon binding of uPA to uPAR, may also promote migration through degradation of ECM components and adhesion molecules, resulting in release of the trailing edge [5].

uPAR and Integrins

Integrins are transmembrane cell surface receptors that mediate cell-ECM and cell-cell contact and transduce signals from the extracellular environment to the cell interior. Ligand-activated uPAR influences integrin-dependent cell adhesion and migration [74] and these functions are blocked, not only by anti-integrin Ab, but also by anti-uPAR Ab [7]. Co-clustering of the antigen receptor complex with β1 or β2-integrins on T cells increases uPAR mRNA and protein expression and promotes migration of T cells *in vitro* [56]. In addition, removal of uPAR from the leukocyte surface reduces β2-integrin-mediated leukocyte adhesion to the endothelium in vitro [76] and uPAR-deficient mice have impaired β2-integrin-mediated leukocyte recruitment to sites of inflammation [76,82,83].

Studies of uPAR-deficient mice have demonstrated that uPAR is important for leukocyte recruitment to sites of inflammation/infection and for the antibacterial host defence. Thus, uPAR-deficient mice have impaired recruitment of neutrophils, monocytes and T cells to inflamed peritoneum [76] and impaired lymphocyte recruitment to inflamed lung [83]. uPAR-deficient mice with pulmonary Pseudomonas (P.) aeruginosa [82] or S. pneumoniae [84] infection have impaired neutrophil [82,84], macrophage and lymphocyte [84] recruitment, impaired pathogen clearance [82,84], enhanced dissemination of the infection and a poor survival [84]. In addition, neutrophil phagocytosis and superoxide generation is impaired in uPAR-deficient mice [85]. Since neutrophil recruitment to the pulmonary parenchyma is β2-integrin dependent in P. aeruginosa infection [82] and β-2-integrin independent in S. pneumoniae infection [84], an abolished uPAR/integrin-interaction cannot alone explain the impaired neutrophil recruitment in uPAR-deficient mice.

The uPAR-integrin interaction is most likely mediated by at least two mechanisms: simple interactions at the cell surface (activation of integrins) or interactions resulting in complex formation between integrins, caveolin and uPAR, which function as adhesive and signalling units at the cell surface [78].

The uPAR/integrin interactions have most often been demonstrated within the same cell membrane [74,75,79]. However, it has also been reported that the uPAR/integrin interaction can modulate cell-cell interaction [86]. The interaction most likely requires uPAR(I-III) as cleavage between uPAR(I) and uPAR(II) prevents co-localization of uPAR and integrins [75].

uPAR And Lipid Rafts

Lipid rafts are membrane microdomains that are enriched with lipids and cholesterol, glycolipids, sphingolipids and the cholesterol-binding protein caveolin [7].

GPI-anchored receptors have high affinity towards lipid rafts and uPAR is no exception [100]. Cunningham and co-workers found that uPAR exists in both monomeric and dimeric forms, and that dimeric uPAR partitions preferentially to lipid rafts. The dimerization of uPAR is a prerequisite for the high-affinity interaction between uPAR and vitronectin [51,100].

uPAR-mediated adhesion to vitronectin correlates with the formation of multimeric membrane complexes consisting of integrins, caveolin and uPAR and is associated with the activation of intracellular signalling pathways and the cytoskeleton system involved in cell adhesion and migration [74,78,79].

uPAR and G-Protein Coupled Receptors

The previous finding that chemotaxis induced by the chemotactic epitope in suPAR(II-III) could be blocked by Bordetella pertussis toxin (inhibits some G-proteins), indicated that suPAR (II-III) induced chemotaxis is mediated through a G-protein coupled receptor [87]. This was later shown to be the low-affinity G-protein coupled receptor, FPRL1 [88], and co-expression of uPAR and FPLR1 is required for cell responsiveness to suPAR(II-III) [75,88]. In addition to integrins, caveolin and a G-protein coupled receptor, other transmembrane adaptor molecules also interact with uPAR and may modulate cell adhesion and migration: gp130 (activated upon uPAR clustering), LRP (internalizes the uPAR/uPA/PAI-1 complex), insulin like growth factor II receptor (binds and degrades suPAR(II-III)) [7] and urokinase-receptor-associated protein [39,89].

uPAR, Vitronectin and PAI-1

The interaction uPAR/vitronectin/PAI-1 also regulates cell adhesion and migration. uPAR and PAI-1 share binding regions on vitronectin and thus bind competitively [49,80]. An excess of PAI-1 will replace uPAR from vitronectin resulting in detachment of cells from vitronectin and inhibition of cell migration. Conversely, an excess of uPA will promote attachment through enhanced binding of vitronectin to uPAR and detachment through plasmin-catalyzed disruption of the uPAR-vitronectin binding, thereby promoting cell migration [42,49,78]. Thus, the function of uPA and PAI-1 at the leading edge of migrating cells may not only be to enhance or inhibit plasminogen activation, respectively, but also to modulate cell migration. Overall, uPAR participates in cell migration through proteolytic as well as non-proteolytic functions. It is possible that proteolytic mechanisms dominate at the trailing edge whereas non-proteolytic mechanisms dominate at the leading edge during normal cell migration [5]. This is opposite tumour cell invasion, in which proteolytic mechanisms seem to be of major importance for degradation of basement membrane barriers at the leading edge [5].

Chemotaxis

uPA (or pro-uPA or ATF) binding to uPAR and intra-domain cleavage of uPAR(I-III) both cause a conformational change in uPAR. This can result in exposure of a chemotactic epitope located in the protease-sensitive linker region between uPAR(I) and uPAR(II) (minimum required sequence SRSRY, amino-acid residues 88-92) [87]. Exposure of the chemotactic epitope in vitro not only depends on interaction with uPA as the linker region is sensitive to other proteases and suPAR(I-III)-bound uPA does not expose the chemotactic epitope [8,41,42,64]. Thus, chymotrypsin-catalyzed cleavage of suPAR(I-III) between uPAR(I) and uPAR(II) generates a soluble chemotactic factor, suPAR(II-III) [87,90]. The chemotactic epitope of uPAR interacts with FPRL1 [88] which is expressed by monocytes, lymphocytes and neutrophils and upregulated by various cytokines and growth factors [91]. FPRL1 is also present on many other cells including vascular endothelial cells, epithelial cells, hepatocytes and tumour cells [91] and the widespread expression of FPRL1 is in accordance with the broad range of cells that respond to uPA/uPAR chemotactic signals.

In addition to inducing chemotaxis, suPAR(II-III) decreases the activity of the FPRL1-ligand, fMLP (formyl methionyl leucyl proline) [88] and inhibits chemokine-induced chemotaxis in response to MCP-1 and RANTES [92]. suPAR(II-III) inhibits MCP-1 and RANTES-induced chemotaxis by preventing rapid integrin-dependent cell adhesion.

FPRL1 regulates β2-integrin activities, which is important for monocyte motility. The suPAR(II-III) induced decreased chemotaxis is therefore not due to direct suPAR(II-III)-integrin binding, but is caused by suPAR(II-III) binding to FPRL1. uPA-uPAR complexes inhibits chemokine induced monocyte chemotaxis in the same manner whereas neither suPAR(I-III) nor suPAR(I) regulate chemotaxis, since they do not expose a chemotactic sequence.

The uPAR-derived peptide uPAR$_{84-95}$, containing the chemotactic epitope, has also been found to chemoattract CD34$^+$ leukaemia cells and CD34$^+$ haematopoietic stem cells (HSCs) and inhibit the stromal-derived factor (SDF) 1-induced migration of CD34$^+$ HSCs by binding to FPRL1. Chemotactically active suPAR hereby seems to be able to mobilise HSCs from the bone marrow and prevent the SDF1-mediated bone marrow retention of HSCs. The authors suggested this to be mediated through heterologous desensitization of the SDF1 receptor CXCR4, but another explanation could be that chemotactically active suPAR inhibits SDF1-induced migration by affecting integrin activation, as observed in monocytes [96,97].

Other Functions of uPAR

uPAR is often over-expressed by human tumour cells, and uPAR-expression and integrin interaction promotes proliferation of certain tumour cells in vitro [7]. Expression of uPAR(I-III) is required for integrin interaction and induction of proliferation as uPAR(II-III) does not interact with integrins [75].

Binding of uPAR to vitronectin is essential for adhesion and hence differentiation of monocytes into macrophages in vitro [7]. In addition, expression of uPAR on maturating monocytes, granulocytes or bone marrow stromal cells may interact with and modify integrin function, thereby contributing to release of monocytes and granulocytes from the bone marrow [63].

suPAR MEASUREMENT, ORIGIN AND FUNCTION

suPAR Measurements

Many studies of suPAR in human are based on ELISA measurements of "bulk" suPAR (bulk-suPAR), i.e. quantifying the sum of uPAR(I-III), uPAR(II-III) and uPAR(I-III)-ligand complexes.

Earlier studies only detected suPAR(I-III) and suPAR(II-III) in plasma [71] and serum [70] from healthy individuals in contrast to the recent detection of all suPAR forms (suPAR(I-III), suPAR(II-III), suPAR(I)) in normal plasma by time-resolved fluorescence immunoassay (TRFIA) [12,72,93] – a discrepancy probably attributed to better sensitivity of the newer techniques. As descript later, both suPAR(I-III), suPAR(II-III), but not suPAR(I) carries prognostic value in HIV infection. However, the combined measurement of suPAR(I-III), suPAR(II-III) carries the strongest prognostic value.

Most studies on suPAR have been carried out using in-house suPAR assay's and suPAR values obtained from different groups are not directly comparable. In 2007, the first commercial CE/IVD approved suPAR assay (suPARnostic, ViroGates, Denmark) became available. The monoclonal-monoclonal detection assay quantifies suPAR(I-III) and suPAR(II-III) and the assay has, in contrast to previous suPAR assays, been developed on clinical value and not on best binding antibodies. This was done by developing 28 monoclonal hybridoma cell lines of anti-suPAR antibodies. These were combined into 8 ELISA's and plasma samples from HIV infected individuals with known outcomes were analysed. While all antibody combinations gave significant prognostic value, one set of antibodies (termed VG-1 and VG-2) gave superior prognostic value and forms the basis for the suPARnostic assay. The availability of a commercial assay will allow cross-study comparison of suPAR values in different diseases.

suPAR Origin

The origin of suPAR in blood of healthy individuals is mainly unknown [94] although there are several potential sources. Senescence of uPAR-expressing leukocytes [95], differentiation of megakaryocytes into platelets [57], hematopoietic stem cell maturation [63] or mobilization from the bone marrow [96,97], clot formation [98] and resolution [31,99], constitutive release from ECs and/or leukocytes [12,16,59,70] and leukocyte adhesion/migration [61].

For long time the origin of the high circulating suPAR levels in cancer patients was unknown and only recently it was demonstrated that mice carrying transplanted human xenograft tumours have human suPAR in their blood that correlates positively with tumour volume [95]. In line with this, a recent study demonstrated that the circulating suPAR level correlates positively with the number of circulating tumour cells and the amount of uPAR in tumour cell lysates from patients with acute leukaemia [71].

The origin of the high circulating suPAR levels in patients with severe infections or inflammatory diseases is yet unknown.

suPAR Functions

Only one study has documented in vivo function of suPAR by injecting suPAR84-95 to mice where it induced leukocytosis and CD34+ hematopoietic stem/progenitor cell mobilization in magnitude similar to granulocyte-colony-stimulating factor (G-CSF) [97].

Although the function of suPAR in the blood is mainly unknown, many studies in vitro have indicated that suPAR has biological activities either by directly modulating cell adhesion and migration, by competitive inhibition of cell-bound uPAR and/or by substituting functions of cell-bound uPAR.

Modulation of Cell Adhesion and Migration

suPAR may modulate cell adhesion and migration, through binding to vitronectin and inhibition of uPAR binding, by interaction with integrins and by induction of chemotaxis. Also, interaction with cell-bound uPAR through formation of uPAR/uPAR or uPAR/suPAR dimers results in preference for lipid rafts and increased affinity for vitronectin binding [100].

suPAR(I-III) can bind to the active conformation of the β2-integrin Mac-1 (CD11b/CD18) [74] and suPAR(II-III) and suPAR(I) can bind to integrins expressed on the cell surface [86]. suPAR(I-III), suPAR(II-III) and suPAR(I) all support adhesion of integrin expressing cells [86] and suPAR(I-III) and suPAR(II-III) promote adhesion of macrophages to vitronectin and fibronectin *in vitro* [101]. Thus, (activated) integrins are target for direct interaction and regulation by suPAR.

The chemotactic epitope of suPAR(II-III) is a strong inducer of chemotaxis in monocyte-like cells [90]. suPAR(II-III) may however rather modulate than stimulate leukocyte recruitment to sites of inflammation since suPAR(II-III) interferes with the chemokine-induced rapid integrin-dependent cell adhesion and chemotaxis [92]. Also, binding of suPAR (II-III) to the 7-transmembrane G-protein coupled receptor FPRL-1 results in desensitisation of chemokine receptors such as CCR5 [92] and thus influencing cellular trafficking.

Competitive Inhibition of Cell-Bound uPAR

In vitro, suPAR(I-III) can competitively inhibit the binding of uPA to cell-bound uPAR on haematopoietic cells [102], vascular endothelial cells [59] and various tumour cells [103,104]. By competing with cell-bound uPAR, suPAR(I-III) may function as a scavenger for uPA by inhibiting cell-associated plasminogen activation [102,104] and tumour cell proliferation and invasion in vitro [103]. In addition, tumours with over-expression of suPAR in vivo (mice carrying transplanted human xenograft breast tumours [104] or ovarian tumours [105] transfected with expression plasmids encoding suPAR) have reduced growth and colonization potential [104,105] compared to normal tumours. These findings indicate that high local levels of suPAR may restrict invasion and proliferation of tumour cells. Notably, suPAR in plasma from sepsis patients and in extra-vascular exudates contains increased uPA binding capacity [16].

Substituting Functions for Cell-Bound uPAR

suPAR(I-III) (but not suPAR(II-III)) can reconstitute integrin-associated adhesion of uPAR-deficient leukocytes [76] because suPAR(I-III) modulates integrin function similarly to cell-bound uPAR(I-III) [74]. suPAR(I-III) can also increase uPA binding in uPAR-deficient cells [59] and addition of suPAR(I-III) to tumour cells with low uPAR-expression (transfected with anti-sense uPAR mRNA) restores extracellular regulated kinase (ERK) activation which may stimulate proliferation [106]. suPAR(II-III) can induce chemotaxis in uPAR-deficient cells and it can activate the tyrosine kinase p56/p59hck in cells with normal uPAR-expression [90]. suPAR(I-III) in complex with uPA can bind to ECM-bound vitronectin and become distributed at sites distant from its production [81] and suPAR(I-III) can redistribute the presentation of uPA on the cell surface through vitronectin binding [59]. Pro-uPA-mediated fibrinolysis is enhanced by complex-formation with suPAR(I-III) [31] through IgG-mediated stimulation and reduced inactivation by PAI-1 [99]. Pro-uPA-mediated fibrinolysis is not enhanced by complex-formation with suPAR(I) or suPAR(II-III) [99].

Thus, suPAR may both serve as a physiological inhibitor of cell surface proteolysis by competitive inhibition of cell-bound uPAR or as an alternative non-cell-bound plasminogen activation site [68].

uPA, uPAR AND suPAR IN HIV INFECTION

uPAR and HIV-1

Several studies have demonstrated that HIV influences uPAR-expression in immune cells. The first indication of a link between uPAR and HIV came in 1994 when Nykaer *et al.* showed that CD3+ lymphocytes from healthy donors exhibited no significant uPAR expression whereas antiretroviral-untreated HIV-1 infected patients showed distinct uPAR expression in up to 80% of all T cells – and especially on activated HLA-DR+CD25+T cells [55].

This finding was later confirmed by in vitro studies reporting increased uPAR-expression (mRNA, protein) in T cells, monocytes and PBMC infected by HIV-1 *in vitro* [107,108]. In addition, it was shown that HIV-1-induced upregulation of uPAR was attributed to enhanced transcription rate of uPAR rather than stabilization of uPAR mRNA [107]. Also, autopsies from HIV infected patients with AIDS dementia complex or opportunistic CNS infections have revealed high uPAR-expression in HIV infected microglia cells, multinucleated giant cells and macrophages [109,110]. In contrast, granulocytes from HIV infected patients have reduced cell surface expression of uPAR that correlates positively with CD4-count [111]. Despite low uPAR-expression, granulocytes from HIV-1-infected patients displayed normal upregulation of uPAR in response to chemoattractants [111]. Also, children with AIDS have reduced levels of uPAR/uPA-expressing monocytes (but normal levels of uPAR/uPA-expressing lymphocytes in contrast to [55]) coinciding with increased uPA levels that increase with disease progression [112].

uPA and HIV-1

In addition to interaction between HIV-1 and uPAR, several studies have demonstrated interactions between HIV-1 and uPA.

In 1996, Handley and co-workers showed that uPA can bind to HIV-1 particles and cleave recombinant gp120 at the V3 loop of HIV-1, resulting in increased viral replication in vitro through enhanced HIV infectivity of macrophages and production of HIV-1 particles [113].

In contrast, several studies performed by two independent groups have demonstrated inhibitory effects of uPA on late steps of HIV replication [35-38].

In 2001, Wada and co-workers were trying to identify HIV antiviral factors in a CD8+ cell line supernatant (referred to as CAF), and found that one of the most potent antiviral protein among other candidates was ATF, the receptor-binding moiety of uPA [35]. The difference in uPA modulation of HIV infection is most likely due to the different cell models applied. While Handley used HIV virions and macrophages, Wada's model system was based on the cocultivation of promonocytic U937 cells (bearing CD4 and CXCR4 on their cell surface) with a well-known chronically infected cell line (named U1) derived from acutely infected U937 cells. In the later system, HIV is generated from two integrated HIV DNA strands following activation with phorbol 12, myristate-13, acetate (PMA) or other extracellular stimuli including proinflammatory cytokines [114].

Alfano and co-workers [36] also used the U1 cell system and showed that uPA inhibits PMA induced HIV-1 expression through the trapping of virions in endosomes and not at the transcription level (Fig. **3**).

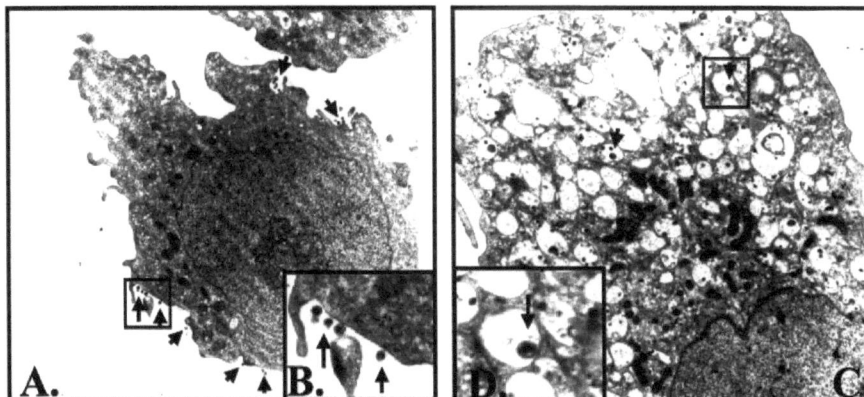

Figure 3. Accumulation of HIV-1 virions in intracytoplasmatic vacuoles in PMA-stimulated U1 cells in the presence of pro-uPA. U1 cells were stimulated for 48 h with (*A*) PMA (magnification ×11,000) or (*B*) PMA plus pro-uPA (10 nM) (magnification ×15,000). Pictures kindly provided by M. Alfano [36].

In 2007, Eila and coworker [37] found that the uPA mediated intracellular trapping of HIV virions in U1 cells was dependent of vitronectin, which binds the uPA/uPA receptor complex, resulting in cell adhesion to the culture disk surface. The authors suggest that macrophage cell adhesion per se curtails HIV replication.

In addition to binding uPA and vitronectin, uPAR interacts with Mac-1 (CD11b/CD18), a cell surface interaction that can be blocked using M25, a peptide homologous to a portion of CD11b

Recently, Alfano and co-workers [38] showed that siRNA against uPAR as well as antibodies against Mac-1 abolished the anti-HIV effects of uPA in the U1 cell line. Also, addition of M25 inhibited HIV virion release in PMA-stimulated U1 cells. Altogether, either uPA/uPAR interaction, Mac-1 activation or prevention of its association with uPAR triggers a signalling pathway leading to the inefficient release of HIV-1 from monocytic cells.

In addition to a direct effect on HIV-1 replication, uPA can activate the precursor chemokine HCC-1 into a potent truncated form [40] that can block entry of HIV-1 strains that use CCR5 as a co-receptor [115].

suPAR AND HIV DISEASE PROGRESSION

Several independent studies of HIV infected patients have demonstrated that the blood level of suPAR is intimately associated with disease stage and a strong and independent predictor of disease progression and mortality in antiretroviral-untreated patients.

Thus, the circulating level of bulk-suPAR [12,109,116], suPAR(I-III), suPAR(II-III) and suPAR(I) [12,93] are increased in moderate/advanced antiretroviral-untreated HIV infection and increases with HIV disease progression [11,12].

The blood level of bulk-suPAR is an independent predictor of mortality in early (seroconversion) [15] and late [11-14] HIV-1 and HIV-2 [13] infection. Also, the circulating level of suPAR(I-III) and suPAR(II-III) independently predicts mortality in antiretroviral-untreated HIV infected patients [12].

Besides high suPAR level, the level of uPAR/uPA-complexes is also increased in chronic HIV infection as previously suggested [12] and later confirmed [110]. In healthy individuals, part of the circulating suPAR(I-III) is associated with other molecules (ligands) [70] and altered levels of suPAR-ligand complexes is also observed in other diseases with systemic inflammation [16,117] emphasizing that this phenomenon is not specific for HIV infection. Since uPA-cleavage mainly occurs at sites with concomitant high uPA and uPAR expression [65], the concurrent high levels of suPAR(I) [12,93] and uPAR/uPA-complexes [12,110] most likely reflect increased local uPA and/or plasmin-generation with enhanced cleavage and release of uPAR and uPAR/uPA-complexes [33,65,118]. Hypothetically, high local uPA/plasmin-generation could be attributed to both HIV [35,112] and inflammation/immune activation [8].

Based on the notion that uPA exerts a significant inhibitory effect on HIV replication *in vitro* [35-38], it is suggested that the negative predictive value of high bulk-suPAR levels is attributed to suPAR(I-III)-mediated competitive inhibition of uPA binding to membrane-bound uPAR(I-III), with subsequent enhanced HIV replication and disease progression [37,110].

At present, there is accumulating evidence indicating that suPAR(I-III) alone cannot account for the negative predictive value of high bulk-suPAR levels in HIV infection.

The observation that suPAR and VL correlate only weakly [11] or do not correlate [12,14,93,116] in antiretroviral-untreated HIV infection indicates that suPAR and viral replication are not intimately associated.

Also, the finding that circulating suPAR(II-III) – which is devoid of uPA binding capacity – is an independent predictor of mortality in HIV infection [12] further argues against an exclusive role of suPAR(I-III).

uPA, uPAR and suPAR IN INFLAMMATION

Inflammation is the reaction of a vascularized tissue to a pathogenic insult i.e., trauma, infectious agent, foreign particle, ischemia or neoplasm. It is characterized by the generation of inflammatory mediators, by increased vascular permeability and by migration of leukocytes into extravascular tissues. The primary purpose of the inflammatory response is to eliminate the pathogenic insult and remove injured tissue components. Ideally, the result of the inflammatory response is resolution in which the pathogenic insult is eliminated, the inflammatory response is resolved and normal tissue architecture and physiological function is restored. Thus, tissue repair and remodelling always accompany the inflammatory response. If the immune cells fail to eliminate the source of tissue injury, the inflammatory reaction persists, leading to chronic inflammation.

The inflammatory response begins as the result of direct injury or stimulation of the cellular and structural components of the tissue, including parenchymal cells, microvasculature, tissue macrophages and mast cells, fibroblasts, smooth muscle cells and the ECM. Inflammatory mediators produced at the site of injury regulate the response of the vasculature to injury (by production of vasoactive molecules) and the recruitment of leukocytes (by production of chemotactic factors). uPA, uPAR and suPAR are all intimately involved in the inflammatory response and may therefore be good markers of the inflammatory state of the individual.

Inflammatory Mediators

Inflammatory mediators produced in response to tissue injury include vasoactive mediators, chemotactic mediators and cytokines that regulate expression and release of uPAR in immune cells and tissue cells.

Many bacterial components (LPS, muramyl dipeptide, lipoteichoic acid, Staphylococcal enterotoxin B, heat killed Staphylococcus aureus, lipoarabinomannan, Tuberculin purifed protein derivate, viable/heat killed Borrelia Burgdorferi) and HIV-1 enhance uPAR-expression in vitro in monocyte-like cells [23,107,119-122], granulocytes [121] and T cells [55,107]. Furthermore, LPS, lipoteichoic acid and B. Burgdorferi enhance uPAR-release in monocyte-like cells [120,122]. Endotoxemia induced by IV injection of endotoxin enhances uPAR-expression in vivo in monocytes [23,121] and granulocytes [121] and increases the level of suPAR in plasma [17,23,118] and urine [17]. Even low-dose endotoxemia enhances uPAR-release from cultured PBMC [22]. However, it should be noted that suPAR does not show acute phase protein dynamics such as C-reactive protein (CRP). While CRP is a highly inducible acute phase protein, suPAR does not show major variation in blood. Infusion with 2 ng/kg LPS in human subjects lead to less than 2-fold increase in plasma suPAR level [22] and in contrast to many pro-inflammatory cytokines, circadian suPAR levels (measured every 20 minutes for 24 hours) have been shown to be quite constant [123]. C5a enhances uPAR-expression in vitro in monocyte-like cells [124] and many cytokines (TNF-α, IFN-γ, IL-1β, IL-2, IL-6, IL-7, IL-8) enhance uPAR-expression in vitro in monocyte-like cells [23,124-126], granulocytes [111,127], T cells [55], NK cells [128] and vascular endothelial cells [60]. Furthermore, TNF-α and IL-1β enhance uPAR-release in vitro in monocyte-like cells, granulocytes and vascular endothelial cells [60,126,127]. In contrast, IL-4 and TGF-β can downregulate uPAR-expression in vitro in T cells [55] and IL-4, IL-10 and IL-13 can downregulate uPAR-expression and release in vitro in monocyte-like cells [129]. It should be noted that studies investigating uPA binding capacity as a marker of the amount of uPAR protein at the cell surface [55,124,125] may underestimate uPAR-expression because the cleaved receptor (uPAR(II-III)) is unable to bind uPA.

Vascular Permeability

The vascular mediators exert their effect by binding to specific receptors on vascular endothelial and smooth muscle cells. Vascular mediators induce vasodilatation and contraction of endothelial cells resulting in endothelial gap formation and increased permeability of the endothelial cell barrier. The loss of endothelial cell integrity leads to leakage of fluid and plasma components and emigration of erythrocytes and leukocytes from the vascular compartment to the extravascular compartment.

Expression of uPAR on endothelial cells may modulate vascular permeability as uPA binding and plasmin generation at the surface of endothelial cells induces loss of cell-cell contacts, retraction of endothelial cells and increased permeability [130]. Also, uPAR is indirectly involved in generation of uPA-catalyzed vasoactive mediators (plasmin, degradation products of fibrin). Several vasoactive mediators affect uPAR by enhancing uPAR-expression in immune cells (C5a) [124] or by cleaving the receptor between uPAR(I) and uPAR(II) (plasmin) [64].

Tissue Repair and Remodelling

Tissue repair is part of the inflammatory response and represents an attempt to maintain normal structure and function. Protease activity is essential for the tissue remodelling process [2,3,7,78,131,132]. Thus, plasminogen-deficient mice have impaired wound healing [131] and inhibition of MMPs in plasminogen-deficient mice completely arrests wound healing and wound closure [132].

As a cellular receptor for uPA, uPAR is involved in ECM degradation during physiological processes with tissue remodelling and tumour cell invasion. Accordingly, in mice, uPAR is highly expressed in tissues undergoing extensive remodelling such as trophoblast cells in placenta, migrating keratinocytes at the edge of incisional wounds and granulocytes infiltrating the area beneath the wound crust [131,133-135]. In addition to ECM degradation, plasmin and uPA both activate and release various growth factors, cytokines and chemokines of importance for tissue repair, remodelling and cell recruitment [3,5,6,8,40,63,136] and (s)uPAR(II-III) may recruit immune cells to the site of injury thus enhancing the tissue remodelling process [8].

INFLAMMATION IN HIV-1 INFECTION

HIV infection is characterized by CD4+ T cell immunodeficiency in the context of generalized immune activation and dysregulation with widespread explosive infection and massive depletion of memory CD4+ T cells in acute HIV infection [137-140] and gradual loss of remaining CD4+ T cells due to persistent immune hyperactivation and insufficient regeneration and replenishment of the lost cells in chronic HIV infection [141,142].

The idea that immune activation contributes significantly to HIV pathogenesis emerged only few years after the discovery of HIV. The first evidence came from clinical studies of chronically infected patients, demonstrating that soluble [143,144] and CD8+ T cell [145-148] markers of immune activation were strong independent predictors of disease progression and mortality. Many later studies have supported and extended these findings and also the pre-infection [149] and early p.i. [150] systemic level of immune activation strongly predict HIV disease progression rate. Studies of SIV infection have revealed that immune activation is the principal factor responsible for the immunopathology accompanying pathogenic SIV [151] and HIV infection [142,152,153]. The recent demonstration that induction of immune activation in non-pathogenic SIV infection increases viral replication and CD4+ T cell loss in GALT serves as a proof-of-concept of a causal relationship between immune activation, viral replication and CD4+ T cell depletion in HIV/SIV infection [154].

Thus, the prevailing view today is that – following the first "hit" by HIV – the immunopathologic rather than cytopathic properties of HIV account for the progressive immunodeficiency and ultimate immune collapse.

Although the critical role of immune activation is perceived – the mechanisms by which chronic immune activation translates into profound immunodeficiency and immune collapse are only beginning to emerge. A prevailing view is that immune hyperactivation, in the context of pathogen (HIV) persistence and immunodeficiency, drives turnover of CD4+ T_{EM} with downstream immune activation and upstream depletion of CD4+ T_{CM} and naive cells [155,156] ultimately leading to immune exhaustion [152,153] and immune collapse when the frequency of CD4+ T_{EM} in lymphoid and extralymphoid tissues fall below the threshold required for effective resistance against pathogens [142].

There is strong evidence that immune activation and high suPAR levels are intimately linked in HIV infection. In chronic antiretroviral-untreated HIV infection, suPAR is consistently positively associated with circulating TNF-α/sTNFrII [12,93,116] and negatively associated with CD4-count [11,12,14,93,116] – whereas the negative correlation between suPAR and CD4-count is absent in less progressed [15] and HAART-treated HIV infection [93,116,157]. Also, the level of soluble immune activation markers are independent predictors of all circulating suPAR forms in HIV infection [12]. The observation that bulk-suPAR accumulates in ng levels per ml over several days in stimulated and non-stimulated whole-blood cultures [118] – similar in amount to circulating levels and reported release from cultures of mononuclear immune cells [61,70] – emphasizes that blood cells have a high constitutive and induced capacity to release uPAR. The lack of correlations between circulating suPAR forms and blood counts of immune cells in HIV infected patients [12] does not exclude that circulating immune cells contribute to high suPAR levels. In sepsis, the neutrophil count is negatively/not correlated with circulating suPAR [16,20] and in human endotoxemia the increase in circulating suPAR and uPAR-expressing monocytes coincides with low monocyte cell count [23], indicating that immune cell adhesion and/or emigration (and hence disappearance from blood) may enhance uPAR-release in vivo and thereby contribute to high suPAR levels. This notion is supported by vitro studies in which adherence of PBMC or platelets to ECs enhances uPAR-release from PBMC and/or ECs [61] and co-clustering of TCR and β1 or β2-integrins increases uPAR-expression in T cells and promote their migration [56]. Finally, many pathogenic hallmarks of chronic HIV infection may, through different mechanisms, enhance uPAR-release from tissue/immune cells in vivo and thus contribute to high circulating suPAR levels. HIV itself [107,108], microbial translocation and high endotoxin levels [17,22,23,121], co-infections [13,26-30], bystander activation of immune cells [158] and bystander/antigen-driven extensive differentiation of naive T cells (low uPAR-expression) into effector/memory T cells (high uPAR-expression) [55,56,153], ongoing repopulation of GALT with extensive migration of CD4+ T_{EM} may contribute to enhanced uPAR-release and lymphoid tissue/GALT remodelling and/or collagen deposition [159,160] probably involves enhanced local uPAR-expression and release, as uPAR is highly expressed in tissues undergoing repair and/or extensive remodelling due to the critical involvement of protease activity in this process [7,8,133,134].

The potential association between suPAR and several hallmarks of chronic HIV infection, i.e. pathogen/bystander-induced activation, turnover, adhesion and migration of immune cells, EC activation and lymphoid tissue remodelling (and indirectly CD4+ T cell depletion in GALT), may explain both the strong predictive value of suPAR and support the notion that suPAR reflects multiple pathogenic events including HIV replication [35-38].

HAART AND suPAR IN HIV-1 INFECTION

The profound decline in blood and tissue VL after starting HAART accounts for the ensuing deactivation of the immune system evidenced by reductions in circulating/tissue levels of soluble and cellular immune activation markers [93,116,161-164].

Starting HAART immediately reduces circulating bulk-suPAR [109,116], suPAR(I), suPAR(II-III) and suPAR(I-III) [93] and CSF bulk-suPAR [109]. This reduction is in accordance with therapy-induced reductions in circulating suPAR in pulmonary tuberculosis [13], acute malaria [30], acute myeloid leukemia [71] and therapy-induced reductions in urine-suPAR in uro-sepsis [17]. The finding of unchanged suPAR levels in patients with low/normal suPAR levels pre-HAART [116] is comparable to the diminished therapy-response observed in pulmonary tuberculosis [13] or acute myeloid leukemia [71] patients with low/normal pre-therapy suPAR levels.

The disparate suPAR change in HIV-1 infected patients with high vs. low circulating suPAR may be attributed to e.g., differences in HIV disease severity [11,12,14,93,109,116], comorbidity [116], dysmetabolism [123,157] and/or genetic polymorphism(s) – although there is no published evidence yet for associations between the suPAR level and polymorphism(s) in promoters of uPAR [15] or other genes.

It remains to be determined if the blood level of suPAR or changes in this post-HAART may be able to predict ensuing viral or immunologic non-response or failure and studies are ongoing to enlighten these issues.

FUTURE PERSPECTIVES

The involvement of uPA/uPAR in trapping HIV virions within the cell has drug target potential.

Also, as suPAR is a strong marker of HIV disease progression, the addition of suPAR to other markers of progression such as CD4 T cell counts and HIV viral load may be relevant. It has been shown that the immune activation level measured by suPAR is associated with increased viral replication, CD4 T-cell depletion and disease progression.

This should be determined in a randomised study where the decision making on when to initiate HAART is based on suPAR and CD4 count. The hypothesis would be that individuals with high suPAR should initiate HAART at higher CD4 count according to (Fig. **4**).

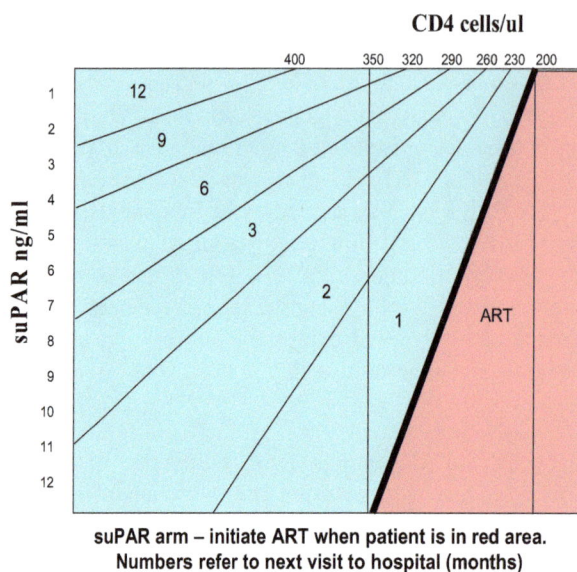

Figure 4: Algorithm of suPAR and CD4 count guided initiation of ART.

Current recommendations on when to start antiretroviral therapy (ART) were discussed by an expert panel at the International AIDS conference in Mexico 2008 and the conclusions were, in agreement with WHO guidelines:

1. Start therapy in any patient with symptomatic HIV disease, regardless of CD4 count or viral load, and asymptomatic patients with less than 200/μL CD4 cell count.

2. Initiation of therapy in patients within the 200 to 350/μL CD4 cell count range should be strongly considered and individualized.

Hence, in the CD4 window between 350 and 200 cells per μl, the measurement of suPAR can be used to guide clinical decision making. If the hypothesis is proven through a randomised study, that is if knowledge of the inflammatory state of the HIV positive patient gives the clinician better grounds for deciding when to initiate ART and whether the patients is responding to the treatment regime, the use of suPAR and CD4 count could enhance treatment efficacy in particular in areas of the world where measurement of viral load is currently unavailable due to cost and technical demands.

CONCLUSIONS

The uPA/uPAR/suPAR molecules are involved in several immune functions including migration, adhesion, angiogenesis, fibrinolysis and cell proliferation. These are also important functions involved in the regulation of a viral infection as demonstrated in recent years research on uPA/uPAR/suPAR in HIV infection. The uPA involvement in HIV trapping, the dependence of this mechanism of cell adhesion, and the strong prognostic value of suPAR in HIV disease progression. Future research will determine whether this knowledge can be implemented in HIV drug development and in the use of suPAR for initiating antiretroviral therapy and for monitoring treatment efficacy.

CONFLICT OF INTEREST

Jesper Eugen-Olsen is co-founder and shareholder in ViroGates A/S, the company that produces the suPARnostic assay. No other authors have any conflict of interest.

REFERENCES

[1]   Collen D. On the regulation and control of fibrinolysis. Edward Kowalski Memorial Lecture. Thromb Haemost 1980; 43: 77-89.

[2]   Dano K, Andreasen PA, Grondahl-Hansen J, Kristensen P, Nielsen LS, Skriver L. Plasminogen activators, tissue degradation, and cancer. Adv Cancer Res 1985; 44: 139-266.

[3]   Collen D. The plasminogen (fibrinolytic) system. Thromb Haemost 1999; 82: 259-70.

[4]   Irigoyen JP, Munoz-Canoves P, Montero L, Koziczak M, Nagamine Y. The plasminogen activator system: biology and regulation. Cell Mol Life Sci 1999; 56: 104-32.

[5]   Andreasen PA, Egelund R, Petersen HH. The plasminogen activation system in tumor growth, invasion, and metastasis. Cell Mol Life Sci 2000; 57: 25-40.

[6]   Werb Z. ECM and cell surface proteolysis: regulating cellular ecology. Cell 1997; 91: 439-42.

[7]   Blasi F, Carmeliet P. uPAR: a versatile signalling orchestrator. Nat Rev Mol Cell Biol 2002; 3: 932-43.

[8]   Mondino A, Blasi F. uPA and uPAR in fibrinolysis, immunity and pathology. Trends Immunol 2004; 25: 450-5.

[9]   Montuori N, Visconte V, Rossi G, Ragno P. Soluble and cleaved forms of the urokinase-receptor: degradation products or active molecules? Thromb Haemost 2005; 93: 192-8.

[10]   Ragno P. The urokinase receptor: a ligand or a receptor? Story of a sociable molecule. Cell Mol Life Sci 2006; 63: 1028-37.

[11]   Sidenius N, Sier CF, Ullum H, *et al.* Serum level of soluble urokinase-type plasminogen activator receptor is a strong and independent predictor of survival in human immunodeficiency virus infection. Blood 2000; 96: 4091-5.

[12]   Ostrowski SR, Piironen T, Hoyer-Hansen G, Gerstoft J, Pedersen BK, Ullum H. High Plasma Levels of Intact and Cleaved Soluble Urokinase Receptor Reflect Immune Activation and Are Independent Predictors of Mortality in HIV-1-Infected Patients. J Acquir Immune Defic Syndr 2005; 39: 23-31.

[13]   Eugen-Olsen J, Gustafson P, Sidenius N, *et al.* The serum level of soluble urokinase receptor is elevated in tuberculosis patients and predicts mortality during treatment: a community study from Guinea-Bissau. Int J Tuberc Lung Dis 2002; 6: 686-92.

[14]   Lawn SD, Myer L, Bangani N, Vogt M, Wood R. Plasma levels of soluble urokinase-type plasminogen activator receptor (suPAR) and early mortality risk among patients enrolling for antiretroviral treatment in South Africa. BMC Infect Dis 2007; 7: doi:10.1186/1471-2334-7-41.

[15]   Schneider UV, Nielsen RL, Pedersen C, Eugen-Olsen J. The prognostic value of the suPARnostic ELISA in HIV-1 infected individuals is not affected by uPAR promoter polymorphisms. BMC Infect Dis 2007; 7:134.: 134.

[16]   Mizukami IF, Faulkner NE, Gyetko MR, Sitrin RG, Todd RF. Enzyme-linked immunoabsorbent assay detection of a soluble form of urokinase plasminogen activator receptor in vivo. Blood 1995; 86: 203-11.

[17]   Florquin S, van den Berg JG, Olszyna DP, *et al.* Release of urokinase plasminogen activator receptor during urosepsis and endotoxemia. Kidney Int 2001; 59: 2054-61.

[18]   Kofoed K, Schneider UV, Scheel T, Andersen O, Eugen-Olsen J. Development and validation of a multiplex add-on assay for Sepsis Biomarkers using xMAP technology. Clin Chem 2006; 52: 1284-93.

[19]   Kofoed K, Andersen O, Kronborg G, *et al.* Use of plasma C-reactive protein, procalcitonin, neutrophils, macrophage migration inhibitory factor, soluble urokinase-type plasminogen activator receptor, and soluble triggering receptor expressed on myeloid cells-1 in combination to diagnose infections: a prospective study. Crit Care 2007; 11: doi:10.1186/cc5723.

[20]   Wittenhagen P, Kronborg G, Weis N, *et al.* The plasma level of soluble urokinase receptor is elevated in patients with Streptococcus pneumoniae bacteraemia and predicts mortality. Clin Microbiol Infect 2004; 10: 409-15.

[21]   Moller HJ, Moestrup SK, Weis N, *et al.* Macrophage serum markers in pneumococcal bacteremia: Prediction of survival by soluble CD163. Crit Care Med 2006; 34: 2561-6.

[22]   Ostrowski SR, Plomgaard P, Fischer CP, *et al.* Interleukin-6 infusion during human endotoxemia inhibits in vitro release of the urokinase receptor from peripheral blood mononuclear cells. Scand J Immunol 2005; 61: 197-206.

[23]   Dekkers PE, ten Hove T, te Velde AA, van Deventer SJ, van Der PT. Upregulation of monocyte urokinase plasminogen activator receptor during human endotoxemia. Infect Immun 2000; 68: 2156-60.

[24]   Kofoed K, Eugen-Olsen J, Petersen J, Larsen K, Andersen O. Predicting mortality in patients with systemic inflammatory response syndrome: an evaluation of two prognostic models, two soluble receptors, and a macrophage migration inhibitory factor. Eur J Clin Microbiol Infect Dis 2008; 27: 375-83.

[25]   Garcia-Monco JC, Coleman JL, Benach JL. Soluble urokinase receptor (uPAR, CD 87) is present in serum and cerebrospinal fluid in patients with neurologic diseases. J Neuroimmunol 2002; 129: 216-23.

[26] Ostrowski SR, Ravn P, Hoyer-Hansen G, Ullum H, Andersen AB. Elevated levels of soluble urokinase receptor in serum from mycobacteria infected patients: Still looking for a marker of treatment efficacy. Scand J Infect Dis 2006; 38: 1028-32.

[27] Zhou H, Wu X, Lu X, Chen G, Ye X, Huang J. Evaluation of plasma urokinase-type plasminogen activator and urokinase-type plasminogen-activator receptor in patients with acute and chronic hepatitis B. Thromb Res 2009; 123:537-42.

[28] Ostrowski SR, Ullum H, Goka BQ, et al. Plasma concentrations of soluble urokinase-type plasminogen activator receptor are increased in patients with malaria and are associated with a poor clinical or a fatal outcome. J Infect Dis 2005; 191: 1331-441.

[29] Ostrowski SR, Shulman CE, Peshu N, et al. Elevated plasma urokinase receptor predicts low birth weight in maternal malaria. Parasite Immunol 2007; 29: 37-46.

[30] Perch M, Kofoed PE, Fischer TK, et al. Serum levels of soluble urokinase plasminogen activator receptor is associated with parasitemia in children with acute *Plasmodium falciparum* malaria infection. Parasite Immunol 2004; 26: 207-11.

[31] Pawlak K, Pawlak D, Mysliwiec M. Excess soluble urokinase-type plasminogen activator receptor in the plasma of dialysis patients correlates with increased fibrinolytic activity. Thromb Res 2007; 119: 475-80.

[32] Slot O, Brunner N, Locht H, Oxholm P, Stephens RW. Soluble urokinase plasminogen activator receptor in plasma of patients with inflammatory rheumatic disorders: increased concentrations in rheumatoid arthritis. Ann Rheum Dis 1999; 58: 488-92.

[33] Hoyer-Hansen G, Lund IK. Urokinase receptor variants in tissue and body fluids. Adv Clin Chem 2007; 44: 65-102.

[34] Rasch MG, Lund IK, Almasi CE, Hoyer-Hansen G. Intact and cleaved uPAR forms: diagnostic and prognostic value in cancer. Front Biosci 2008; 13: 6752-62.

[35] Wada M, Wada NA, Shirono H, Taniguchi K, Tsuchie H, Koga J. Amino-terminal fragment of urokinase-type plasminogen activator inhibits hiv-1 replication. Biochem Biophys Res Commun 2001; 284: 346-51.

[36] Alfano M, Sidenius N, Panzeri B, Blasi F, Poli G. Urokinase-urokinase receptor interaction mediates an inhibitory signal for HIV-1 replication. Proc Natl Acad Sci U S A 2002; 99: 8862-7.

[37] Elia C, Cassol E, Sidenius N, et al. Inhibition of HIV replication by the plasminogen activator is dependent on vitronectin-mediated cell adhesion. J Leukoc Biol 2007; 82: 1212-20.

[38] Alfano M, Mariani SA, Elia C, Pardi R, Blasi F, Poli G. Ligand-engaged urokinase-type plasminogen activator receptor (uPAR) and activation of the CD11b/CD18 (Mac1) integrin inhibit late events of HIV expression in monocytic cells. Blood 2009; 113:1699-709.

[39] Behrendt N. The urokinase receptor (uPAR) and the uPAR-associated protein (uPARAP/Endo180): membrane proteins engaged in matrix turnover during tissue remodeling. Biol Chem 2004; 385: 103-36.

[40] Vakili J, Standker L, Detheux M, Vassart G, Forssmann WG, Parmentier M. Urokinase plasminogen activator and plasmin efficiently convert hemofiltrate CC chemokine 1 into its active [9-74] processed variant. J Immunol 2001; 167: 3406-13.

[41] Stephens RW, Brunner N, Janicke F, Schmitt M. The urokinase plasminogen activator system as a target for prognostic studies in breast cancer. Breast Cancer Res Treat 1998; 52: 99-111.

[42] Ploug M. Structure-function relationships in the interaction between the urokinase-type plasminogen activator and its receptor. Curr Pharm Des 2003; 9: 1499-528.

[43] Behrendt N, Ronne E, Ploug M, et al. The human receptor for urokinase plasminogen activator. NH2-terminal amino acid sequence and glycosylation variants. J Biol Chem 1990; 265: 6453-60.

[44] Behrendt N, Ploug M, Patthy L, Houen G, Blasi F, Dano K. The ligand-binding domain of the cell surface receptor for urokinase-type plasminogen activator. J Biol Chem 1991; 266: 7842-7.

[45] Ploug M, Ronne E, Behrendt N, Jensen AL, Blasi F, Dano K. Cellular receptor for urokinase plasminogen activator. Carboxyl-terminal processing and membrane anchoring by glycosyl-phosphatidylinositol. J Biol Chem 1991; 266: 1926-33.

[46] Behrendt N, Ronne E, Dano K. Domain interplay in the urokinase receptor. Requirement for the third domain in high affinity ligand binding and demonstration of ligand contact sites in distinct receptor domains. J Biol Chem 1996; 271: 22885-94.

[47] Hoyer-Hansen G, Behrendt N, Ploug M, Dano K, Preissner KT. The intact urokinase receptor is required for efficient vitronectin binding: receptor cleavage prevents ligand interaction. FEBS Lett 1997; 420: 79-85.

[48] Wei Y, Waltz DA, Rao N, Drummond RJ, Rosenberg S, Chapman HA. Identification of the urokinase receptor as an adhesion receptor for vitronectin. J Biol Chem 1994; 269: 32380-8.

[49]   Deng G, Curriden SA, Wang S, Rosenberg S, Loskutoff DJ. Is plasminogen activator inhibitor-1 the molecular switch that governs urokinase receptor-mediated cell adhesion and release? J Cell Biol 1996; 134: 1563-71.

[50]   Kanse SM, Kost C, Wilhelm OG, Andreasen PA, Preissner KT. The urokinase receptor is a major vitronectin-binding protein on endothelial cells. Exp Cell Res 1996; 224: 344-53.

[51]   Sidenius N, Andolfo A, Fesche R, Blasi F. Urokinase regulates vitronectin binding by controlling urokinase receptor oligomerization. J Biol Chem 2002; 277: 27982-90.

[52]   Plesner T, Ralfkiaer E, Wittrup M, *et al.* Expression of the receptor for urokinase-type plasminogen activator in normal and neoplastic blood cells and hematopoietic tissue. Am J Clin Pathol 1994; 102: 835-41.

[53]   Ferrero E, Vettoretto K, Bondanza A, *et al.* uPA/uPAR system is active in immature dendritic cells derived from CD14+CD34+ precursors and is down-regulated upon maturation. J Immunol 2000; 164: 712-8.

[54]   Nykjaer A, Petersen CM, Moller B, Andreasen PA, Gliemann J. Identification and characterization of urokinase receptors in natural killer cells and T-cell-derived lymphokine activated killer cells. FEBS Lett 1992; 300: 13-7.

[55]   Nykjaer A, Moller B, Todd RF, *et al.* Urokinase receptor. An activation antigen in human T lymphocytes. J Immunol 1994; 152: 505-16.

[56]   Bianchi E, Ferrero E, Fazioli F, *et al.* Integrin-dependent induction of functional urokinase receptors in primary T lymphocytes. J Clin Invest 1996; 98: 1133-41.

[57]   Wohn KD, Kanse SM, Deutsch V, Schmidt T, Eldor A, Preissner KT. The urokinase-receptor (CD87) is expressed in cells of the megakaryoblastic lineage. Thromb Haemost 1997; 77: 540-7.

[58]   Haddock RC, Spell ML, Baker CD III, *et al.* Urokinase binding and receptor identification in cultured endothelial cells. J Biol Chem 1991; 266: 21466-73.

[59]   Chavakis T, Kanse SM, Yutzy B, Lijnen HR, Preissner KT. Vitronectin concentrates proteolytic activity on the cell surface and extracellular matrix by trapping soluble urokinase receptor-urokinase complexes. Blood 1998; 91: 2305-12.

[60]   Chavakis T, Willuweit AK, Lupu F, Preissner KT, Kanse SM. Release of soluble urokinase receptor from vascular cells. Thromb Haemost 2001; 86: 686-93.

[61]   Mustjoki S, Sidenius N, Vaheri A. Enhanced release of soluble urokinase receptor by endothelial cells in contact with peripheral blood cells. FEBS Lett 2000; 486: 237-42.

[62]   Piguet PF, Vesin C, Donati Y, Tacchini-Cottier F, Belin D, Barazzone C. Urokinase receptor (uPAR, CD87) is a platelet receptor important for kinetics and TNF-induced endothelial adhesion in mice. Circulation 1999; 99: 3315-21.

[63]   Plesner T, Behrendt N, Ploug M. Structure, function and expression on blood and bone marrow cells of the urokinase-type plasminogen activator receptor, uPAR. Stem Cells 1997; 15: 398-408.

[64]   Hoyer-Hansen G, Ronne E, Solberg H, *et al.* Urokinase plasminogen activator cleaves its cell surface receptor releasing the ligand-binding domain. J Biol Chem 1992; 267: 18224-9.

[65]   Hoyer-Hansen G, Ploug M, Behrendt N, Ronne E, Dano K. Cell-surface acceleration of urokinase-catalyzed receptor cleavage. Eur J Biochem 1997; 243: 21-6.

[66]   Wilhelm OG, Wilhelm S, Escott GM, *et al.* Cellular glycosylphosphatidylinositol-specific phospholipase D regulates urokinase receptor shedding and cell surface expression. J Cell Physiol 1999; 180: 225-35.

[67]   Pliyev BK. Activated human neutrophils rapidly release the chemotactically active D2D3 form of the urokinase-type plasminogen activator receptor (uPAR/CD87). Mol Cell Biochem 2009; 321: 111-22.

[68]   Pyke C, Eriksen J, Solberg H, *et al.* An alternatively spliced variant of mRNA for the human receptor for urokinase plasminogen activator. FEBS Lett 1993; 326: 69-74.

[69]   Wahlberg K, Hoyer-Hansen G, Casslen B. Soluble receptor for urokinase plasminogen activator in both full-length and a cleaved form is present in high concentration in cystic fluid from ovarian cancer. Cancer Res 1998; 58: 3294-8.

[70]   Sidenius N, Sier CF, Blasi F. Shedding and cleavage of the urokinase receptor (uPAR): identification and characterisation of uPAR fragments in vitro and in vivo. FEBS Lett 2000; 475: 52-6.

[71]   Mustjoki S, Sidenius N, Sier CF, *et al.* Soluble urokinase receptor levels correlate with number of circulating tumor cells in acute myeloid leukemia and decrease rapidly during chemotherapy. Cancer Res 2000; 60: 7126-32.

[72]   Piironen T, Laursen B, Paas J, *et al.* Specific Immunoassays for Detection of Intact and Cleaved Forms of the Urokinase Receptor. Clin Chem 2004; 50: 2059-68.

[73]   Nykjaer A, Conese M, Christensen EI, *et al.* Recycling of the urokinase receptor upon internalization of the uPA:serpin complexes. EMBO J 1997; 16: 2610-20.

[74]   Wei Y, Lukashev M, Simon DI, *et al.* Regulation of integrin function by the urokinase receptor. Science 1996; 273: 1551-5.

[75]   Montuori N, Carriero MV, Salzano S, Rossi G, Ragno P. The cleavage of the urokinase receptor regulates its multiple functions. J Biol Chem 2002; 277: 46932-9.

[76]   May AE, Kanse SM, Lund LR, Gisler RH, Imhof BA, Preissner KT. Urokinase receptor (CD87) regulates leukocyte recruitment via beta 2 integrins in vivo. J Exp Med 1998; 188: 1029-37.

[77]   Ossowski L, Aguirre-Ghiso JA. Urokinase receptor and integrin partnership: coordination of signaling for cell adhesion, migration and growth. Curr Opin Cell Biol 2000; 12: 613-20.

[78]   Chapman HA. Plasminogen activators, integrins, and the coordinated regulation of cell adhesion and migration. Curr Opin Cell Biol 1997; 9: 714-24.

[79]   Chapman HA, Wei Y, Simon DI, Waltz DA. Role of urokinase receptor and caveolin in regulation of integrin signaling. Thromb Haemost 1999; 82: 291-7.

[80]   Preissner KT, Seiffert D. Role of vitronectin and its receptors in haemostasis and vascular remodeling. Thromb Res 1998; 89: 1-21.

[81]   Preissner KT, Kanse SM, May AE. Urokinase receptor: a molecular organizer in cellular communication. Curr Opin Cell Biol 2000; 12: 621-8.

[82]   Gyetko MR, Sud S, Kendall T, Fuller JA, Newstead MW, Standiford TJ. Urokinase receptor-deficient mice have impaired neutrophil recruitment in response to pulmonary Pseudomonas aeruginosa infection. J Immunol 2000; 165: 1513-9.

[83]   Gyetko MR, Sud S, Sonstein J, Polak T, Sud A, Curtis JL. Cutting Edge: Antigen-Driven Lymphocyte Recruitment to the Lung Is Diminished in the Absence of Urokinase-Type Plasminogen Activator (uPA) Receptor, but Is Independent of uPA. J Immunol 2001; 167: 5539-42.

[84]   Rijneveld AW, Levi M, Florquin S, Speelman P, Carmeliet P, van Der PT. Urokinase receptor is necessary for adequate host defense against pneumococcal pneumonia. J Immunol 2002; 168: 3507-11.

[85]   Gyetko MR, Aizenberg D, Mayo-Bond L. Urokinase-deficient and urokinase receptor-deficient mice have impaired neutrophil antimicrobial activation in vitro. J Leukoc Biol 2004; 76: 648-56.

[86]   Tarui T, Mazar AP, Cines DB, Takada Y. Urokinase-type plasminogen activator receptor (CD87) is a ligand for integrins and mediates cell-cell interaction. J Biol Chem 2001; 276: 3983-90.

[87]   Fazioli F, Resnati M, Sidenius N, Higashimoto Y, Appella E, Blasi F. A urokinase-sensitive region of the human urokinase receptor is responsible for its chemotactic activity. EMBO J 1997; 16: 7279-86.

[88]   Resnati M, Pallavicini I, Wang JM, et al. The fibrinolytic receptor for urokinase activates the G protein-coupled chemotactic receptor FPRL1/LXA4R. Proc Natl Acad Sci USA 2002; 99: 1359-64.

[89]   Behrendt N, Jensen ON, Engelholm LH, Mortz E, Mann M, Dano K. A urokinase receptor-associated protein with specific collagen binding properties. J Biol Chem 2000; 275: 1993-2002.

[90]   Resnati M, Guttinger M, Valcamonica S, Sidenius N, Blasi F, Fazioli F. Proteolytic cleavage of the urokinase receptor substitutes for the agonist-induced chemotactic effect. EMBO J 1996; 15: 1572-82.

[91]   Le Y, Li B, Gong W, et al. Novel pathophysiological role of classical chemotactic peptide receptors and their communications with chemokine receptors. Immunol Rev 2000; 177:185-94.: 185-94.

[92]   Furlan F, Orlando S, Laudanna C, et al. The soluble D2D3(88-274) fragment of the urokinase receptor inhibits monocyte chemotaxis and integrin-dependent cell adhesion. J Cell Sci 2004; 117: 2909-16.

[93]   Ostrowski SR, Katzenstein TL, Pedersen M, et al. Plasma levels of intact and cleaved urokinase receptor decrease in HIV-1-infected patients initiating highly active antiretroviral therapy. Scand J Immunol 2006; 63: 478-86.

[94]   Behrendt N, Stephens RW. The urokinase receptor. Fibrinolysis & Proteolysis 1998; 12: 191-204.

[95]   Holst-Hansen C, Hamers MJ, Johannessen BE, Brunner N, Stephens RW. Soluble urokinase receptor released from human carcinoma cells: a plasma parameter for xenograft tumour studies. Br J Cancer 1999; 81: 203-11.

[96]   Selleri C, Montuori N, Ricci P, et al. Involvement of the Urokinase-type plasminogen activator receptor in hematopoietic stem cell mobilization. Blood 2005; 105: 2198-205.

[97]   Selleri C, Montuori N, Ricci P, et al. In vivo activity of the cleaved form of soluble urokinase receptor: a new hematopoietic stem/progenitor cell mobilizer. Cancer Res 2006; 66: 10885-90.

[98]   Riisbro R, Piironen T, Brünner N, et al. Measurements of soluble urokinase plasminogen activator receptor in serum. J Clin Ligand Assay 2002; 25: 53-6.

[99]   Higazi AA, Bdeir K, Hiss E, et al. Lysis of plasma clots by urokinase-soluble urokinase receptor complexes. Blood 1998; 92: 2075-83.

[100]   Cunningham O, Andolfo A, Santovito ML, Iuzzolino L, Blasi F, Sidenius N. Dimerization controls the lipid raft partitioning of uPAR/CD87 and regulates its biological functions. EMBO J 2003; 22: 5994-6003.

[101]   Trigwell S, Wood L, Jones P. Soluble urokinase receptor promotes cell adhesion and requires tyrosine-92 for activation of p56/59(hck). Biochem Biophys Res Commun 2000; 278: 440-6.

[102]   Mizukami IF, Todd RF. A soluble form of the urokinase plasminogen activator receptor (suPAR) can bind to hematopoietic cells. J Leukoc Biol 1998; 64: 203-13.

[103] Wilhelm O, Weidle U, Hohl S, Rettenberger P, Schmitt M, Graeff H. Recombinant soluble urokinase receptor as a scavenger for urokinase-type plasminogen activator (uPA). Inhibition of proliferation and invasion of human ovarian cancer cells. FEBS Lett 1994; 337: 131-4.

[104] Kruger A, Soeltl R, Lutz V, et al. Reduction of breast carcinoma tumor growth and lung colonization by overexpression of the soluble urokinase-type plasminogen activator receptor (CD87). Cancer Gene Ther 2000; 7: 292-9.

[105] Lutz V, Reuning U, Kruger A, et al. High level synthesis of recombinant soluble urokinase receptor (CD87) by ovarian cancer cells reduces intraperitoneal tumor growth and spread in nude mice. Biol Chem 2001; 382: 789-98.

[106] Aguirre Ghiso JA, Kovalski K, Ossowski L. Tumor dormancy induced by downregulation of urokinase receptor in human carcinoma involves integrin and MAPK signaling. J Cell Biol 1999; 147: 89-104.

[107] Speth C, Pichler I, Stockl G, Mair M, Dierich MP. Urokinase plasminogen activator receptor (uPAR; CD87) expression on monocytic cells and T cells is modulated by HIV-1 infection. Immunobiology 1998; 199: 152-62.

[108] Frank I, Stoiber H, Godar S, et al. Acquisition of host cell-surface-derived molecules by HIV-1. AIDS 1996; 10: 1611-20.

[109] Cinque P, Nebuloni M, Santovito ML, et al. The urokinase receptor is overexpressed in the AIDS dementia complex and other neurological manifestations. Ann Neurol 2004; 55: 687-94.

[110] Sidenius N, Nebuloni M, Sala S, et al. Expression of the urokinase plasminogen activator and its receptor in HIV-1-associated central nervous system disease. J Neuroimmunol 2004; 157: 133-9.

[111] Storgaard M, Obel N, Black FT, Moller BK. Decreased urokinase receptor expression on granulocytes in HIV-infected patients. Scand J Immunol 2002; 55: 409-13.

[112] Murali R, Wolfe JH, Erber R, et al. Altered levels of urokinase on monocytes and in serum of children with AIDS; effects on lymphocyte activation and surface marker expression. J Leukoc Biol 1998; 64: 198-202.

[113] Handley MA, Steigbigel RT, Morrison SA. A role for urokinase-type plasminogen activator in human immunodeficiency virus type 1 infection of macrophages. J Virol 1996; 70: 4451-6.

[114] Folks TM, Justement J, Kinter A, Dinarello CA, Fauci AS. Cytokine-induced expression of HIV-1 in a chronically infected promonocyte cell line. Science 1987; 238: 800-2.

[115] Detheux M, Standker L, Vakili J, et al. Natural proteolytic processing of hemofiltrate CC chemokine 1 generates a potent CC chemokine receptor (CCR)1 and CCR5 agonist with anti-HIV properties. J Exp Med 2000; 192: 1501-8.

[116] Ostrowski SR, Katzenstein TL, Piironen T, Gerstoft J, Pedersen BK, Ullum H. Soluble Urokinase Receptor Levels in Plasma During 5 Years of Highly Active Antiretroviral Therapy in HIV-1-Infected Patients. J Acquir Immune Defic Syndr 2004; 35: 337-42.

[117] De Witte H, Sweep F, Brunner N, et al. Complexes between urokinase-type plasminogen activator and its receptor in blood as determined by enzyme-linked immunosorbent assay. Int J Cancer 1998; 77: 236-42.

[118] Ostrowski SR, Piironen T, Høyer-Hansen G, Gerstoft J, Pedersen BK, Ullum H. Reduced release of intact and cleaved urokinase receptor in stimulated whole-blood cultures from human immunodeficiency virus-1-infected patients. Scand J Immunol 2005; 61: 347-56.

[119] Todd RF, III, Alvarez PA, Brott DA, Liu DY. Bacterial lipopolysaccharide, phorbol myristate acetate, and muramyl dipeptide stimulate the expression of a human monocyte surface antigen, Mo3e. J Immunol 1985; 135: 3869-77.

[120] Coleman JL, Gebbia JA, Benach JL. Borrelia burgdorferi and other bacterial products induce expression and release of the urokinase receptor (CD87). J Immunol 2001; 166: 473-80.

[121] Juffermans NP, Dekkers PE, Verbon A, Speelman P, van Deventer SJ, van Der PT. Concurrent upregulation of urokinase plasminogen activator receptor and CD11b during tuberculosis and experimental endotoxemia. Infect Immun 2001; 69: 5182-5.

[122] Coleman JL, Benach JL. The urokinase receptor can be induced by Borrelia burgdorferi through receptors of the innate immune system. Infect Immun 2003; 71: 5556-64.

[123] Andersen O, Eugen-Olsen J, Kofoed K, Iversen J, Haugaard SB. Soluble urokinase plasminogen activator receptor is a marker of dysmetabolism in HIV-infected patients receiving highly active antiretroviral therapy. J Med Virol 2008; 80: 209-16.

[124] Yoshida E, Tsuchiya K, Sugiki M, Sumi H, Mihara H, Maruyama M. Modulation of the receptor for urokinase-type plasminogen activator in macrophage-like U937 cells by inflammatory mediators. Inflammation 1996; 20: 319-26.

[125] Kirchheimer JC, Nong YH, Remold HG. IFN-gamma, tumor necrosis factor-alpha, and urokinase regulate the expression of urokinase receptors on human monocytes. J Immunol 1988; 141: 4229-34.

[126] Sitrin RG, Todd RF, III, Mizukami IF, Gross TJ, Shollenberger SB, Gyetko MR. Cytokine-specific regulation of urokinase receptor (CD87) expression by U937 mononuclear phagocytes. Blood 1994; 84: 1268-75.

[127] Plesner T, Ploug M, Ellis V, *et al.* The receptor for urokinase-type plasminogen activator and urokinase is translocated from two distinct intracellular compartments to the plasma membrane on stimulation of human neutrophils. Blood 1994; 83: 808-15.

[128] Al Atrash G, Shetty S, Idell S, *et al.* IL-2-mediated upregulation of uPA and uPAR in natural killer cells. Biochem Biophys Res Commun 2002; 292: 184-9.

[129] Paysant J, Vasse M, Soria J, *et al.* Regulation of the uPAR/uPA system expressed on monocytes by the deactivating cytokines, IL-4, IL-10 and IL-13: consequences on cell adhesion to vitronectin and fibrinogen. Br J Haematol 1998; 100: 45-51.

[130] Conforti G, Dominguez-Jimenez C, Ronne E, Hoyer-Hansen G, Dejana E. Cell-surface plasminogen activation causes a retraction of in vitro cultured human umbilical vein endothelial cell monolayer. Blood 1994; 83: 994-1005.

[131] Romer J, Bugge TH, Pyke C, *et al.* Impaired wound healing in mice with a disrupted plasminogen gene. Nat Med 1996; 2: 287-92.

[132] Lund LR, Romer J, Bugge TH, *et al.* Functional overlap between two classes of matrix-degrading proteases in wound healing. EMBO J 1999; 18: 4645-56.

[133] Almus-Jacobs F, Varki N, Sawdey MS, Loskutoff DJ. Endotoxin stimulates expression of the murine urokinase receptor gene in vivo. Am J Pathol 1995; 147: 688-98.

[134] Solberg H, Ploug M, Hoyer-Hansen G, Nielsen BS, Lund LR. The murine receptor for urokinase-type plasminogen activator is primarily expressed in tissues actively undergoing remodeling. J Histochem Cytochem 2001; 49: 237-46.

[135] Romer J, Lund LR, Eriksen J, Pyke C, Kristensen P, Dano K. The receptor for urokinase-type plasminogen activator is expressed by keratinocytes at the leading edge during re-epithelialization of mouse skin wounds. J Invest Dermatol 1994; 102: 519-22.

[136] Rubin E, Farcet JP. Pathology. Third ed. Philadelphia, US: Lippincott-Raven Publishers, 1999.

[137] Guadalupe M, Reay E, Sankaran S, *et al.* Severe CD4+ T-cell depletion in gut lymphoid tissue during primary human immunodeficiency virus type 1 infection and substantial delay in restoration following highly active antiretroviral therapy. J Virol 2003; 77: 11708-17.

[138] Mehandru S, Poles MA, Tenner-Racz K, *et al.* Primary HIV-1 infection is associated with preferential depletion of CD4+ T lymphocytes from effector sites in the gastrointestinal tract. J Exp Med 2004; 200: 761-70.

[139] Brenchley JM, Schacker TW, Ruff LE, *et al.* CD4+ T cell depletion during all stages of HIV disease occurs predominantly in the gastrointestinal tract. J Exp Med 2004; 200: 749-59.

[140] Sankaran S, George MD, Reay E, *et al.* Rapid onset of intestinal epithelial barrier dysfunction in primary human immunodeficiency virus infection is driven by an imbalance between immune response and mucosal repair and regeneration. J Virol 2008; 82: 538-45.

[141] Picker LJ, Watkins DI. HIV pathogenesis: the first cut is the deepest. Nat Immunol 2005; 6: 430-2.

[142] Grossman Z, Meier-Schellersheim M, Paul WE, Picker LJ. Pathogenesis of HIV infection: what the virus spares is as important as what it destroys. Nat Med 2006; 12: 289-95.

[143] Fahey JL, Taylor JM, Detels R, *et al.* The prognostic value of cellular and serologic markers in infection with human immunodeficiency virus type 1. N Engl J Med 1990; 322: 166-72.

[144] Fahey JL, Taylor JM, Manna B, *et al.* Prognostic significance of plasma markers of immune activation, HIV viral load and CD4 T-cell measurements. AIDS 1998; 12: 1581-90.

[145] Liu Z, Cumberland WG, Hultin LE, Prince HE, Detels R, Giorgi JV. Elevated CD38 antigen expression on CD8+ T cells is a stronger marker for the risk of chronic HIV disease progression to AIDS and death in the Multicenter AIDS Cohort Study than CD4+ cell count, soluble immune activation markers, or combinations of HLA-DR and CD38 expression. J Acquir Immune Defic Syndr Hum Retrovirol 1997; 16: 83-92.

[146] Liu Z, Cumberland WG, Hultin LE, Kaplan AH, Detels R, Giorgi JV. CD8+ T-lymphocyte activation in HIV-1 disease reflects an aspect of pathogenesis distinct from viral burden and immunodeficiency. J Acquir Immune Defic Syndr Hum Retrovirol 1998; 18: 332-40.

[147] Giorgi JV, Hultin LE, McKeating JA, *et al.* Shorter survival in advanced human immunodeficiency virus type 1 infection is more closely associated with T lymphocyte activation than with plasma virus burden or virus chemokine coreceptor usage. J Infect Dis 1999; 179: 859-70.

[148] Mocroft A, Bofill M, Lipman M, *et al.* CD8+,CD38+ lymphocyte percent: a useful immunological marker for monitoring HIV-1-infected patients. J Acquir Immune Defic Syndr Hum Retrovirol 1997; 14: 158-62.

[149] Hazenberg MD, Otto SA, van Benthem BH, *et al.* Persistent immune activation in HIV-1 infection is associated with progression to AIDS. AIDS 2003; 17: 1881-8.

[150] Deeks SG, Kitchen CM, Liu L, *et al.* Immune activation set point during early HIV infection predicts subsequent CD4+ T-cell changes independent of viral load. Blood 2004; 104: 942-7.

[151] Pandrea I, Sodora DL, Silvestri G, Apetrei C. Into the wild: simian immunodeficiency virus (SIV) infection in natural hosts. Trends Immunol 2008; 29: 419-28.

[152] Grossman Z, Meier-Schellersheim M, Sousa AE, Victorino RM, Paul WE. CD4+ T-cell depletion in HIV infection: are we closer to understanding the cause? Nat Med 2002; 8: 319-23.

[153] Hazenberg MD, Hamann D, Schuitemaker H, Miedema F. T cell depletion in HIV-1 infection: how CD4+ T cells go out of stock. Nat Immunol 2000; 1: 285-9.

[154] Pandrea I, Gaufin T, Brenchley JM, *et al.* Cutting Edge: Experimentally Induced Immune Activation in Natural Hosts of Simian Immunodeficiency Virus Induces significant Increases in Viral Replication and CD4 T Cell Depletion. J Immunol 2008; 181: 6687-91.

[155] Hellerstein MK, Hoh RA, Hanley MB, *et al.* Subpopulations of long-lived and short-lived T cells in advanced HIV-1 infection. J Clin Invest 2003; 112: 956-66.

[156] Wherry EJ, Teichgraber V, Becker TC, *et al.* Lineage relationship and protective immunity of memory CD8 T cell subsets. Nat Immunol 2003; 4: 225-34.

[157] Andersen O, Eugen-Olsen J, Kofoed K, Iversen J, Haugaard SB. suPAR associates to glucose metabolic aberration during glucose stimulation in HIV-infected patients on HAART. J Infect 2008; 57: 55-63.

[158] Lawn SD, Butera ST, Folks TM. Contribution of immune activation to the pathogenesis and transmission of human immunodeficiency virus type 1 infection. Clin Microbiol Rev 2001; 14: 753-77.

[159] Schacker TW, Nguyen PL, Beilman GJ, *et al.* Collagen deposition in HIV-1 infected lymphatic tissues and T cell homeostasis. J Clin Invest 2002; 110: 1133-9.

[160] Estes J, Baker JV, Brenchley JM, *et al.* Collagen deposition limits immune reconstitution in the gut. J Infect Dis 2008; 198: 456-64.

[161] Autran B, Carcelain G, Li TS, *et al.* Positive effects of combined antiretroviral therapy on CD4+ T cell homeostasis and function in advanced HIV disease. Science 1997; 277: 112-6.

[162] Cohen Stuart JW, Hazebergh MD, Hamann D, *et al.* The dominant source of CD4+ and CD8+ T-cell activation in HIV infection is antigenic stimulation. J Acquir Immune Defic Syndr 2000; 25: 203-11.

[163] Aukrust P, Muller F, Lien E, *et al.* Tumor necrosis factor (TNF) system levels in human immunodeficiency virus-infected patients during highly active antiretroviral therapy: persistent TNF activation is associated with virologic and immunologic treatment failure. J Infect Dis 1999; 179: 74-82.

[164] Stylianou E, Aukrust P, Kvale D, Muller F, Froland SS. IL-10 in HIV infection: increasing serum IL-10 levels with disease progression--down-regulatory effect of potent anti-retroviral therapy. Clin Exp Immunol 1999; 116: 115-20.

α_1Antitrypsin Therapy Increases CD4$^+$ Lymphocytes to Normal Values in HIV-1 Patients

Cynthia L. Bristow[1,2,*], Jose Cortes[3], Roya Mukhtarzad[4], Maylis Trucy[2], Aaron Franklin[5], Val Romberg[6], Ronald Winston[2].

[1]*Weill Medical College of Cornell University, New York, NY 10065;* [2] *Institute for Human Genetics and Biochemistry, New York, NY 10065;* [3]*Beth Israel Medical Center, New York, New York 10003;* [4]*Kingsbrook Jewish Medical Center, Brooklyn, NY 11203;* [5]*University of Toledo College of Medicine, Toledo, OH 43614;* [6]*CSL Behring, Bern, Switzerland CH3000.*

Abstract: Adult thymopoiesis is a multi-step process that in adult mice is highlighted by a 21-day cycle of coordinated journeying of progenitor cells between adult bone marrow and thymus. In the analogous human system, cell surface human leukocyte elastase (HLE$_{CS}$), the chemokine receptor CXCR4, and its ligand stromal-derived factor-1 (SDF-1, CXCL12) are required for progenitor cells to vacate bone marrow. We have recently observed that the number of circulating CD4$^+$ lymphocytes is correlated with the HLE$_{CS}$ ligand, $\alpha_1$antitrypsin ($\alpha_1$proteinase inhibitor, α_1PI). In HIV-1 disease, α_1PI levels are deficient and rate limiting for CD4$^+$ lymphocytes. We demonstrate herein that α_1PI therapy increases the number of CD4$^+$ lymphocytes in blood. In HIV-1 patients the number of CD4$^+$ lymphocytes is increased to normal values after 2 weeks of therapy. Importantly, the 23-day periodicity of appearance of CD4$^+$ lymphocytes suggests that α_1PI regulates adult human thymopoiesis.

INTRODUCTION

The three predominant blood cell subtypes are erythrocytes, granulocytes, and CD4$^+$ lymphocytes. Growth factors such as erythropoietin and G-CSF are currently used therapeutically to mobilize erythroid and myeloid progenitor cells. Emerging information related to stem cell mobilization suggested to us that a fundamental and previously unrecognized function of the blood protein α_1PI is mobilization of CD4$^+$ progenitor cells. Active α_1PI binds to a receptor complex central to cell migration that includes the chemokine stromal-derived factor-1 (SDF1, CXCL12), its receptor CXCR4, and the α_1PI receptor, HLE$_{CS}$ [1-3].

Blood cell migration occurs as the result of two discrete steps. First, the relevant receptors polarize at the leading edge of the cell, and second, these receptors are endocytosed at the trailing edge [4]. When integrins are involved in the receptor complex, cells attach to the tissue matrix. Subsequent endocytosis of the receptor complex at the trailing edge releases the cells from the tissue matrix [4]. Plasma membrane-associated proteinases at the attachment point do not act as proteinases, rather bind to their relevant proteinase inhibitors as receptor and ligand. When these proteinase receptors are in complex with their ligands, e.g. α_1PI-complexed HLE$_{CS}$, conformational changes expose novel domains that attract nearby low-density lipoporotein (LDL) receptor complexes [4, 5]. Binding of the LDL receptor complex to the proteinase inhibitor complex induces their endocytosis which causes the cell to advance forward [4, 5].

In earlier work, we established that antibodies reactive with HIV-1 gp120 also bind and inactivate human α_1PI, producing IgG-α_1PI immune complexes [6]. IgG-α_1PI immune complexes produce functional α_1PI deficiency in HIV-1 infected individuals. A single amino acid differentiates chimpanzee α_1PI from human α_1PI, and this difference is in the HIV-1 gp120 homologous domain, perhaps explaining the lack of progression of HIV-1 infected chimpanzees to AIDS [7]. Further, comparison of the amino acid sequences of human α_1PI, HIV-1, HIV-2, SIV, HTLV-1, and HTLV-2 reveals that all share homology with the hydrophobic core of the fusion domain of HIV-1 gp41 (LFLGFL), but only HIV-1 gp120 shares homology with α_1PI [6]. We hypothesized that the insufficient α_1PI that attends HIV-1 disease might secondarily cause

---

*Address Correspondence to this Author Cynthia L. Bristow at: [1]Weill Medical College of Cornell University, New York, NY 10065, USA; E-mail: cyb2005@med.cornell.edu

Massimo Alfano (Ed)

$CD4^+$ lymphocytes to become trapped in tissue, unable to complete the second step of cell migration and be released into blood. We demonstrate herein that α_1PI augmentation induces substantial increases in $CD4^+$ lymphocytes that cycle with a 23±3.5 day periodicity.

METHODS

Human Subjects

It was determined using the empirical correlation between α_1PI and $CD4^+$ lymphocytes that a sample size of 2 HIV-1$^+$ patients would be adequate two achieve a significance level with alpha = 0.05 and power of test = 0.8 between pre- and post-treatment $CD4^+$ lymphocytes levels. Inclusion criteria for treatment were: i) active α_1PI below 11 μM; ii) one year history with $CD4^+$ lymphocytes at levels ranging between 150 and 300 cells/μl; iii) absence of symptoms suggestive of HIV-1 disease progression; iv) adequate suppression of virus (<50 HIV RNA/ml); and v) history of compliance with antiretroviral medication. Due to the small size of the study and to avoid other complications of pregnancy, only male HIV-1 patients were enrolled. The half-life of Zemaira® (purified α_1PI) after infusion is 4.5 days, reaching steady state after 3-4 wks therapy [8]. CSL Behring contributed a sufficient quantity of Zemaira® (lot# C405702) for administration of 8 weekly infusions at a dose of 120mg/kg.

Written informed consent was received from 4 HIV-1 patients designated Alpha, Beta, Gamma, and Delta. For comparison, blood was collected from 2 non-HIV-1 patients, both female, with a diagnosis of emphysema in the context of genetic α_1PI deficiency (PI$_{ZZ}$-1 and PI$_{ZZ}$-2, ages 52 and 53, respectively). In all cases, patients had never before received α_1PI augmentation therapy. After initiating therapy, an assessment of dosage and the quantity of donated Zemaira® allowed for the extended treatment of patient Alpha for a total of 12 weeks.

Due to an insufficient number of serum samples from patient PI$_{ZZ}$-2, only functional analyses of $CD4^+$ lymphocytes are presented. Patient Gamma who was PPD positive and elderly had become PPD negative 2 yrs prior to the treatment presented here which is clinically interpreted as a loss of immune function. Patient Delta reported to the first infusion stating that due to unforeseen circumstances, his antiretroviral medication was interrupted for 4 days. Although there was no fever present or other indication of infection at the time of the first infusion, in follow-up analysis, this patient was found to have pre-treatment serum IL-2 levels of 51 pg/ml (normal is undetectable) and other atypical baseline measures indicative of an inflammatory response and exceeding study inclusion criteria including 454 $CD4^+$ cells/μl, 205 HIV RNA copies/ml, and 14 μM α_1PI. Thus, blood from patient Delta was analyzed for the purpose of assessing treatment response in the presence of systemic inflammation. Only pre- and post-treatment NFκB activation, cytokine release, and lymphocyte phenotype were determined for this patient. Blood was collected at each session and was sent to a contractor medical laboratory which provided independent measurement of the complete blood cell count (CBC) with differential, lipid panel, blood chemistry, lymphocyte panel, and HIV RNA. Periodically, kidney (BUN and creatinine) and liver function tests (ALT, AST) were monitored for potential immune complex disease, and all measurements were within the normal range. Lymphocyte function and phenotype analysis were performed by our laboratory. The study protocol was approved by CSL Behring and by the institutional review board of Cabrini Medical Center. No adverse effects were reported by any patient.

Serum α_1PI Levels

Active α_1PI was determined in once-thawed serum samples by our laboratory as previously described with the modification that end-point, rather than kinetic, analysis was measured [9]. Briefly, the inhibition of porcine pancreatic elastase (PPE, Sigma, St. Louis, MO) that was specifically attributable to serum α_1PI was quantitated in the context of the serum concentration of $\alpha_2$macroglobulin and its higher affinity for PPE relative to α_1PI.

Lymphocyte Phenotype Analysis

Surface staining on whole blood was performed by incubating for 15 min at 23 °C with ASR type, fluorescently conjugated antibodies recognizing CD4, CD3, CD8, CD45RA, CD45RO, CXCR4, CCR5, CD34. CD25, and isotype controls (BD Biosciences). Cells were subsequently stained to detect HLE$_{CS}$ by incubating whole blood for an additional 15 min at 23 °C with rabbit anti-HLE (Biodesign, Kennebunkport, ME) or negative control rabbit IgG (Chemicon, Temecula, CA) which had been conjugated to Alexa Fluor 647 (Molecular Probes). At least 10,000 cells from each sample were acquired using a FACSCalibur flow cytometer. Markers on cells in the lymphocyte gate were quantitated, and CD4$^+$ cells in the lymphocyte gate were validated using a contractor medical laboratory. Cell staining was analyzed using CellQuest (BD Biosciences) or FlowJo software (Tree Star, Inc., Ashland, OR).

Table 1: HIV-1 population at baseline. [1]All patients were at different stages of HIV-1 disease progression and were on antiretroviral medication with adequate suppression of virus. [2]Infected for many years, and first tested 01/03/2005. [3]Serum levels.

Patient [1]	NRT/NNRT/PI	Age	HIV-1$^+$ since	α_1PI[3] (μM)	CD4[3] cells/μl	HIV RNA[3] copies/ml
Alpha	Epivir/Sustiva/none	47	2001	9	297	<400
Beta	Combivir/Sustiva/none	53	1982	7	276	<400
Gamma	Combivir/Viramune/Kaletra	70	Unknown[2]	4	148	<400
Delta	Truvada/Sustiva/none	51	1982	14	445	205

CD4$^+$ Lymphocyte Functional Analysis

CD4$^+$ lymphocytes were negatively selected from PBMC using magnetic cell sorting as recommended by the manufacturer (Miltenyi Biotec, Auburn, CA). Isolated cells (1x10^6 cells/ml) were cultured in medium containing 10% FBS in 24-well tissue culture plates for 3 days at 37 °C, 5% CO_2, in the presence or absence of stimulation antibodies reactive with CD2, CD3, and CD28 as recommended by the manufacturer (Miltenyi Biotec). Culture supernatants were measured by ELISA as recommended by the manufacturer (R&D Systems, Minneapolis, MN) for IL-2, IL-4, IL-10, and IFNγ. Harvested CD4$^+$ lymphocytes were examined for NFκB phospho-epitope staining by flow cytometry as previously described [10]. Briefly, 1x10^6 cells/well in 96 well plates were fixed using 1.5% paraformaldehyde, washed with PBS containing 1% BSA, and incubated at 4 °C for 10 min in 100μl ice-cold methanol. Cells were washed and incubated at 23 °C for 20 min with phosphoprotein-specific antibodies (BD Pharmingen and BD PhosFlow, San Diego, CA) directly conjugated with Alexa Fluor 647 (Molecular Probes Invitrogen, Carlsbad, CA).

RESULTS

CD4$^+$ Lymphocytes Increase and CD8$^+$ Lymphocytes Decrease in Response to α_1PI Replacement Therapy

To examine the interrelationship between α_1PI concentration and CD4$^+$ lymphocyte numbers, data were examined from a blinded study conducted to monitor hematologic changes following weekly infusions of α_1PI (60 mg/kg) in 11 individuals with genetic α_1PI deficiency (PI$_{ZZ}$) who had never before received α_1PI therapy. Treatment with α_1PI caused an increase in lymphocytes in 10 of these individuals (data not shown), suggesting that such treatment might benefit HIV-1$^+$ patients.

Two HIV-1 patients, Alpha and Beta at different stages of disease (Table **1**) received weekly infusions of 120 mg/kg α_1PI augmentation. Two additional HIV-1 patients, Gamma and Delta, with *a priori* evidence of abnormal immune status received the same therapy. The ability of Gamma to respond to antigen was impaired (positive PPD followed by negative PPD), and Delta exhibited systemic inflammation. Finally, 2 non-HIV-1 patients were included in the study, PI$_{ZZ}$-1 and PI$_{ZZ}$-2, who manifested normal numbers of CD4$^+$ lymphocytes and a diagnosis of emphysema in the context of genetic α_1PI deficiency. The PI$_{ZZ}$ patients received half-dose weekly infusions of 60 mg/kg α_1PI augmentation. Patients Delta and PI$_{ZZ}$-2 were included only in CD4$^+$ lymphocyte functional analyses (see Methods).

HIV-1$^+$ patients Alpha, Beta, and Gamma (Fig. **1**) and both PI$_{ZZ}$ patients (not depicted) responded to therapy with an initial burst of lymphocytes. After 2 wks of therapy, patients Alpha and Beta achieved normal numbers of CD4$^+$ lymphocytes with increases from 297 to 710 and from 276 to 393 cells/μl, respectively.

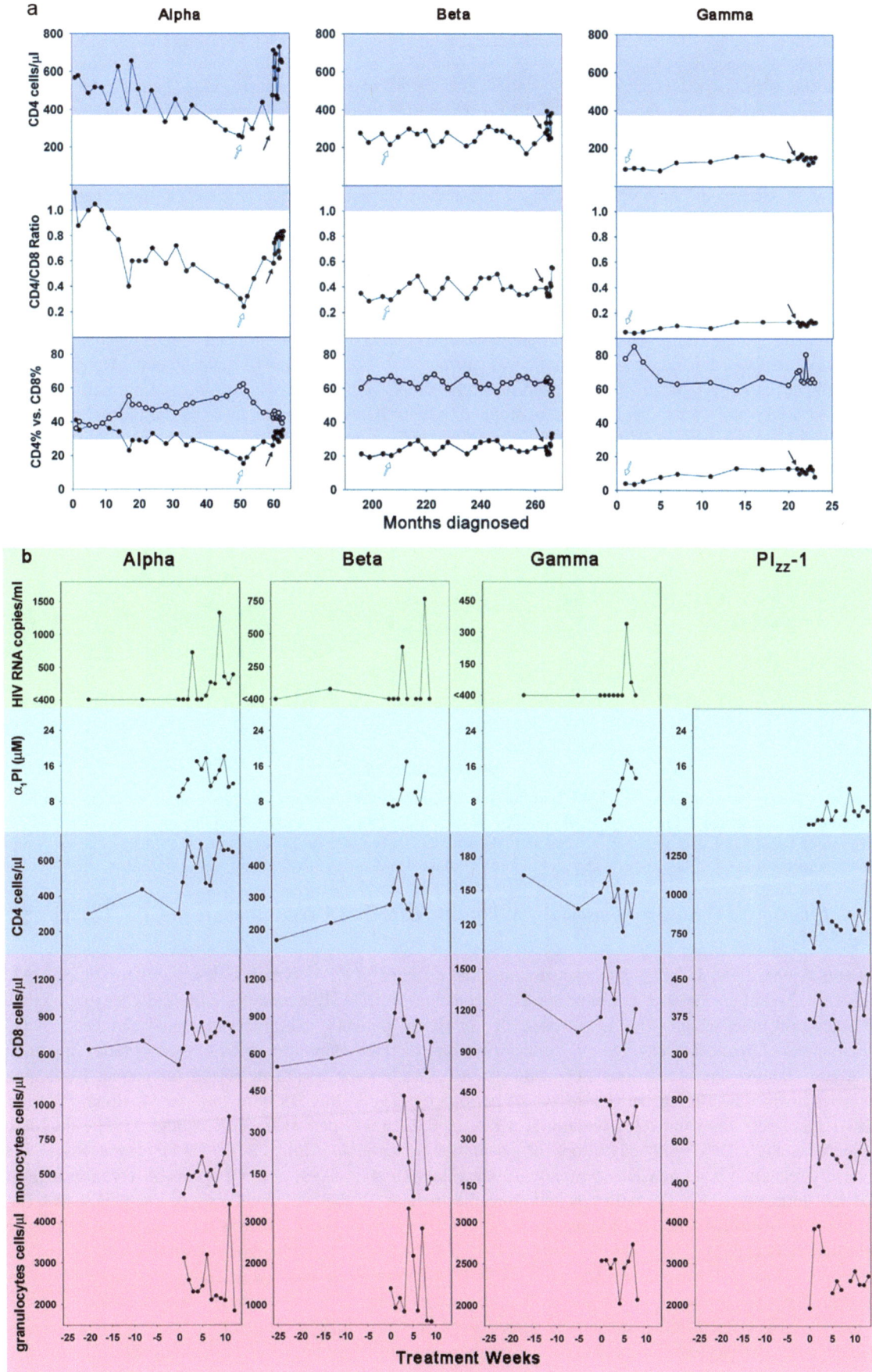

Figure 1: Corresponding cyclic variation in blood cells, α_1PI, and viral load in patients treated with α_1PI augmentation. Baseline CD4$^+$ lymphocyte levels were determined in patients Alpha, Beta, and Gamma to be 297, 276, and 148 cells/μl, respectively. Blood was collected prior to infusion, and each data point represents patient status at 7 days post-infusion such that wk 9 represents patient status after the 8th wk of treatment. **(a)** CD4$^+$ lymphocytes, CD4/CD8 ratios, and CD4% ($\bullet$) vs. the corresponding CD8% (o) are presented with respect to months of disease diagnosis. Shaded areas represent normal reference ranges for CD4, CD4/CD8 ratio, and CD4%. Black arrows designate initiation of Zemaira$^{®}$ treatment. White arrows designate initiation of antiretroviral therapy. **(b)** Patients Alpha, Beta, Gamma, and PI$_{ZZ}$-1 were monitored weekly for changes in blood cell subtypes and serum levels of α_1PI. HIV-1$^+$ patients were monitored for changes in HIV RNA. Treatment wk 0 represents baseline pre-treatment values. In some instances, blood samples were not acceptable for measuring blood cells, HIV RNA, or α_1PI due to delay in sample delivery or hemolysis, and these are depicted as gaps in the line graphs.

Patients PI$_{ZZ}$-1 and PI$_{ZZ}$-2 increased from 743 to 954 and from 899 to 1024 cells/μl, respectively. Patient Beta, who had never exhibited CD4$^+$ lymphocytes in the normal range in more than 20 years, even continued to exhibit the normal range of CD4$^+$ lymphocytes 2 wks after treatment stopped with 382 cells/μl. Using regression analysis, this duration of benefit was attributed to α_1PI therapy (Fig. **2**). Patient Alpha who was first infected 5 years prior to the study had not exhibited CD4$^+$ lymphocytes within the normal range in 2 years. At 5 wks and 14 wks after treatment stopped, patient Alpha continued to be in the normal range with 470 cells/μl. By regression analysis, this duration of benefit appeared to be related to antiretroviral medication as well as α_1PI therapy (Fig. **2**). Patient Gamma, who was known to have lost immune function, showed an increase from 148 to 167 cells/μl and never achieved normal numbers of CD4$^+$ lymphocytes.

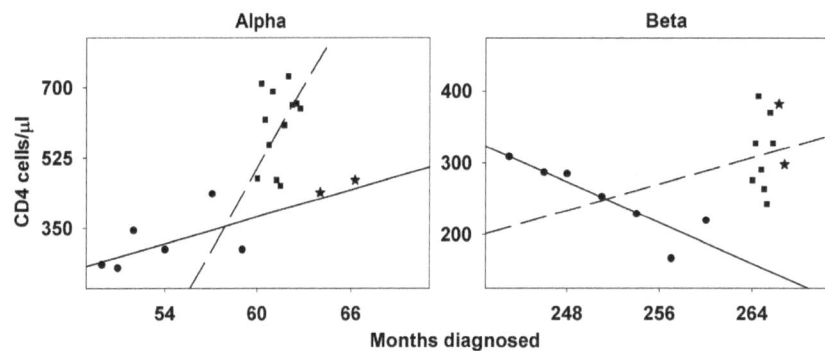

Figure 2: Duration of increase in CD4$^+$ lymphocytes following α_1PI therapy. Comparison of the change in CD4$^+$ lymphocytes represented in Fig. **1** before ($\bullet$), during ($\blacksquare$), and after ($\bigstar$) α_1PI augmentation therapy demonstrates that the duration of benefit is 1 or 2 weeks post-treatment (Patient Beta), but not 5 or 14 weeks post-treatment (Patient Alpha). Linear regression of CD4$^+$ lymphocyte changes before (solid line) and during (dashed line) show significant improvement.

CD4$^+$ Lymphocyte Cycling is Sinusoidal. All Patients Exhibited Cyclic Changes in CD4$^+$ Lymphocytes (Fig. 3).

Patients Alpha, Beta, and PI$_{ZZ}$-1 exhibited sinusoidal changes in CD4$^+$ lymphocytes with periodicity 23±3.5 days (Fig. **3**). Patient Gamma exhibited sinusoidal changes in CD4$^+$ lymphocytes with periodicity of 15 days. Of important note, patient PI$_{ZZ}$-1, but none of the HIV-1 patients, exhibited sinusoidal changes in CD8$^+$ lymphocytes. In patient Alpha, the sinusoidal wave was damped exhibiting decreased amplitude. In patients Beta and Gamma, the oscillations sloped downward. The 5 week treatment period for patient PIzz-2 was insufficient for determining the occurrence of periodicity. The CD4/CD8 ratio in patients Alpha, Beta, and PIzz-1 increased following α1PI therapy at a rate of 0.02±0.008 per week (Figs. **1** and **3**). The degree of increase in the CD4+ lymphocyte axis of oscillation in patients Alpha, Beta, Gamma, and PI$_{ZZ}$-1 was inversely related to baseline CD8+ lymphocyte percentage (n=4, r^2=0.99, p<0.008). This observation suggests that the improved CD4/CD8 ratio resulted from the increase in the horizontal axis of oscillation of CD4+ lymphocytes as well as the longitudinal decrease in CD8+ lymphocytes. There was no sustained increase or decrease in B cells (CD19+ lymphocytes), NK cells (CD16+/56+ lymphocytes), granulocytes, monocytes, eosinophils, basophils, or platelets (data not shown). However, there were cyclic changes in all cell types, as illustrated by the levels of monocytes and granulocytes (Fig. **1**, lower panels). Granulocytes, NK cells, basophils, eosinophils, and platelets, all derive from myeloid-lineage progenitors and cycled in tandem. Monocytes are of myeloid lineage, but cycled independently of lymphocytes and granulocytes.

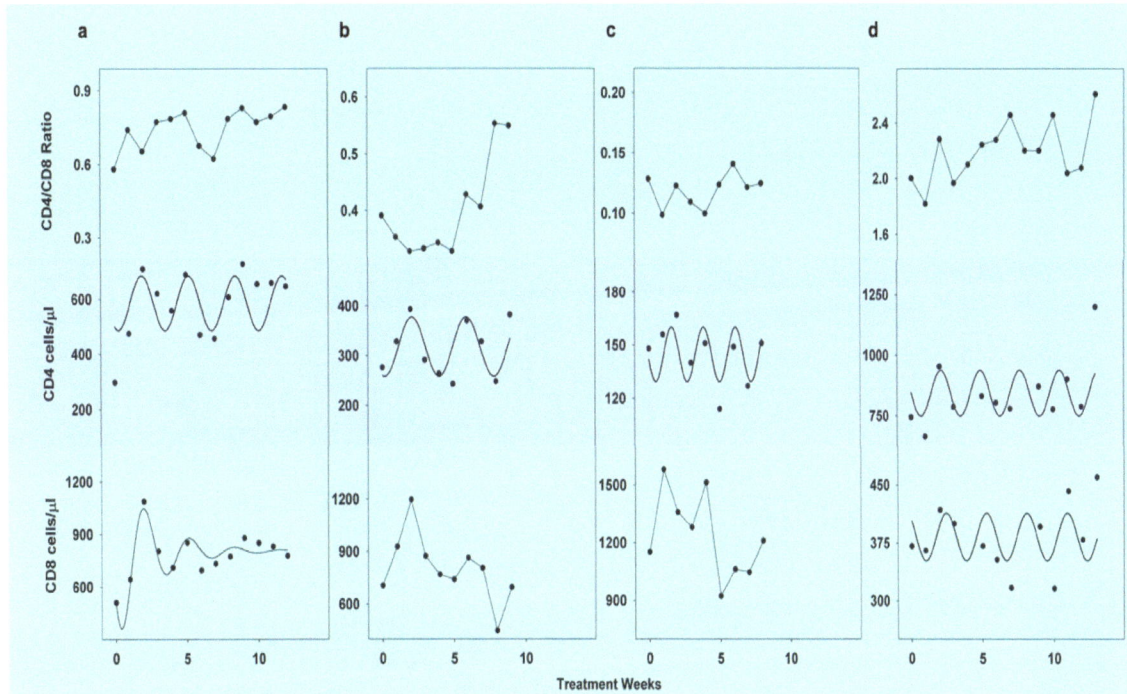

Figure 3: Sinusoidal analysis of CD4⁺ and CD8⁺ lymphocytes and the corresponding increase in CD4/CD8 ratio.
Sinusoidal curve fit analyses were performed using CD4 and CD8 data from patients Alpha **(a)**, Beta **(b)**, Gamma **(c)** and
PI_{ZZ}-1 **(d)** over the course of Zemaira® therapy. CD4⁺ lymphocyte oscillation is defined by $f(x) = y_0 + a * \sin[(2\pi x/b)+c]$
where y_0 = axis of oscillation, a = amplitude, x = days in treatment, b = wavelength, and c = phase shift from day 0. Each
sine curve has a fit of $r^2 > 0.99$, $\alpha = 0.05$, power of test = 1.0, and each variable contributed to the equation with $p < 0.02$ with
the exception of patient Gamma's CD4 data where amplitude contributed to the equation with $p < 0.07$. CD8 data for
patients Beta and Gamma did not fit a sine curve. CD4 sine wave values determined for each patient (y_0,a): Alpha
(585,100), Beta (318,59), Gamma (145,15), PI_{ZZ}-1 (814,92). By sigmoidal regression, greater amplitude is correlated with
a greater axis of oscillation, $r^2 = 0.999$, and a greater pre-treatment CD4/CD8 ratio is correlated with a greater post-
treatment axis of oscillation, $r^2 = 0.999$.

Expanded CD4⁺ Lymphocytes are Phenotypcially Mature and Respond to Stimulation.

Glucocorticoids cause the release of granulocytes and lymphocytes from tissue, but the peak increase occurs
within 6 hrs and dissipates within 24 hrs [11]. Glucocorticoid-induced demarginalized lymphocytes are
unresponsive to stimulation. To determine whether α_1PI-mobilized CD4⁺ lymphocyte populations were
functional, CD4⁺ lymphocytes were isolated from blood and cultured in stimulation media. Harvested culture
supernatants were quantitated for a panel of cytokines representing subpopulations of CD4⁺ lymphocytes,
specifically IL-2 (Th1), IL-4 (Th2 + NKT), IL-10 (Th2), and IFNγ (Th1 + NKT).

Harvested cells were examined for NFκB activation. Whether isolated from HIV-1 uninfected volunteers or
from HIV-1 patients pre-treatment or under treatment, CD4⁺ lymphocyte populations were equivalently
capable of being stimulated (Table **2**, Fig. **4**).

CD4⁺ lymphocytes in whole blood were analyzed by FACS analysis for phenotypic markers characteristic of
mature and immature, activated and quiescent cells including CD34 (stem cells), CD8 (double positive and
double negative immature cells), CD45RA (naïve cells), CD45RO (memory cells), CD25 (IL-2Rα activated
cells and thymocytes), CXCR4 and CCR5 (HIV-1 tropism-determining chemokine receptors). Patients Alpha
and PIzz-1 expressed significantly greater CD4⁺CD45RA⁺ naïve cells than did the HIV-1
uninfectedvolunteers (Fig. **4b**). In parallel, patient Alpha and PIzz-1 as well as PI_{ZZ}-2 expressed significantly
lower CD4⁺CD45RO⁺ memory cells than the HIV-1 uninfected volunteers. However, these differences did
not appear to be related to α_1PI therapy since the percentage of naïve and memory cells remained steady in
each patient throughout therapy. All other surface markers measured were normal (not depicted). These
results suggest that the phenotypic profile of CD4⁺ lymphocytes unique to each individual was maintained
within the new generation of lymphocytes.

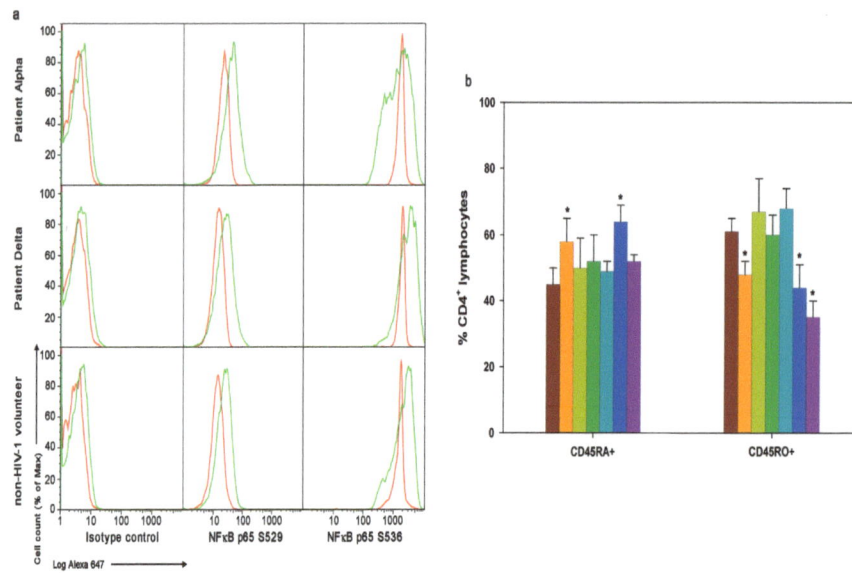

Figure 4: Functional characteristics of expanded CD4$^+$ lymphocytes. a) NFκB phosphorylataion in response to stimulation of the T cell antigen receptor complex. Isolated CD4$^+$ T cells were cultured at 10^6 cells/ml for 3 days in the presence of antibodies reactive with CD2, CD3, and CD28. Cells from patient Alpha were isolated after 11 weeks of Zemaira$^®$ therapy. Cells from patient Delta were isolated at baseline. Culture supernatants were simultaneously measured for cytokine release (Table **2**). b) Percentage of immature, naïve (CD4$^+$CD45RA$^+$), and memory (CD4$^+$CD45RO$^+$) T cells. Phenotypic analysis was performed at 3-8 different time points during therapy using blood collected from patients Alpha (■), Beta (■), Gamma (■), Delta (■), PI$_{ZZ}$-1 (■), PI$_{ZZ}$-2 (■), and non-HIV-1 controls (■). Values represent mean and standard deviation. Stars (✳) indicate statistical differences with respect to non-HIV-1 control values, $p<0.001$ and power of test $\alpha > 0.99$.

DISCUSSION

The processes that renew the adult human CD4$^+$ lymphocyte population are poorly understood and the sinusoidal changes we observed may offer insight into the renewal mechanisms. While cyclic variation in circulating CD4$^+$ lymphocytes has not been previously described, cyclic neutropenia occurs with an average 21-28 day periodicity and is caused by mutations in the α_1PI receptor, HLE$_{CS}$ [12]. The α_1PI-induced *in situ* proliferation of CD4$^+$ lymphocytes (24-48 h) [13] or the release of functional CD4$^+$ lymphocytes from lymph tissue into circulation as occurs in an acute phase reaction (4-24 h) [14] may explain cycling, but neither of these explanations account for the 2 wk lag in appearance and 23 day periodicity. Rather, a multi-step process is implied.

In adult mice, thymopoiesis is a multi-step process defined by a 21-day cycle. The process involves the cyclic accumulation of progenitor cells in the adult bone marrow (3-5 wk), export of progenitor cells from the bone marrow thereby vacating the bone marrow niche (~1 wk), temporally coordinated importation of progenitor cells into the finite niche of the thymus, positive selection, release of mature T cells and progenitor cells into blood, and repopulation of the bone marrow niche at the end of the cycle [15].

Table 2: Stimulated T cell cytokine release. Cytokines were measured in culture supernatants harvested from isolated CD4$^+$ T cells stimulated by antibodies reactive with CD2, CD3, and CD28. Harvested CD4$^+$ T cells were simultaneously monitored for NFκB activation (Fig. **4**). In two attempts, the number of CD4$^+$ lymphocytes isolated from Patient Gamma was insufficient for stimulation analysis. Cytokines were undetectable in serum or culture supernatants from unstimulated CD4$^+$ T cells with the exception of Patient Delta who exhibited 51 pg IL-2/ml in his baseline serum sample, and Patient Beta who exhibited 14 pg IL-10/ml in serum at treatment week 8. ^{2}not determined.

Patient	Treatment Week	IL-2 (pg/ml)	IL-4 (pg/ml)	IL-10 (pg/ml)	INFγ (pg/ml)
Alpha	11	>800	<31.2	148	>500
Beta	6	792	<31.2	<7.8	>500
Delta	untreated	>800	<31.2	n.d.^{2}	>500
non-HIV-1	untreated	>800	<31.2	239	>500

When positive selection of $CD4^+$ thymocytes is impaired, the number of $CD4^+$ lymphocytes diminishes by up to 80% [16], and as a consequence the number of $CD8^+$ lymphocytes increases thereby producing a decreased CD4/CD8 ratio [16, 17].

In the analogous human system, HLE_{CS}, CXCR4, and CXCL12 are required for progenitor cells to vacate bone marrow [2, 18].

In the present study, a lower pre-treatment CD8 percentage was inversely correlated with α_1PI–induced expansion of $CD4^+$ lymphocytes as would be expected if treatment had re-established positive selection.

Thus, we propose that the observed α_1PI–induced changes in $CD4^+$ and $CD8^+$ lymphocyte numbers resulted from the binding of α_1PI to the $CXCR4/HLE_{CS}/CXCL12$ complex during cell migration thereby facilitating adult thymopoiesis. In contrast to all other patients in the study who exhibited a 3-week cycle, patient Gamma exhibited a 2-week cycle suggesting some parts of the thymopoiesis cycle were intact, but that at least one step was impaired. This patient was documented to have lost the ability to respond to PPD which is a T lymphocyte-mediated response and is clinically interpreted to mean loss of immune function. In support of this hypothesis, there was no evidence of increased numbers of T lymphocytes in this patient suggesting that progenitor cells were being released from bone marrow, but not establishing residence in the stem cell niche of the thymus.

The phenomenon that PI_{ZZ} patients exhibit deficient hepatocyte-synthesized α_1PI from birth, yet manifest normal numbers of $CD4^+$ lymphocytes suggests there are additional considerations during fetal thymic selection, possibly the thymic or stromal supply of α_1PI.

Both myeloid and lymphoid cells are known to synthesize α_1PI in bone marrow [19, 20] Alternatively, the role of α_1PI in hematopoiesis might be supplanted by other proteinase inhibitors during fetal development.

The duration of benefit for 2 wks, but not 5 wks, post-treatment suggests α_1PI augmentation might be effective with less frequent than weekly administration. Our results predict that α_1PI augmentation may overcome a localized pathologic system thereby allowing the immune system to recover and regain production of normal numbers of $CD4^+$ lymphocytes in a subset of $HIV-1^+$ patients who are on antiretroviral therapy and have functioning lymphatic and hematopoietic tissue.

ACKNOWLDEGEMENTS

We wish to thank CSL Behring for contributing Zemaira®; BioReferences Laboratories for performing routine patient analyses; M.A. Reeves for data analysis; P Quartararo and Dr. M. Murtiashaw for manuscript advice; the many volunteers and patients who participated by contributing their time and blood for this study; the Infusion/Transfusion Unit nurses and Drs. A. Distenfeld, E. Medina, and M. LaBrunda for assisting with patient follow-up. This study was supported by the Harry Winston Research Foundation.

AUTHOR INFORMATION

V.R. is Senior Vice President of Research and Development, CSL Behring. All other authors declare no competing financial interest.

REFERENCES

[1]   Cepinskas G, Sandig M, Kvietys PR. PAF-induced elastase-dependent neutrophil transendothelial migration is associated with the mobilization of elastase to the neutrophil surface and localization to the migrating front. J Cell Sci. 1999;112 (Pt 12):1937-1945.

[2]   Lapidot T, Petit I. Current understanding of stem cell mobilization: the roles of chemokines, proteolytic enzymes, adhesion molecules, cytokines, and stromal cells. Experimental hematology. 2002;30(9):973-981.

[3]   Bristow CL, Mercatante DR, Kole R. HIV-1 preferentially binds receptors copatched with cell-surface elastase. Blood. 2003;102(13):4479-4486.

[4]   Cao C, Lawrence DA, Li Y, Von Arnim CA, Herz J, Su EJ, *et al.* Endocytic receptor LRP together with tPA and PAI-1 coordinates Mac-1-dependent macrophage migration. The EMBO journal. 2006;25(9):1860-1870.

[5]   Kounnas MZ, Church FC, Argraves WS, Strickland DK. Cellular internalization and degradation of antithrombin III-thrombin, heparin cofactor II-thrombin, and alpha 1-antitrypsin-trypsin complexes is mediated by the low density lipoprotein receptor-related protein. The Journal of biological chemistry. 1996;271(11):6523-6529.

[6]   Bristow CL, Patel H, Arnold RR. Self antigen prognostic for human immunodeficiency virus disease progression. Clinical and diagnostic laboratory immunology. 2001;8(5):937-942.

[7]   Huber R, Carrell RW. Implications of the three-dimensional structure of alpha 1-antitrypsin for structure and function of serpins. Biochemistry. 1989;28(23):8951-8966.

[8]   Bayer H. Prolastin Product Monograph.: www.talecris.com 2003.

[9]   Bristow CL, Di Meo F, Arnold RR. Specific activity of alpha1proteinase inhibitor and alpha2macroglobulin in human serum: application to insulin-dependent diabetes mellitus. Clinical immunology and immunopathology. 1998;89(3):247-259.

[10] Krutzik PO, Nolan GP. Fluorescent cell barcoding in flow cytometry allows high-throughput drug screening and signaling profiling. Nature methods. 2006;3(5):361-368.

[11] Chrousos G. Adrenocorticoids & Adrenocortical Antagonists. In: Katzung B, ed. *Basic & Clinical Pharmacology*: McGraw-Hill Companies. 2007.

[12] Horwitz M, Benson KF, Person RE, Aprikyan AG, Dale DC. Mutations in ELA2, encoding neutrophil elastase, define a 21-day biological clock in cyclic haematopoiesis. Nature genetics. 1999;23(4):433-436.

[13] Congote LF, Temmel N. The C-terminal 26-residue peptide of serpin A1 stimulates proliferation of breast and liver cancer cells: role of protein kinase C and CD47. FEBS letters. 2004;576(3):343-347.

[14] Mehigan BJ, Hartley JE, Drew PJ, Saleh A, Dore PC, Lee PW, *et al.* Changes in T cell subsets, interleukin-6 and C-reactive protein after laparoscopic and open colorectal resection for malignancy. Surgical endoscopy. 2001;15(11):1289-1293.

[15] Donskoy E, Foss D, Goldschneider I. Gated importation of prothymocytes by adult mouse thymus is coordinated with their periodic mobilization from bone marrow. J Immunol. 2003;171(7):3568-3575.

[16] Nakagawa T, Roth W, Wong P, Nelson A, Farr A, Deussing J, *et al.* Cathepsin L: critical role in Ii degradation and CD4 T cell selection in the thymus. Science. 1998;280(5362):450-453.

[17] He X, Kappes DJ. CD4/CD8 lineage commitment: light at the end of the tunnel? Current opinion in immunology. 2006;18(2):135-142.

[18] Tavor S, Petit I, Porozov S, Goichberg P, Avigdor A, Sagiv S, *et al.* Motility, proliferation, and egress to the circulation of human AML cells are elastase dependent in NOD/SCID chimeric mice. Blood. 2005;106(6):2120-2127.

[19] Bashir MS, Morrison K, Wright DH, Jones DB. Alpha-1 antitrypsin gene exon use in stimulated lymphocytes. Journal of clinical pathology. 1992;45(9):776-780.

[20] Winkler IG, Hendy J, Coughlin P, Horvath A, Levesque JP. Serine protease inhibitors serpina1 and serpina3 are down-regulated in bone marrow during hematopoietic progenitor mobilization. The Journal of experimental medicine. 2005;201(7):1077-1088.

CHAPTER 7

Vitamin D and HIV Infection

Joan Fibla[1,*] and Antonio Caruz[2]

[1]*Human Genetics Unit, Department of Basic Medical Sciences. Universitat de Lleida. IRB-LLEIDA. Montserrat Roig, 2 25199-Lleida, Catalonia, Spain and* [2]*Immunogenetics Unit, Faculty of Sciences, Universidad de Jaén, Pasaje Las Lagunillas s/n 23071-Jaén, Spain.*

Abstract: Among environmental factors related to pathogen infection, vitamin D is largely considered to be protective and promoter of good health. For these reasons, a general concern exists about vitamin D insufficiency that has been found around world reaching epidemic dimensions. In the last few years, interest about the role of vitamin D on immune response has been increased after encouraging data illustrated the well-known contribution of the binomial sunlight exposure/vitamin D on protection to mycobacterium infections. The vitamin D mediated induction of microbicide factors against bacterial infections runs in parallel with the vitamin D immunosuppressant activity induced to control the exacerbation of the cellular immune response. These complementary effects can be modulated to guarantee a correct vitamin D action. Concerning HIV infection a protective role can be expected from the vitamin D mediated microbicide activity, but no single effects can be deduced from the vitamin D immunosuppressant activity. In addition, the direct effects of vitamin D by promoting HIV replication can act as a confounding factor when trying to understand the role of vitamin D in HIV infection. In the present review we have evaluated available bibliography of vitamin D action on the immune system response crossing it with data on HIV immunopathology trying to find common pathways that can shed light on the role of vitamin D on HIV infection and disease progression to AIDS.

INTRODUCTION

In addition to its role on mineral metabolism, vitamin D has pleiotropic effects on the control of cell proliferation and on the modulation of immune responses [1-3]. Following the activation of vitamin D precursors in the skin by the exposure to sunlight and their biochemical transformation in the liver, vitamin D acquires full active form after been converted to 1-α-25-dihydroxyvitamin D3 (1,25(OH)$_2$D3) by the kidney enzyme 25-hydroxyvitamin D3 1-α-hydroxylase (CYP27B1) [4]. At the molecular level vitamin D interacts with the nuclear receptor, vitamin D receptor (VDR) that acts as a transcription factor activating or repressing specific genes [5].

Although the immunomodulatory response triggered by active vitamin D was first reported more than 25 years ago, a growing body of experimental evidence has been obtained in the last decade, supporting a key role of vitamin D in the control of both innate and acquired immune responses [6-8]. Both CYP27B1 and VDR are expressed by several immune cells, such as macrophages (MAC), dendritic cells (DC) and lymphocytes. This allows these cells to synthesize and respond to vitamin D in an autocrine/paracrine circuit involved in the modulation of the immune response [6]. The active vitamin D hormone stimulates the innate immune response in MAC and DC, while at the same time acts to squelch any excessive reaction in the adaptive immune response to the antigen. These contrasting effects confer to the vitamin D endocrine system, a central role in the modulation of the immune responses, being responsible of a proper and well-dimensioned response.

In the present review we have emphasized the involvement of vitamin D on infectious diseases, and specifically on HIV infection and disease progression to AIDS. A potential role of vitamin D on HIV infection has been previously considered, either evaluating sun light exposure [9] or taking into consideration HIV infected patients characterized by vitamin D insufficiency [10-14]. A growing body of evidence supports the role of vitamin D as a protection factor in intracellular pathogen infection, such as mycobacterium, through

---

***Address Correspondence to this Author Dr. Joan Fibla at:** Human Genetics Unit, Department of Basic Medical Sciences. Universitat de Lleida. IRB-LLEIDA. Montserrat Roig, 2 25199-Lleida, Catalonia, Spain E-mail: joan.fibla@cmb.udl.cat*

activation of innate immune response [15], despite vitamin D has been found detrimental in *Leishmania* infection by interfering with key functions of interferon (IFN)-γ activated macrophages [16]. In addition, direct effects of vitamin D promoting HIV replication have been described [17,18] and associated studies of *VDR* gene polymorphism seem to indicate that gene variants that hamper VDR-mediated activity are associated with susceptibility to infection and disease progression to AIDS [19- 22].

VITAMIN D SOURCES AND ENDOGENOUS SYNTHESIS

Vitamin D is a secosteroid hormone that has pleiotropic effects on the regulation of mineral metabolism and the modulation of the immune response [1, 2]. Sources of vitamin D come from dietary intake of foods that are rich in vitamin D, such as fish liver oils and egg yolks, and from endogenous synthesis by photolysis reaction in the skin (Fig. **1**).

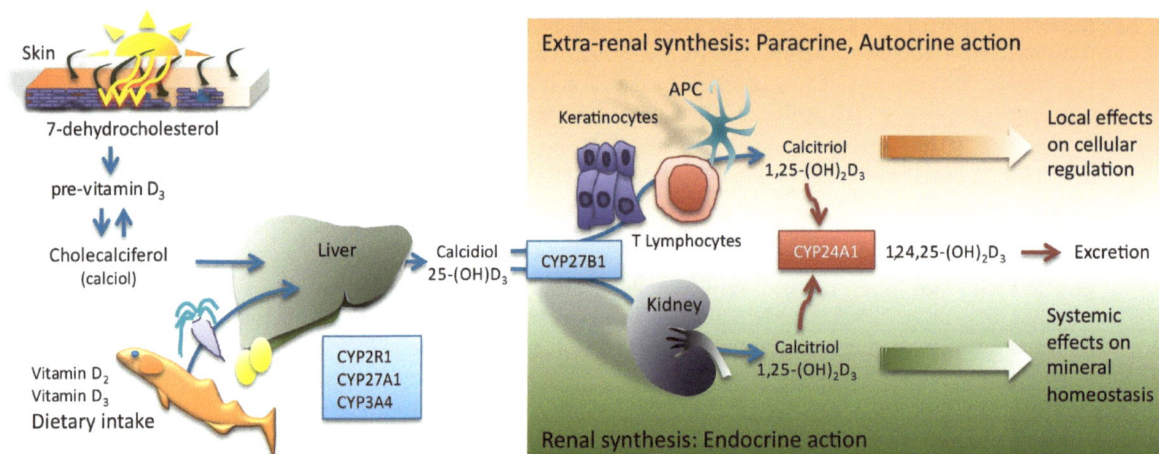

Figure 1: Vitamin D synthesis. Ultraviolet radiation acts on 7-dehydrocholesterol in human skin to form the pre-vitamin D3, that after thermogenic isomerisation forms cholecalciferol (calciol). In addition, vitamin D2 and vitamin D3 can be supplied via food intake. Active vitamin D3 is formed by two sequential hydroxylations in the liver and kidney, to produce 25(OH)D3 (calcidiol) and 1,25(OH)$_2$D3 (calcitriol), respectively. In addition to renal vitamin D synthesis, other tissues and cell types, such as keratinocytes, APC (MAC and DC) and other immune system cells have the capability to produce the active hormone. Vitamin D produced in extra-renal tissues acts locally in a paracrine/autocrine manner and usually does not contribute to the hormone levels in circulation.

There are two main forms of vitamin D used by the human body, vitamin D2 and vitamin D3, which have a chemical structure closely related to the cholesterol molecule. Ultraviolet radiation (UVB), at the 290-315 nm wavelength, alters the cholesterol-based precursor 7-dehydrocholesterol in human skin by breaking C-9 and C-10 of the B ring to form the pre-vitamin D3. Following this, naturally occurring thermogenic isomerisation give rise to the unhydroxylated vitamin D3 form cholecalciferol (calciol) that is biologically inactive. In a similar way, vitamin D2 is formed from the irradiation of ergosterol, a plant sterol that can be ingested within the diet. Endogenously produced vitamin D3 can be selectively transported in the bloodstream by vitamin D binding protein (DBP) to target cells of the vitamin D endocrine system for metabolism. In addition, vitamin D3 supplied by the diet can be absorbed through the duodenum and transported into the lymph via chylomicrons. To reach its active form vitamin D3 undergoes two sequential hydroxylations. First, hydroxylated onto the C-25 group by the monooxygenases, mainly P450 cytochrome sterol 27-hydroxylase (CYP27A1), to produce the major circulating vitamin D form, 25-hydroxycholecalciferol (25(OH)D3) also known as calcidiol. This 25(OH) D3 is then transported to the kidney by DBP where it is further hydroxylated onto C-1.

This key step is performed in the proximal tubular cells of the nephron by P450 cytochrome 25-hydroxyvitamin D3 1-α-hydroxylase (CYP27B1) enzyme to produce (1,25(OH)$_2$D3), also known as calcitriol, that corresponds to the "active" or "hormonal" form of vitamin D. Calcitriol plays an essential role in stimulating an intestinal absorption of calcium and phosphorus ions, in the mobilization of calcium from bone, and in renal resorption of calcium [23]. While the liver conversion of vitamin D3 to 25(OH)D3 is not actively regulated, the conversion of 25(OH)D3 to the active $1,25(OH)_2D3$ form is tightly regulated in the kidney by parathyroid hormone (PTH), calcium and phosphorus levels. In response to low calcium and elevated phosphorous, PTH is released by the parathyroid gland to stimulate calcium resorption and to activate CYP27B1 to synthesize more $1,25(OH)_2D3$. Over-production of $1,25(OH)_2D3$ is regulated by a negative feedback loop, in that $1,25(OH)_2D3$ inhibits PTH synthesis and induces 1,25-dihydroxyvitamin D3 24-hydroxylase (CYP24A1) activity in a very sensitive manner [24]. CYP24A1 participates in the $1,25(OH)_2D3$ catabolism by incorporating a hydroxyl group on C-24 allowing its secretion in the bile.

In addition to renal vitamin D synthesis, other tissues and cell types have the capability to convert 25(OH)D3 to the active $1,25(OH)_2D3$ form. This conversion is due to the activity of CYP27B1, the same enzyme that is present in the kidney. Extra-renal synthesis was first reported in studies of granulomatous diseases such as sarcoidosis, characterised by an ectopic over production of $1,25(OH)_2D3$. Primary cultures of pulmonary alveolar MAC of patients with sarcoidosis showed a significant level of conversion of 25(OH)D3 to $1,25(OH)_2D3$, but, in contrast to renal conversion, macrophage CYP27B1 activity did not respond to the $1,25(OH)_2D3$ dependent negative regulation, being sensitive to the up-regulation by IFN-γ [25]. This explains that the observed overproduction of $1,25(OH)_2D3$ and the associated hypocalcaemia that characterises the severe forms of this disease, besides indicate a distinct regulation for the extra-renal enzyme. Extra-renal sites for CYP27B1 expression include skin, endothelium, lymphoid organs, decidua, parathyroid, pancreas, adrenal medulla, colon and cerebellum [26]. Expression of CYP27B1 activity has also been described in normal MAC [27] and other antigen presenting cells such as DC [28] and Langerhan cell (LC) [29]. In addition, T lymphocytes obtained by bronchoalveolar lavage of patients suffering from granulomatous disease such as tuberculosis [30] and T Cell Lymphotrophic Virus-I-transformed Lymphocytes [31] have been shown to produce $1,25(OH)_2D3$. The functional hormone produced in extra-renal target tissues acts locally in a paracrine/autocrine manner and usually does not contribute to the hormone levels in circulation.

Autonomous synthesis of vitamin D, from 7-dehydrocholesterol to $1,25(OH)_2D3$, can be achieved in the skin keratinocytes as they can perform the sequential hydroxylation at both C-25 on previtamin D3 to be converted to 25(OH)D3 and at C-1 to transform it to the $1,25(OH)_2D3$ active form [32]. This autonomous vitamin D3 pathway has also been reported in intestinal CaCo-2 and myeloid THP-1 cell lines [33]. Recently, it has been described that also human primary MAC and DC are also able to perform both hydroxylation steps on vitamin D3 precursor, allowing these cells to develop an autonomous production of active vitamin D [34].

This autonomous production of the hormone could be of vital importance for tissues with limited availability of 25(OH)D3 and $1,25(OH)_2D3$. To reach keratinocytes in the deeper layers of the epidermis 25(OH)D3-carrier complexes must cross from low vascularised stratums. Under these circumstances the low concentration of 25(OH)D3 could impair enough synthesis of the functional hormone. Total serum concentrations of $1,25(OH)_2D3$ are in the range of 10^{-11} to 10^{-10} M, being too low to induce hormonal response on target cells, such as skin keratinocytes in peripheral tissues [35]. Even more if we consider that nearly 99% of serum calcitriol is bound to carrier, which means that less than 1% of serum calcitriol, corresponding to a "functional" concentration of 10^{-13} M, remains free and is able to induce hormonal response.

The autonomous capacity of keratinocytes to produce functional hormone from vitamin D3 precursor can overcome this limitation. High levels of vitamin D precursors are present in the skin (from UVB photochemical activation) that could be incorporated in the autonomous production of functional $1,25(OH)_2D3$ in keratinocytes, dermal MAC and DC. In addition, ingested vitamin D precursors can serve as substrate for the autonomous production of functional $1,25(OH)_2D3$ in MAC and DC from the gastrointestinal tract. Therefore, the direct local conversion of vitamin D precursors to functional hormone in the skin and gut could overcome the limited access to the systemic hormone. This could be essential for these two "barrier" systems to enable an appropriate vitamin D dependent innate immune response.

GENOMIC AND RAPID RESPONSE PATHWAY TO VITAMIN D

Genomic and rapid response pathways to vitamin D have been described on target cells. While slow response normally takes hours to days to reach full manifestation, being dependent on new protein synthesis, rapid response to $1,25(OH)_2D3$ only needs seconds to minutes to become manifested, being unaffected by inhibitors of transcription and translation. Genomic responses are initiated upon the interaction between vitamin D compound and nuclear VDR, whereas the rapid response pathway has been related to a putative $1,25(OH)_2D3$ membrane-associated rapid response steroid-binding protein (MARRS).

Evidence for a Vitamin D membrane Receptor

The rapid-acting response has been observed in several contexts as fast intestinal absorption of calcium, secretion of insulin by pancreatic cells, rapid migration of endothelial cells and opening of $Ca2^+$ and Cl⁻ voltage-gated channels in osteoclasts. This rapid and non-genomic related response seems to be mediated by the activation of signal transduction pathways, including protein kinase C, cAMP, intracellular calcium and MAP kinase [36] in target cells through a putative cell membrane-associated receptor for $1,25(OH)_2D3$. The nature of the membrane receptor for vitamin D has been extensively debated with some authors arguing that the "classical" nuclear VDR could act as the membrane receptor being responsible for the vitamin D rapid response [37]. Recent reports also proposed that an alternate pocket conformation in the ligand-binding domain of the nuclear VDR is involved in the rapid response [38]. A candidate for the rapid response-related membrane binding protein/receptor for $1,25(OH)_2D3$ was isolated from chicken intestinal basolateral membrane [39] and also detected in mammalian cell membranes [40, 41], termed MARRS for membrane-associated rapid-response to steroid. The $1,25(OH)_2D3$-MARRS protein has no sequence similarity with the nuclear VDR. Characterisation of chicken MARRS cDNA sequence reveals it to be identical to the multifunctional protein ERp57, also known as Protein disulfide-isomerase A3 precursor (PDIA3) [40], a protein conserved among several species. ERp57/PDIA3/1,25D3-MARRS receptor is a member of the protein disulphide-isomerase (PDI) family of oxidoreductases that contains two redox domains. ERp57 works in a variety of cellular processes and functions. PDIs are involved in native disulphide bond formation of glycoproteins in the endoplasmic reticulum (ER), acting as chaperone proteins. PDIs participate in the antigen presentation process facilitating the formation of disulphide bonds in the nascent MHC class I heavy chains [42,43] and the mentioned 1,25D3-MARRS receptor function [44]. Besides ER, PDIs are present in plasma membrane rafts, cytosol and nucleus [45]. The reducing activity on disulfide bonds mediated by the cell surface PDIs seems to be related with the infective capacity of certain viruses, such as the Sindbis virus [46] and HIV [47]. Thiol-disulfide exchange reactions have been described to be crucial during cell penetration by virus disrupting the rigid protein-protein associations of the envelope and facilitating membrane fusion and release of the viral genome into the cell [46].

Antibodies against PDI and inhibitors of disulphide isomerase activity have been described to interfere with virus-host membrane fusion. It has been proved that thiol-disulphide interchange mediates HIV-target cell fusion. Reduction of critical disulphides in viral envelope glycoproteins may be the initial event that triggers conformational changes required for HIV entry [47]. Although, it has yet to be determined whether, and to what extent, these PDI mediated phenomena are affected by the interaction with vitamin D endocrine system.

Nuclear Vitamin D Receptor

Genomic actions of the vitamin D on target cells are mediated by the nuclear VDR, which belongs to the family of steroid-hormone receptors [48]. Full length VDR protein has a molecular weight of 48 kDa that shows nuclear localization motif and several functional domains such as ligand-binding domain to the hormone, DNA-binding domain that binds to the vitamin D response elements (VDREs) located in the promoter region of target genes, dimerization domain which allows its binding with partner retinoic X receptor and transactivation domain that mediates transcriptional activation (Fig. **2**).

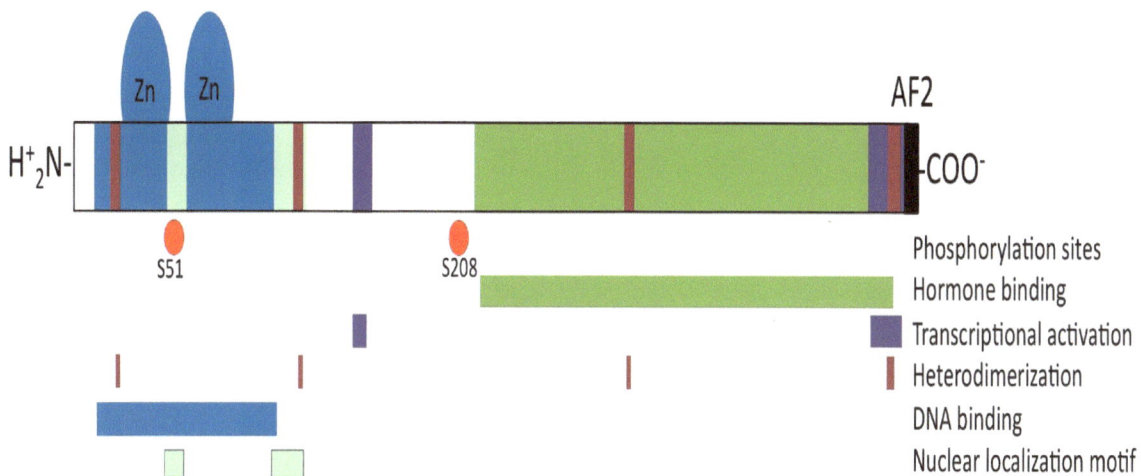

Figure 2: Schematic structure of the vitamin D receptor. VDR protein holds several functional domains. Nuclear localization motifs and DNA binding domain with two zinc fingers motifs are located at the N-terminal region. Hormone-binding domain is located along C-terminal half of the molecule including the activation function (AF)-2 domain on the C-terminal extreme. Scattered regions define the heterodimerization domain that allows binding with partner retinoic X receptor.

Interaction of $1,25(OH)_2D3$ with VDR induces translocation from the cytosol to the nucleus, where it heterodimerizes with its partner retinoic X receptor (RXR), to form a protein complex that acts as a transcription factor involved in the expression of target genes. Promoter region of vitamin D responsive genes shows sequence motifs acting as vitamin D responsive elements (VDRE) composed of direct repeats of consensus PuG(G/T)TCA motifs [49] that are recognised by the $1,25(OH)_2D3$-VDR-RXR complex. $1,25(OH)_2D3$-VDR-RXR complex recognition a VDRE activating motif facilitates the assembly of the transcription initiation complex by the release of corepressors and the recruitment of basal transcription factors and co-regulator molecules, including members of the steroid receptor coactivator (SRC) family and the VDR activating proteins (DRIP) that modulates chromatin remodelling to increase RNA-polymerase II gene transcription rate. Alternatively, when the ligand-VDR-RXR complex is engaged to the inhibitory VDRE, corepressors are recruited to inhibit gene transcription. In addition, VDRE independent regulation of gene transcription by $1,25(OH)_2D3$-VDR complex has been described. In this way, $1,25(OH)_2D3$ exerts regulatory role by interfering with the signal of key immune related transcription factors such as activating protein-1 (AP-1), nuclear factor of activated T-cell (NFAT), specific protein-1 (Sp1) and nuclear factor kappa-light-chain-enhancer of activated B cells (NF-KB). The biological actions resulting from $1,25(OH)_2D3$-VDR transcriptional regulation have pleiotropic effects affecting genes involved on the vitamin D hormone synthesis/catabolism and calcium homeostasis [50], cell differentiation and suppression of cell proliferation [51], neuroprotection in the central nervous system [52] and modulation of innate and adaptative immune response [53].

Human VDR gene expands over 100 kb of the chromosome 12q13.11 and consists of 14 exons distributed among 5'UTR region (upstream exons 1a to 1e), protein coding region (exons 2 to 9) and 3'UTR region (exon 9) (Fig. **3**). VDR gene expression is under complex transcriptional control by multiple promoters. Distal promoter (1f) and proximal promoters (1a and 1d) generate multiple variant VDR transcripts showing tissue and cell type specificity [54]. Naturally occurring mutations of VDR gene are responsible for the hereditary $1,25(OH)_2D3$ dependent rickets (vitamin D dependent rickets type II; VDDR II), that are characterised by defective bone mineralization, low intestinal calcium absorption, hypocalcaemia and elevated serum levels of $1,25(OH)_2D3$. All VDDR II related VDR mutations are inactivating mutations disturbing VDR DNA binding ability as well as transcriptional transactivation. VDR knockout mice have been obtained, and represent an animal model for the study of VDDR II [55,56].

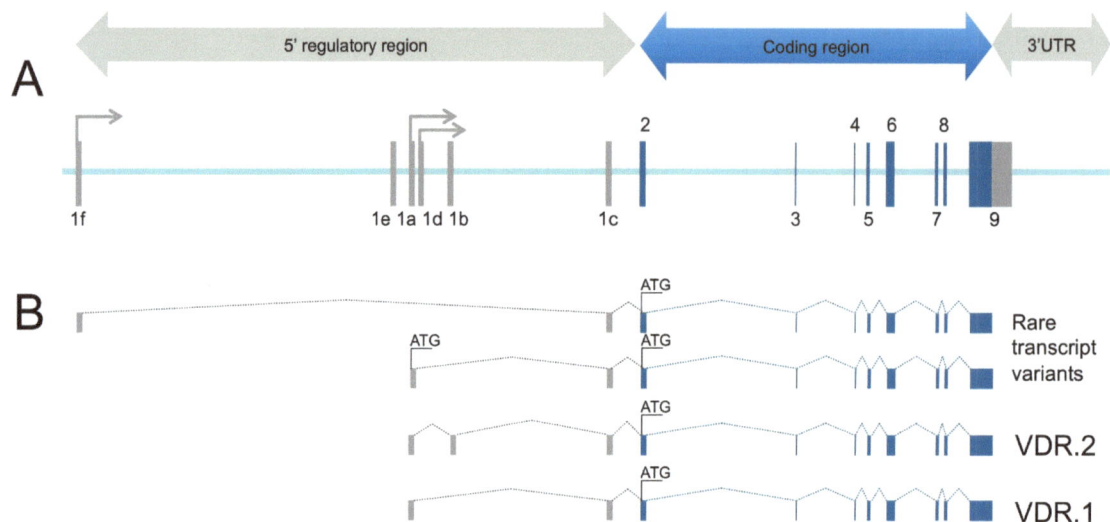

Figure 3: Genomic architecture of the human *VDR* gene. A, Exon-intron structure of *VDR* gene with non-coding (grey coloured) and coding (blue coloured) exons numbered according [54]. **B**, *VDR* gene expression is under complex transcriptional control by multiple promoters. Distal promoter (1f) and proximal promoters (1a and 1d) generates multiple variant VDR transcripts showing tissue and cell type specificity [54]. Transcript variant 1 (VDR.1) lacks an alternate exon in the 5' UTR (1b) compared to variant 2 (VDR.2). Variants 1 and 2 encode the same protein. Additional rare variants have been described using alternate promoters, at 1f and 1d, and alternative splicing rendering VDR isoforms [54].

1,25(OH)₂D3-VDR Mediated Transcriptional Regulation of Immune Related Genes

As for $1,25(OH)_2$D3-VDR target genes, $1,25(OH)_2$D3-VDR mediated activation/repression of immune genes can be done in a VDRE dependent and independent manner (Table **1**). Increase of tumour necrosis factor-alpha (TNF)-α production by $1,25(OH)_2$D3 treated bone marrow cells is mediated by direct binding of the complex $1,25(OH)_2$D3-VDR-RXR/VDRE in the TNF-α promoter [57]. Moreover, in peripheral blood mononuclear cells of normal and haemodialysis patients [58], in murine MAC cell line P388D1 [59] and in peritoneal MAC of patients treated with continuous ambulatory peritoneal dialysis [60], $1,25(OH)_2$D3 has a potent inhibitory effect on the production of TNF-α, independent of nuclear translocation of (NF-KB) [59] and $1,25(OH)_2$D3–mediated down-regulation of TLR2 and TLR4 [61]. VDRE has been recently found in the promoter region of both the human cathelicidin antimicrobial peptide (*CAMP*) gene and the defensin-β2 (*defβ2*) gene, mediating $1,25(OH)_2$D3 antimicrobial peptide induction in monocytes, MAC and keratinocytes [49, 62].

Negative VDRE-mediated response has also been described for the $1,25(OH)_2$D3-mediated inhibition of IFN-γ [63] and granulocyte/monocyte colony-stimulating factor (GM-CSF) production [64]. In addition, $1,25(OH)_2$D3-VDR also mediates VDRE independent regulation of gene transcription, through a direct or indirect influence on signalling cascades.

By this way, $1,25(OH)_2$D3-VDR complex can interfere, in a dose-dependent manner, with the signalling of key transcription factors involved in the regulation of immune related genes. NF-Kb is a major transcription factor that regulates genes responsible for both the innate and adaptive immune response.

Down-regulation of interleukin (IL)-12 and IL-8 is mediated by ligand-VDR complex that impedes both the activation of NF-Kb transcription factor and the binding on the NF-Kb consensus motif in the promoter sequence of these two genes. Moreover, $1,25(OH)_2$D3 also influences the activity of NF-Kb by interfering i) with the ubiquitination and subsequent degradation of the cytosolic inhibitor of NF-Kb (IKb-α) and ii) by inhibiting NF-Kb nuclear translocation and DNA binding. Thus, enhanced repression of RelB transcription by $1,25(OH)_2$D3-VDR contributes to downregulation of the NF-Kb pathway. Additional pathways are mediated by transcription factors, such as NFAT/AP-1 and MAPK, are involved in the $1,25(OH)_2$D3-VDR mediated inhibition of IL-2, IL-4 and Fas ligand (FasL) genes expression, whereas $1,25(OH)_2$D3-VDR/SP-1 may mediate CD14 upregulation (Table **1**). $1,25(OH)_2$D3 can also regulate transcription of NF-Kb genes such as RelB and c-Rel. A negative VDRE has been described in the promotion region of RelB gene that is constitutively linked to unbound VDR. This VDR-promoter association is enhanced by ligand-binding but reduced by LPS [65].

Table 1: 1,25(OH)$_2$D3-VDR mediated transcriptional regulation of immune related genes.

Regulatory mechanism	Target gene		Mechanism and effect on gene transcription
			VDRE Mediated Regulation
Activating VDRE	1. 2. 3.	TNF-α Cathelicidin Defensin-β2	Direct interaction of ligand-VDR-RXR with VDRE. Increase transcription. [49,57]
Repressing VDRE	4.	GM-CSF	Direct binding of ligand-VDR monomers to VDRE. Increase transcription. [64]
	5.	IFN-γ	Direct binding of ligand-VDR-RXR with VDRE and inhibition of an upstream enhancer element. Inhibition of transcription. [63]
	6.	RelB	Constitutive binding with unliganded-VDR that is increased by ligand and decreased by LPS. Inhibition of transcription. [65]
			Non VDRE Mediated Regulation
NF-kB pathway	7. 8.	IL12p40 IL-8	Indirect inhibition of NF-Kb heterodimer binding to promoter motif. Inhibition of transcription. [66,67]
	9.	TNF-α	Reducing nuclear translocation of NF-Kβ. Inhibition of transcription. [59]
NFATp/AP1 pathway	10. 11.	IL-2 IL-4	Interfering with NFATp/AP-1 complex assembly. Inhibition of transcription. [68]
SP-1 transcription factor	12.	CD14	VDR/SP-1 interaction at promoter SP-1 binding site. Increase transcription. [70]

ROLE OF VITAMIN D ON THE IMMUNE RESPONSE

Expression and regulatory properties of key components of vitamin D endocrine system, CYP27A1, CYP27B1, CYP24A1 and VDR, on immune cells strongly supports the role of vitamin D on immune system modulation. Since the first description of 1,25(OH)$_2$D3/VDR metabolism acting in peripheral mononuclear leukocytes and MAC of healthy individuals and sarcoidosis patients [25,71], vitamin D action on immune system has been mainly considered in the context of both immunosuppressive activity on APC and immunomodulatory effect on polarization of Th lymphocyte. The involvement of vitamin D endocrine system on the induction of innate immune response offers a new and promising picture from which the role of vitamin D on immune system regulation emerges with contrasting and pleiotropic effects.

Regulation of Vitamin D Endocrine System on Immune Cells

VDR is expressed by many cell types of the immune system [71,72], in particular APCs such as MAC, DCs [73] and LCs [74,75], as well as in CD4+ and CD8+ T cells [72]. Constitutive expression of VDR has been observed in MAC and DCs whereas their expression is induced by immune stimulus in B and T lymphocytes. Regulation of VDR expression in APC (monocyte/MAC and DC) depends on maturation status.

Immature APC expresses basal levels of VDR, allowing their responsiveness to agonist stimulus. When infectious agents interact with DC and MAC, these cells mature to capture and present the antigens. Maturation process is characterised by the upregulation of CYP27B1 expression and the downregulation of VDR expression (Fig. **4**). As a consequence, mature APC produces large amounts of 1,25(OH)$_2$D3 while lose its capability to respond to the hormone. As a result, a paracrine circuit is generated in which neighbouring immature APCs respond to the hormone produced by mature APCs (Fig. 4). Afterwards, 1,25(OH)$_2$D3 produced by mature APC inhibits maturation switch of neighbouring immature cells contributing to suppress immune activation [76,77].

Action of Vitamin D on Innate Immune Response

The main features of vitamin D effect on immune system regulation are depicted in Fig. **5** and Table **2**. This interaction is performed by the recognition of pathogen products, named pathogen-associated molecular patterns (PAMPs), a subclass of pattern recognition receptors (PRRs) located in the plasma membrane of these cells. Among membrane-bound PRRs are the transmembrane proteins known as Toll-like receptors

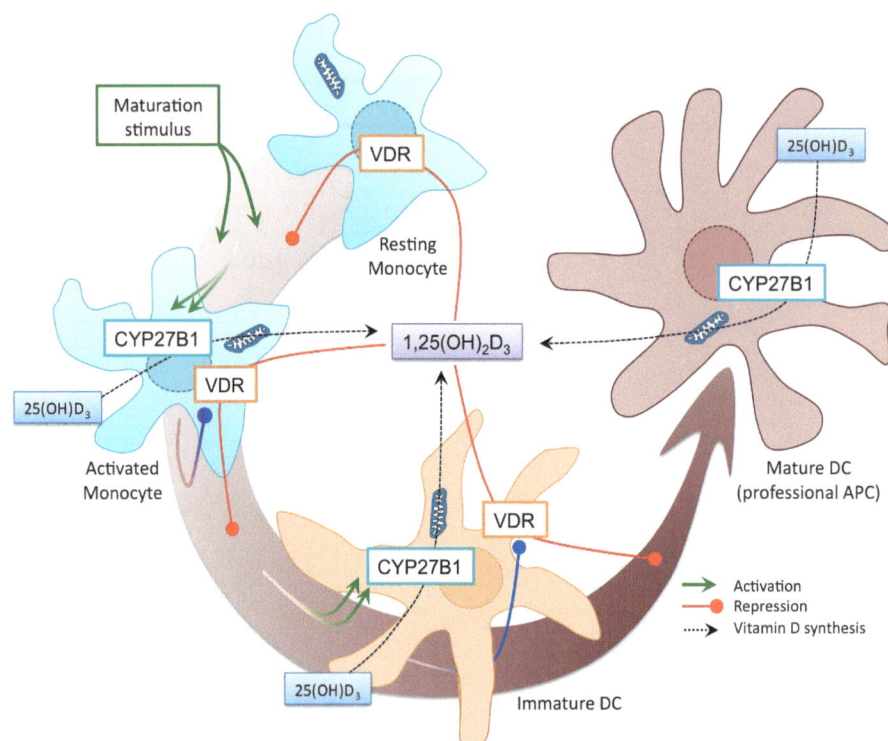

Figure 4: Regulation of vitamin D receptor (VDR) and 25-hydroxyvitamin D3 1-α-hydroxylase (CYP27B1) synthesis during maturation of antigen presenting cells (APC). APC, such as DC and MAC, express basal levels of VDR that allow their responsiveness to ligand stimulus. Activated monocyte (DC and MAC) become induced to mature (green lines). Maturation process is characterised by the upregulation of CYP27B1 expression (green degraded lines) and the downregulation of VDR expression (blue degraded lines). As a result, APC produce large amounts of 1,25(OH)$_2$D3 while lost their capability to respond to the hormone. Neighbouring immature APC can responds to 1,25(OH)$_2$D3 secreted by mature APC, by inhibiting star of maturation through ligand-VDR interaction (red lines). By this paracrine circuit 1,25(OH)$_2$D3 can lead to the suppression of further DC development.

(TLRs) that have the capability to recognize a broad type of molecules, including peptides, lipids and nucleic acids of viral and bacterial origin [78]. These interactions result in the trigger of downstream signalling cascades, many of which terminate in the activation of the transcription factor NF-Kb. The final result is the induction of the innate immunity responses as well as the instruction of the adaptive immune response against pathogen. Mainly, innate immune response is conducted in the form of antigen phagocytosis and pathogen destruction as well as promotion of microbial killing by host antimicrobial peptides (AMPs). Following this, adaptive immune response is instructed by the initiation of cell (cytotoxic activity by T lymphocytes) and/or humoral (antibody production by B lymphocytes)-directed immune response.

Table 2: Action of Vitamin D on target immune cells.

Inhibits	Induces/Favours
T cells	
T cell proliferation [80]	Hyporesponsiveness to self antigens [81, 82]
Th1 polarization [83, 84]	Th2 polarization [83]
NF-kB activation [85]	T-regulatory cells [86]
IL-2 and IFN-γ [63, 66]	CD95 (FasR) [69]
GM-CSF [87]	CD152 (CTLA4) [81]
	GATA-3 [88]
	IL-4, IL-5, IL-10 [81]

Table 2: cont...

Dendritic cells	
Differentiation, maturation [89]	Apoptosis [81]
IL-12 [66]	IL-10 [81]
TNF-α (mature DC) [61]	TNF-α (immature DC) [57]
MHC II mediated antigen presentation [90, 91]	Tolerogenic status of myeloid DC [92, 93]
Costimulatory molecules (CD40, CD40L, CD80, CD80L) [94]	CD14 [91]
DC migration [95]	

MAC/Monocyte	
Effector function of IFN-γ-activated MAC: Listericidal activity and phagocyte oxidase-mediated burst [96]	Chemotactic and phagocytic capacities [92]
Costimulatory molecules (CD40, CD40L, CD80, CD80L) [97]	Cathelicidin [49, 98]
TLR2/4 expression [61]	Defensin-β2 [49]
TNF-α (in mature cells) [58, 99]	TNF-α (in immature cells) [57]
NF-kB activation [59]	CD14 [57]
B cells	
Proliferation of activated B cells [100]	Apoptosis [100]
Ig production [100]	
Cell cycle progression [100]	
Memory B cell differentiation [100]	

Finely tuned mechanisms are engaged to avoid exacerbate innate and adaptive immunity in which vitamin D plays a key role. $1,25(OH)_2D3$ synthesis is upregulated in response to TLRs activation, acting in an autocrine/paracrine fashion to promote APMs synthesis, such as cathelicidin and defensin-β2, while at the same time, checking on the vigour of the adaptive immune response to the pathogen [79]. In this way, the capability of $1,25(OH)_2D3$ to inhibit NF-Kb pathway and to suppress MAC TLR expression supports a key role of the hormone as an autocrine feedback regulator of MAC responses (Fig. **5**). $1,25(OH)_2D3$ mediates innate immune response against *Mycobacterium tuberculosis* in MAC by the induction of antimicrobial peptides such as cathelicidin [15]. CYP27B1 and VDR genes are induced in MAC as a response to an infection by *M. tuberculosis* through the AP-1/NF-Kb pathway, induced after TLR2/4 activation. Following this, hydroxylation of $25(OH)D3$ to $1,25(OH)_2D3$ produces large amounts of active vitamin D hormone that, after interaction with VDR, modulates the expression of vitamin D dependent genes. Among these genes, the defensin-like cathelicidin gene is upregulated through the interaction with the VDRE enhancer located on its promoter [98]. There is no feedback control for the induced $1,25(OH)_2D3$ production in MAC, whereas in other cells the negative feedback is mediated by the $1,25(OH)_2D3$-catabolic enzyme CYP24A1. While CYP24A1 expression is also induced in MAC together with the expression of CYP27B1 and VDR genes, there is no concomitant increase in 24-hydroxylase-enzyme activity.

It has also been shown that CYP24A1 gene in MAC expresses, in addition to the normal CYP24A1 mRNA, an mRNA splice variant that codes for CYP24A1-SV that lacks the mitochondrial targeting domain [101]. It has been proposed that CYP24A1-SV interferes with normal CYP24A1 enzyme attenuating 24-hydroxylase-enzyme activity, which strongly reduces the conversion of active hormone to catabolic products.

Action of vitamin D on T-lymphocyte activation of TLR initiates protective immune responses with both innate and adaptive profile. Thus, the above mentioned induction of $1,25(OH)_2D3$/VDR-mediated AMPs production by MAC goes together with the TLR-mediated activation of NF-Kb in APCs, resulting in the release of proinflammatory cytokines and chemokines as well as the upregulation of co-stimulatory molecules that are essential for T-cell activation (Fig. **5**). Activation of TLR signalling pathway is a critical element for the induction of the innate immune response as well as for the instruction of the adaptive immune response against pathogens [102], although an extensive release of TLR-triggered pro-inflammatory mediators can be capable of harming the host, as in the case of sepsis or autoimmune disorders [61].

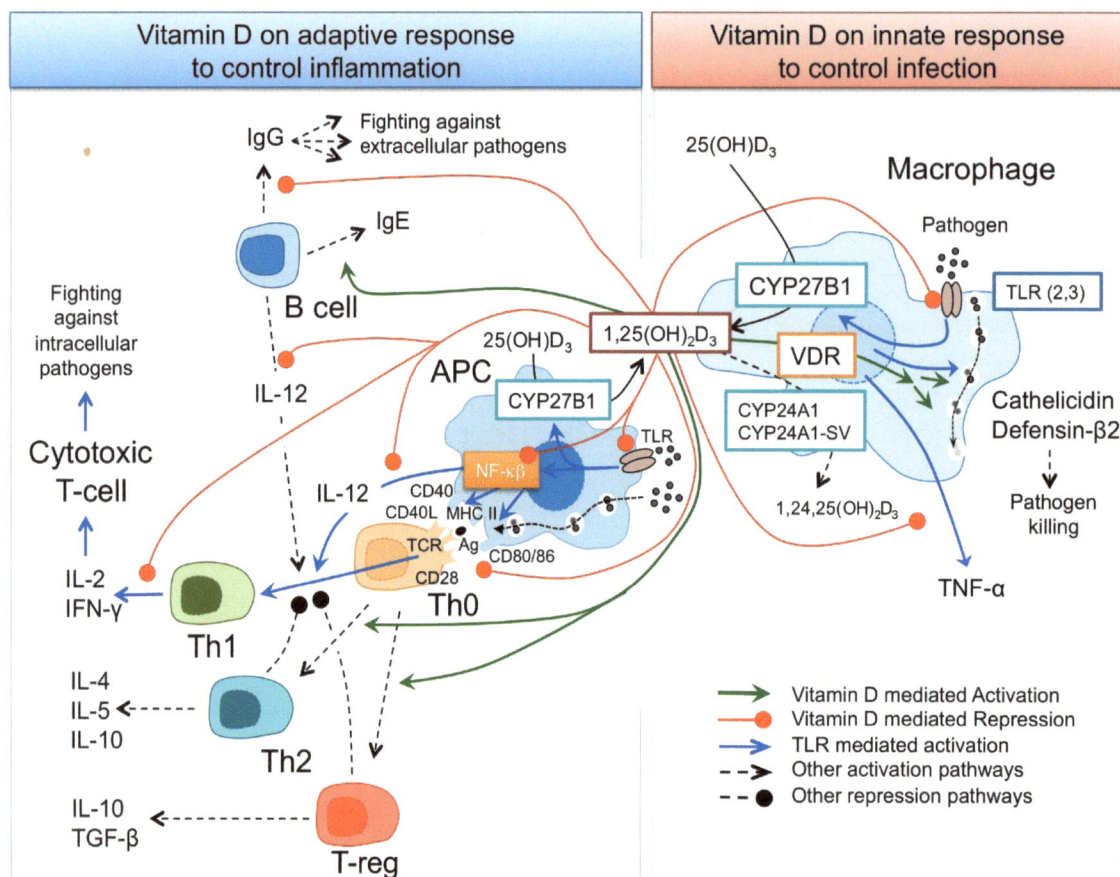

Figure 5: Action of vitamin D on the innate and acquired immune responses. Vitamin D influences innate (right) and adaptive (left) immune responses in a coordinated fashion. Pathogen activated MAC TLR stimulates CYP27B1 synthesis (blue lines) to produce 1,25(OH)₂D3 from the 25(OH)D3 precursor (black lines). 1,25(OH)₂D3, trough interaction with VDR, promotes synthesis of soluble factors killing pathogens, cathelicidin and defensin-β2 (green lines). Afterward, 1,25(OH)₂D3 acts in a paracrine mode to control exacerbated response on APC and T cells. In response to pathogens TLR is also activated in APC that, in addition to activate CYP27B1 synthesis and therefore 1,25(OH)₂D3, acts through activation of NF-Kb to promote antigen presentation and Th1 polarization (blue lines). 1,25(OH)₂D3 produced by MAC and APCs inhibits NF-Kb pathway (red line) modulating APC response. In addition, 1,25(OH)₂D3 inhibited the polarization of Th0 cells to Th1 profile by inhibiting the production of Th1-promoting IL-12 from APC and B cells and down-regulating the expression of Th1 specific cytokines (IL-2 and IFN-γ) (red lines). Finally, locally produced 1,25(OH)₂D3 acts on Th0 cells by promoting Th2 and Treg polarization, on B cells by inhibiting IgG and activating IgE production and on MAC by inhibiting TNF-α production. A control on the innate immune response is also assumed by 1,25(OH)₂D3 by inhibiting TLR synthesis that contributes to shut off the immune response circuit.

It has been proposed that 1,25(OH)₂D3 produced by TLR stimulated MAC or endogenously produced 1,25(OH)₂D3 by APC protects from exacerbated TLR signalling by down-regulating the expression of pro-inflammatory cytokines (IFN-γ and TNF-α), antigen-presenting and costimulatory CD40, CD80/86 molecules, and TLR in MAC and APC [61] *polarization*. The contribution of 1,25(OH)₂D3/VDR on the modulation of immune response is also highlighted by its role on T-lymphocyte polarization (Fig. 5). Although 1,25(OH)₂D3 can act directly on T cell functions, the main immunomodulatory effects on T cell differentiation are monitored indirectly through APC.

Naïve CD4+ T helper (Th) cells, upon stimulation by specific antigen, can differentiate into pluripotent Th0 cells that produce a broad pattern of cytokines.

Under the influence of specific stimulatory soluble factors and costimulatory molecules expressed by APCs, pluripotent Th0 cells further differentiate into Th1, Th2 and T regulatory (Treg) cells that express a limited and specific set of cytokines.

Th1 subset is characterised by the expression of the pro-inflammatory cytokines IL-2 and IFN-γ.

The secretion of IL-4, IL-5 and IL-10 cytokines distinguishes Th2 subset.

Finally, a third subset of T cells may be induced, such as Treg cells, characterised by the secretion of IL-10 and TGF-β [103]. The decision, by which Th0 cells undergoes differentiation to one of these T cell subsets, depends on multiple factors from which APC driven stimulus is crucial. Th1 pro-inflammatory response is promoted in the presence of APC secreting IL-12 and presenting MHC-II coupled antigens and co-stimulatory molecules. Antigen presentation by APC in the absence of IL-12 stimulus promotes Th2 differentiation. Finally, APC lacking co-stimulatory molecules become tolerogenic and, in the presence of IL-10, give rise to regulatory T cells or even induce T cell energy [104]. Both Th2 and Treg cells inhibit Th1 differentiation, reason why Th1 profile is prevented if Th2 or Treg has been induced. Th1/Th2 balance hypothesis has been proposed by which each T-helper subset directs different immune response pathways. Type 1 pathway is directed by Th1 cells and is mainly involved in intracellular microbe control and cellular mediated immunity. Th2 cells drive type 2 pathway, being involved in the control of extracellular parasites and in humoral mediated immunity. Although criticised by some authors, Th1/Th2 balance hypothesis has been considered as a paradigm on co-ordinating immune response. Unbalanced Th1/Th2 response predisposes to immune diseases.

Dominance of Th1 drive response has been associated with autoimmunity, whereas Th2 over-dominance has been related with allergy [103]. 1,25(OH)₂D3/VDR action on APC is characterised by the down-regulation of the expression of the co-stimulatory molecules CD40, CD80 and CD86, reduction of IL-12 and augmentation of IL-10 production. This resulted in a decreased T-cell activation that creates an environment that favours Th2 and, mostly, Treg differentiation [84, 86, 94, 105]. Inhibition of Th1 response and promotion of Th2 and Treg differentiation has been related with 1,25(OH)₂D3-mediated protection against autoimmune diseases [84]. In addition, 1,25(OH)₂D3-promoted tolerogenic status, substantiating its therapeutic use to prevent allograph rejection [92].

Effect of Vitamin D on host Th1 Mediated Immunity

In the context of infection by intracellular pathogens, the balance between i) positive effects of the 1,25(OH)₂D3/VDR pathway by inducing anti-microbial response, ii) the detrimental effect of Th1 inhibition, and iii) induction of a tolerogenic status has to be considered for each disease model. The suppressive effect of 1,25(OH)₂D3/VDR pathway on MAC functions has been revealed detrimental in certain infections. Infection by the intracellular protozoan parasite *Leishmania major*, host defence is focused around activated MAC acting as IFN-γ-effector cells.

Given the suppressive effect of 1,25(OH)₂D3/VDR on Th1-mediated IFN-γ production a detrimental role for 1,25(OH)₂D3 can be expected. In line with this, MAC of VDR-knock-out (VDR-KO) mice has stronger leishmanicidal activity that is reduced when exposed to 1,25(OH)₂D3, supporting a negative role of the hormone [16].

Analogous results were observed in the LP-BM5 mouse model of AIDS; treatment with 1,25-(OH)2D3 enhanced the severity of the disease and increased the mortality rate [106].

Evidences indicate that HIV-1-specific cellular immune responses may play a critical role in antiviral control [107]. Th1 mediated immune response seems to be poorly developed in HIV-1 infected patients at all stages of the disease. In addition, T-cell proliferative responses against virus are inversely correlated with plasma viremia [107].

Importantly, in many seronegative exposed individuals and long-term non-progressors a vigorous HIV-1 specific Th1 and cytotoxic T-lymphocytes (CTL) responses have been observed [108]. Several authors have proposed a shift from Th1 to Th2 immune response that correlates with HIV-1 disease progression [109, 110]. Whatever this Th1>Th2 shift constitutes a viral immune evasion strategy [111], either favoured by opportunistic infections [112] or derived from a selection process against more permissive Th cells [113], the main consequence is that this Th1/Th2 imbalance could preclude to mount humoral and cellular HIV-1 specific immune responses able to control virus infection. According to this, the 1,25(OH)$_2$D3-mediated Th1->Th2 shift could have detrimental effects on both HIV-1 infection and disease progression to AIDS.

ENVIRONMENTAL-MEDIATED AVAILABILITY OF VITAMIN D AND IMMUNE FUNCTION

The influence of either abnormal status or environmental-limiting availability of vitamin D hormone on several disease sustains the critical role of 1,25(OH)$_2$D3/VDR pathway in normal immune system function. Vitamin D deficiency, that tends to induce an over-grounded Th1 response, has been associated with susceptibility to autoimmune diseases such as rheumatoid arthritis, type-1 diabetes, systemic lupus erythematosus, psoriasis, inflammatory bowel disease and multiple sclerosis [114]. On the other hand, the over-induction of 1,25(OH)$_2$D3/VDR pathway that precludes an accurate control of Th1 response and favour a Th2 response and a tolerogenic state, seems to predispose to allergic conditions [115,116]. Concerning 1,25(OH)$_2$D3 involvements on susceptibility to pathogen infection, it has been reported that vitamin D insufficiency predisposes to bacterial and viral infections [7]. Susceptibility to *Mycobacterium* infection has been largely related to vitamin D deficiency [117]. Low levels of vitamin D compromise vitamin D-mediated immune modulations that, in the context of tuberculosis infection, can be detrimental by limiting the capability of MAC function to suppress intracellular growth of tuberculosis bacterium and compromising the production of microbe-killing cathelicidin [15].

Seasonal Variation of Sunlight Exposure, Vitamin D and Immune Functions

Changes in immunological parameters have been described in tourist travelling to sunny countries without prior adaptation to UVB exposure. Subjects receiving substantial doses of UVB, as reflected by response to questionnaires, UVB dosimetry and increase in 25-hydroxyvitamin D3 show significant alterations in the immune system function [118]. A fashion hypothesis proposes a link between sunlight exposure, vitamin D availability and susceptibility to bacterial and virus infection. Following this hypothesis, low sun exposure, due to limiting environmental conditions or in-house social behaviour, predispose to vitamin D insufficiency that could favour the acquisition of bacterial and viral infections. In line with this hypothesis, higher prevalence of tuberculosis infection has been found in Asiatic immigrants living in United Kingdom than in those living in their countries. From such a hypothesis, lowering the availability to sunlight in northern latitudes can preclude enough vitamin D synthesis, which predisposes Asian immigrants in the UK to tuberculosis infection [119]. Also, the seasonal variation of influenza infection has been linked to the seasonal variation of sunlight exposure-related vitamin D deficiency [120]. However, the effect of additional climatic conditions, such as humidity and temperature, as well as the detrimental effect of UV exposure on the survival of viral particles, cannot be ruled out [121]. A recent work evaluating meteorological conditions in relation to respiratory syncytial virus (RSV) infection reveals that RSV activity was inversely related to UVB [122], suggesting that vitamin D insufficiency during winter season increases susceptibility to respiratory infections, and implying that vitamin D supplementation can decrease their severity and occurrence. Nevertheless, a recent report was unable to detect any benefit of vitamin D supplementation in decreasing incidence or severity of respiratory infections during winter season [123]. Influence of seasonal variations in genital infections has also been detected in cervical smears screened for cervical carcinoma in The Netherlands [124]. Seasonal peaks for both *Candida* and *Chlamydia* were detected in fall season. In contrast, infections of *Actinomyces* and *Trichomonas* were more likely to occur in winter season. Concerning to Human Papiloma Virus the seasonal peak was observed in summer season. Complex interactions between host, infectious agent and environmental conditions can be taken into account to explain this pattern of seasonality. The contribution of season-dependent availability of vitamin D, if any, may be pathogen-specific.

Environmental-Mediated Availability of Vitamin D and HIV Infection

There are few data relating sunlight and UVB exposure with HIV-1 infection that can allow us to evaluate their impact on the disease. Early studies were focused on UVB effect on HIV-1 virus replication. Transgenic mice expressing HIV *Tat* gene under the control of the HIV LTR, showed bolstered Tat protein expression in the skin after exposure to UV light [125]. This effect linked to UVB-mediated vitamin D synthesis was not investigated. However, concerns have been raised about potential adverse effects of UV radiation, as used in phototherapy and photo-chemotherapy, on HIV-1 infected persons. Several studies have been addressed to clarify this question that seems to discard any adverse effects of UV radiation on HIV infected patients under UV phototherapy [126,127]. Immunosuppressive effects of sunlight exposure have been also considered detrimental in the context of HIV infection, being proposed as a risk factor for progression to AIDS [9]. Epidemiological studies based on well-established HIV/AIDS cohorts have tried to address this question. Epidemiological data from the Multicenter AIDS Cohort Study (MACS) revealed that sunlight exposure is not associated with a decline in T-helper lymphocyte count or progression to AIDS [128]. Nevertheless, two studies based on the Amsterdam Cohort Study (ACS) on HIV and AIDS show contrasting results. The first study evaluated individual exposure of homosexual men to sunlight by means of a 2-year retrospective questionnaire that was given to some of the participants (n=57). In agreement with the previously mentioned study on MACS, exposure to sunlight does not produce adverse effect on CD4+ T-cell count, CD4+/CD8+ T cell ratio, and T-cell reactivity [129]. The same authors developed a second study by an extended number of subjects (n=557) from which they found lower levels in the mean number of CD4+ T cells and the mean CD4+/CD8+ ratio during summer and spring with seasonal effect being more prominent at a more advanced stage of the HIV/AIDS [130].

The spread of HIV infection in Europe has been mainly observed in intravenous drug users (IDU). In the early HIV epidemic the prevalence of HIV infection in IDU reached the highest values in the Mediterranean area such as Spain (>60%), French (30%) and Italy (23-31%), as well as in North-Atlantic countries such as Scotland (>64%) and Denmark (>20%) [131,132]. Social and political strategies for the prevention of HIV transmission among IDU were implemented from the beginning of the epidemic with encouraging results. As a consequence, a decrease in HIV prevalence has been observed in several countries, but this reduction seems to have stabilised lower prevalence values in the Northern region than in Southern region [131,132]. Based on public data from surveillance of HIV/AIDS infection in Europe [133], we have plotted in Fig. **6** the prevalence of HIV infection in IDU corresponding to selected European country regions: Southern region with latitude <46°N as for Portugal, Spain and Italy, Central region with latitude between 46°N-55°N as for England, Germany and Austria and Northern region with latitude >55°N as for Scotland, Norway and Finland. All these countries belong to the European Union, except for Norway, and share common political, economical and social characteristics. Prevalence trends in the period 2001-2005 were highly stabilised for each region but larger values were observed in Southern (overall 15.3%) than in Central (2.0%) or Northern (0.6%) regions. Taken into account that prevalence of HIV infection in early epidemic was broadly extended in different European areas and that social and political strategies to prevent infection have been applied with equivalent intensities among different countries, the differential set-point pattern achieved was unexpected.

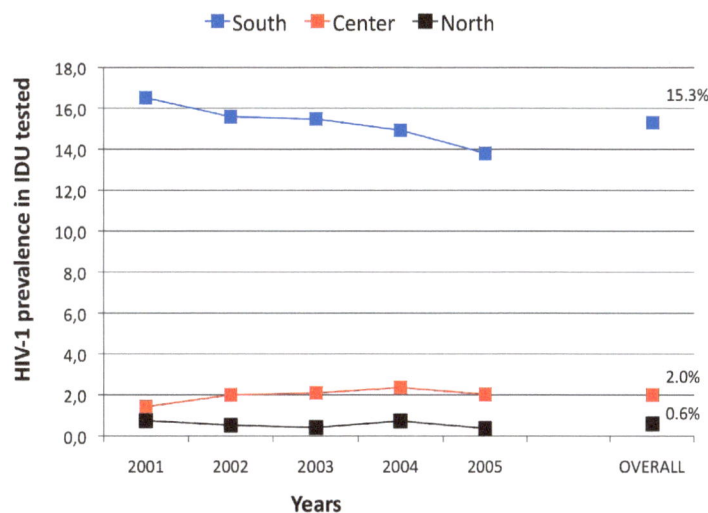

Figure 6: Prevalence of HIV infection among injection drug users in Southern, Centre and Northern European regions. Mean prevalence of HIV infection in IDU subjects corresponding to selected European country regions: South

(latitude <46°N; Portugal, Spain and Italy) (blue line), Central (latitude 46°N-55°N; England, Germany and Austria) (red line) and North (latitude >55°N; Scotland, Norway and Finland) (black line). Data obtained from public surveillance of HIV/AIDS infection in Europe [136] among 2002 to 2005 period. Prevalence trends in 2001-2005 for South Central and North regions were 15.3%, 2.0% and 0.6%, respectively.

Prevalence of HIV infection in Eastern European countries is growing dramatically and no latitudinal distribution can be observed. Probably, in the early spread of the epidemic, such as happened in the western European countries in the 80's, socioeconomic, behavioural and political factors exert the main effect on prevalence. Later, we can expect a plateau on prevalence, such as observed in western countries, in which "intrinsic" factors determined the prevalence set point. The question we address is: what are those "intrinsic" factors? Behavioural and cultural singularities, that characterise each European region, could be critical, although, we cannot exclude that environmental factors such as sunlight exposure/UVB radiation, and the associated bolstering of HIV replication and immunosuppressant effect, can be involved on the determination of the prevalence set point.

It is well known that sensibility to the sunlight/UVB exposure effects varies among human populations depending on geographical location and skin colour. It is considered that evolutionary forces acting on skin colour variability in humans are strongly related with sunlight/UVB exposure [133].

Darker skin subjects are protected from sunburn and UVB-related damages, while they can have compromised vitamin D metabolism, even at high latitude regions. On the contrary, clear skin subjects are vulnerable to sunburn and UVB-related damages, whereas they can reach regular vitamin D metabolism, including in low irradiated regions.

It was stated that cutaneous photolysis of 7-dihydrocholestorol to cholecalciferol in the skin was strongly reduced in winter season in Boston (42°N), while cholecalciferol production occurred throughout the year in Los Angeles (34°N) and San Juan de Puerto Rico (18°N) [134]. Calculation of the time required to have enough amounts of vitamin D for a healthy vitamin D status has been modelled in the customizable web site "http://nadir.nilu.no/~olaeng/fastrt/VitD_quartMED.html" [135]. In the winter season (i.e. December) at 42°N a subject with skin type 1 (Caucasian, very sensitive, always burns easily, never tans, very fair skin tone) needs a minimum of 50 min to reach 1000 IU (daily recommended dose). In contrast, a subject with skin type VI (dark-skinned black) will need 24h of solar exposition to reach this minimal level. Values changed at the summer season (i.e. July) in which subjects with skin type I and VI only need 4 and 18 minutes, respectively, to reach the recommended minimal. At lower latitudes (i.e. 35°N) the capability to synthesise functional vitamin D is not limiting for people with skin type I, that need 25 min in December and 3 minutes in July, and lightly limiting for those with skin type VI, that need 2 hours and 13 min in December and 16 min in July. Lightly coloured skin persons may likely access to any beneficial effect of vitamin D production, while darker coloured persons will be protected from any detrimental effect.

In an attempt to evaluate this proposition we have searched in the literature for epidemiological studies evaluating prevalence of HIV infection on light and dark coloured people living at different latitudes. Unfortunately, there are not many studies of this nature from which we can extract information needed, but a recent epidemiological study of HIV prevalence in civilian applicants for the United States of America military service can help us in this way [137]. This was an exhaustive analysis of the geographical distribution of HIV infection throughout the US territory in which they have studied 5.7 million of subjects (79% White and 21% African-American) who applied for US military service between 1985 and 2003. The authors searched for spatial HIV clustering of data, discriminating between White and African-American groups. They have found three main clusters for the White data, one located in the Northeast area of New York and New Jersey, a second in the Southeast area around Huston, Texas and a third cluster in the Southwest area of Los Angeles, California (Fig. 7). Nevertheless, data from African-American subjects reveals two stronger clusters in the Northeast area of New York-New Jersey and Washington DC and an additional cluster in the Southwest area of Los Angeles, but no cluster was detected in the Southeast area around Houston (Fig. 7). It is remarkable that the two coincident cluster areas between White and African-American correspond to two of the most populated areas in USA, whereas the discordant cluster corresponds to a more rural area. The high population density in these regions and the aggregation behaviour of human beings contribute to the spread of HIV infection among equals. We can interpret that in highly populated areas, social, behavioural and economic factors overcome any additional factor affecting susceptibility to infection. When these factors are less prominent, hidden factors can emerge. Then, environmental factors, such as sunlight exposure, could reveal their protective or detrimental effect on HIV infection in susceptible subjects. The cluster detected in the Southern area around Houston, affecting only White subjects, seems to indicate that, in a highly sunlight exposed and low populated area, white people are more susceptible to infection than African-American. We are conscious that any conclusion derived from an exploratory analysis like this must be taken with caution, but we hope that this could encourage the design of new epidemiological analysis trying to clarify this question.

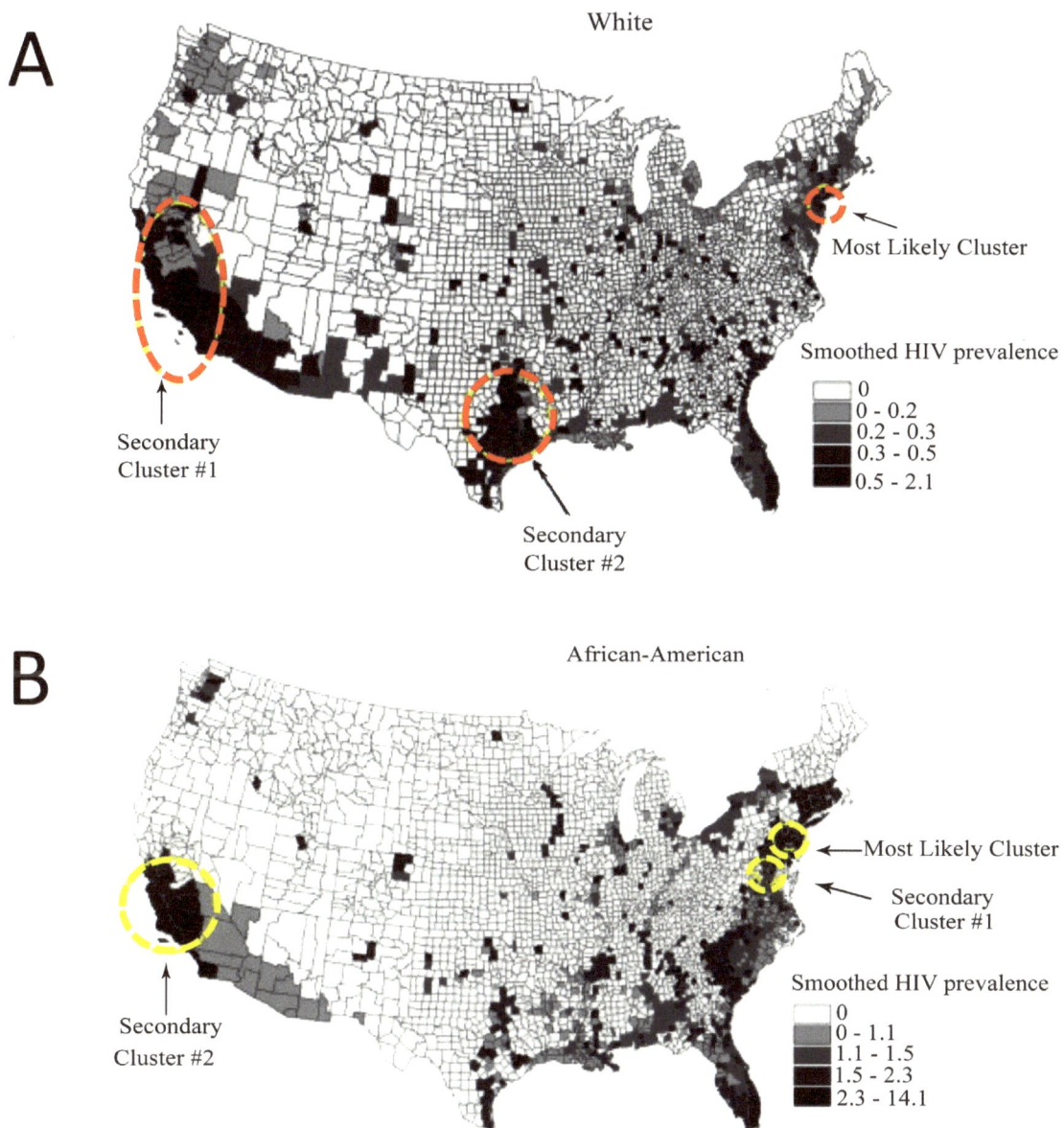

Figure 7: HIV prevalence and clusters among white (A) and African-American (B) civilian applicants for Unites States military service. Reproduced by permission from Bautista CT, Sateren WB, Sanchez JL, Singer DE and Scott P. Geographic mapping of HIV infection among civilian applicants for United States military service. Health & place 2008;14:608-15 [137].

Vitamin D Status and HIV Infection

There is a great concern about vitamin D status in the general population. Vitamin D deficiency has been recognised as a general problem of pandemic dimension. Few foods contain enough quantities of vitamin D and precursors, whereas cultural and social behaviours limit the access to photoproduction of vitamin D precursors in the skin. Following this, synthesis of 25(OH)D3 can be compromised limiting the synthesis of the 1,25(OH)$_2$D3 active form. It is well established that serum levels of 25(OH)D3 but not 1,25(OH)$_2$D3 are indicatives of the vitamin D status.

The circulating concentration of 25(OH)D3 is a good reflection of both exposure to sunlight and dietary intake of vitamin D precursors. Although there is not a general consensus about the optimal serum concentration of 25(OH)D3, vitamin D deficiency is considered when 25(OH)D3 serum levels are below 20 ng per millilitre (50 nmol per litre). However, other authors consider vitamin D insufficiency for serum concentrations between 20 to 30 ng per millilitre (50-75 nmol per litre) and sufficiency for values greater than 30 ng millilitres. Although occurring in rare circumstances, 25(OH)D3 can produce intoxication when serum levels are greater than 150 ng per millilitre (375 nmol per litre) [138].

According to these definitions more than a million people worldwide are affected by deficient/insufficient status [139]. Among them, elderly, postmenopausal women and children are the most significant groups at risk. Environmental factors, sunlight exposure, latitude and season; nutritional factors, diet, fortified foods and dietary intake; behavioural factors, life style (i.e., indoor-outdoor) and clothing; demographic factors, age and finally, healthy factors can affect vitamin D status. HIV infection has been recognised as a risk factor for Vitamin D insufficiency. Deficiency in micronutrients has been early described for HIV/AIDS patients as a common feature, mainly in those with advanced disease [140].

Abnormal levels of 1,25(OH)$_2$D3 have been described in symptomatic HIV infected patients (CDC stage IV) while near to normal levels were observed in asymptomatic (CDC stage II/III). Serum levels of the active hormone were directly correlated with CD4+ cell counts in blood and inversely correlated with survival.

On the other hand, 1,25(OH)$_2$D3 levels have not been correlated with vitamin D deficiency as determined by serum levels of 25OHD3 [141,142]. Disturbances in bone remodelling have been described in patients with advanced disease, mainly related with an increased activity of TNF-α or direct HIV-effect on osteoblasts or osteoclasts precursors. As TNF-α may inhibit the effects of 1,25(OH)$_2$D3 on osteoblasts function [143], decreased levels of 1,25(OH)$_2$D3 may boost TNF- α function and disturbing bone metabolism in HIV infection [144].

Decreased activity of vitamin D metabolic enzymes has been described in patients treated with protease inhibitors (PI). PI inhibits enzymatic activity of 25- and 1,25-hydroxylase enzyme (CYP27A1 and CYP27B1, respectively) and, to a lower extend, 24-hydroxylase (CYP24A1) enzyme activity. In *in vitro* assays with the human monocyte–MAC cell line THP-1 inhibition of 1,25–hydroxylase activity was of 80% by ritonavir, 66% by indinavir and 32% by nelfinavir [145,146]. Impaired vitamin D metabolism during PI-based HAART regimens may be responsible for the higher risk of bone dysfunction in patients under this treatment protocol [147,148].

The true relevance of vitamin D deficient/insufficient status in HIV infected patients must be considered in the context of the general/healthy population. As stated in the epidemiological study based on the Reaching for Excellence in Adolescent Health (REACH) cohort, the prevalence of vitamin D insufficiency in HIV infected urban younger and control-matched subjects were not different [12].

Improvement of vitamin D status in HIV-infected patients by vitamin D supplementation has been studied in several clinical trials, with the aim of improving bone metabolism. Vitamin D supplementation does not show side effects on immune parameters as reflected by the absence of significant changes of CD4+ cell count and percentage after one year of vitamin D supplementation [10,149]. On the other side, in the same HIV individuals it was not possible to estimate the effect of vitamin D treatment on virus replication since all individuals were under anti-retroviral therapy [10,149].

CONTRIBUTION OF VITAMIN D ON PROTECTION/RISK TO HIV INFECTION AND DISEASE PROGRESSION TO AIDS

Both direct effects on HIV replication and indirect effects through innate and adaptive immunity responses affect the complex interactions of vitamin D endocrine system on HIV infection (Table **3**).

Table 3: Contrasting effects of Vitamin D on HIV infection and progression to AIDS.

	Vitamin D confers protection by:	**Vitamin D confers risk by:**
Physiological evidences	Promoting polarization to Treg that facilitates a proper modulation of the initial response	Impairing Th1 cellular immune response
		Promoting a tolerogenic status that favour viral persistence
	Inducing defensin synthesis	Interfering with APOBEC3G synthesis
		Increasing viral replication
Environmental evidences	Solar irradiation favours immune modulation	Lower levels of CD4+ T cells and the mean CD4+/CD8+ ratio in HIV+ patients during summer and spring
		High steady-state prevalence of HIV infection in Southern European countries
Genetic evidences	Less functional VDR-allelic variants that are associated with protection to HIV infection and slow progression to AIDS	

Action of Vitamin D on HIV Replication may Contribute to HIV Infection

Conflicting data have been reported concerning the effects of 1,25(OH)$_2$D3 on HIV-1 replication in primary monocyte-derived MAC as well as myeloid cell lines; both enhancement and inhibition of HIV-1 replication in response to 1,25(OH)$_2$D3 have been reported. Studies of the role of 1,25(OH)$_2$D3 in HIV-1 infection have been hampered by technical and methodological variability, as well as lack of homogeneity in the experimental strategies. Several parameters can have deep influence on the results: cell types, 1,25(OH)$_2$D3 concentration, viral strains (X4 *vs.* R5), 1,25(OH)$_2$D3 treatment before or after infection, co-treatment with other stimuli (such as TNF-α), chronic *vs.* acute infection, days after infection for viral load quantification or infectious dose.

The main used models are cell lines of myeloid origin, although several authors have also analyzed the 1,25(OH)$_2$D3 effects on primary cells.

HL-60 cell line was established from a patient with promyelocytic leukaemia. This cell line acquires morphology and markers of mature granulocytes in the presence of DMSO, retinoic acid, or cAMP, whereas differentiates into a MAC-like phenotype after 1,25(OH)$_2$D3 or phorbol ester (TPA or PMA) stimulation. HL-60 cells are CD4+/CXCR4+/CCR5- and consequently are resistant to R5 but susceptible to X4 HIV-1 strains [150]. However after 1,25(OH)$_2$D3 differentiation (10^{-7} M) for 5 days, this cell line becomes susceptible to HIV-1$_{JR-FL}$ or HIV-1$_{BaL}$ (R5). In this study, the TPA also rendered the cells susceptible to R5 viruses; this observation correlates with the observed induction of CCR5 after PMA treatment of HL-60 [151]. There was no effect of 1,25(OH)$_2$D3 or TPA on HIV-1$_{JR\_FL}$ virus production from HL-60 cells when treated immediately after infection, suggesting a delay time between the stimuli addition and the susceptibility to viral infection. In a model of chronically infected HL-60 cell line (HIV-1$_{JR-FL}$), 1,25(OH)$_2$D3 enhanced virus production more than 10-fold and induced the same phenotypic changes as observed in uninfected cells. HL-60 cells treated with 1,25(OH)$_2$D3 (10 nM) showed increased CXCR4 mRNA expression after 3 days of stimulation [152,153] and 1 mM of 1,25(OH)$_2$D3 increased the viral production of the HTLV$_{IIIB}$ strain (X4) [150]. On the other hand in HL-60 cells a 30% inhibition of CXCR4 surface expression has been reported after 3 days of

1,25(OH)$_2$D3 stimulation at 600 nM without any change in mRNA amount [154]. However, although CXCR4 surface expression was decreased upon treatment with 1,25(OH)$_2$D3, it enhanced the functional G-protein coupling to the receptor as demonstrated by the increase in SDF-1-mediated GTP binding [154].

The U937 cell line was established from a histiocytic lymphoma [155]. This cell line shows a phenotype of myelo-monocytic lineage (CD13+, CD15+, and CD33+). Naïve U937 cells, as HL-60 cells, are CD4+/CXCR4+/CCR5- being vulnerable to infection by X4 strains but resistant to R5 strains [156]. U937 cells exposed to 10^{-6} M 1,25(OH)$_2$D3 for 1 or 2 days prior to infection with HIV-1$_{BRU}$ (X4) displayed 5-fold increase in virus replication; however, shorter 1,25(OH)$_2$D3 stimulation reduced the levels of viral replication and the simultaneous infection plus 1,25(OH)$_2$D3 treatment (10^{-8} M) produced a 75% reduction in the viral load after 3 days of infection [157]. Skolnik *et al.* [158] reported 140-fold increase in viral replication in U937 cells pretreated with 24 nM 1,25(OH)$_2$D3 for 1 day before infection. Opposed results were communicated by Kitano *et al.*, showing that a regime of 10^{-7} M 1,25(OH)$_2$D3 for 5 days prior to infection totally inhibited X4 replication and had no influence on the R5 strains HIV-1$_{JR-FL}$ and HIV-1$_{BaL}$ (no infection at all) [150]. The role of 1,25(OH)$_2$D3 in modulation of HIV-1 production in chronically infected U937 cell line was in agreement with the data reported in HL-60 cell line; 1,25(OH)$_2$D3 at 1mM induced an elevated release of infectious viral particles (14-fold) after 6 days in culture. The authors observed no differences in the amounts of endogenous TNF-α production in control and 1,25(OH)$_2$D3 treated cells, although there was a clear upregulation of the TNF-α receptor [18]. X4 chronically infected U937 cells, named U1 cells, produces HIV-1 particles only after induction with several stimuli such as IFN-γ, IL-6, GM-CSF or TNF-α. The 1,25(OH)$_2$D3 treatment alone (10^{-8} M for 5 days) did not induce any increase in virus replication but co-treatment with TNF-α resulted in 3-fold increase in virus production above that induced by TNF-α alone. In clear contrast, 1,25(OH)$_2$D3 blocked the viral replication induced by INF-γ, IL-6 and GM-CSF [159]. The so-called *plus* clones (UC12, UC14) supported viral replication of X4 strains more efficiently than original U937 cell line; in contrast the *minus* clone (UC11) showed only very limited viral replication [160,161]. The origin of this phenotype is controversial; it appears to be related at least to the density of CXCR4 in cell membrane, and lower in minus clones, although there were no clear differences in mRNA levels and functional Ca^{++} mobilization in response to CXCL12 between the two cell types [162]. Remarkably, stimulation with 1,25(OH)$_2$D3 upregulated HIV-1 X4 replication in *minus* clones to the levels comparable to those observed in *plus* clones, however the *plus* clones did not show any changes in response to the treatment. 1,25(OH)$_2$D3 selectively induces a slight increase in CXCR4 expression on the cell surface in minus clones [163].

The A3.5 cell line was established from human bone cell cultures. This cell line shows a monocyte phenotype (HLA-DR+/CD15+/CD3-) and is susceptible to infection by X4 and R5 HIV-1 strains [158]. A3.5 cells exposed up to 240 nM 1,25(OH)$_2$D3 for 1 day prior to infection with HIV-1$_{IIIB}$ (X4) exhibiting enhanced virus replication in a dose-dependent manner; augmentation was up to 10^4 fold in the presence of 240 nM 1,25(OH)$_2$D3 after 14 days of culture.

THP-1 exposed to 10^{-7} M 1,25(OH)$_2$D3 for 5 days prior to infection with both R5 strains HIV-1$_{JR-FL}$ and HIV-1$_{BaL}$ and X4 strain HIV-1$_{IIIB}$, exhibited a boosted viral replication after 7 days of culture. The effect of 1,25(OH)$_2$D3 treatment on HIV-1 infection of primary monocyte-MAC has been evaluated in three different studies.

Skolnik *et al.* [158] observed up to 12- fold enhancement of R5 replication in cultures treated with 1,25(OH)$_2$D3 (10^{-8} M) after 14 days post-infection.

In contrast, Schuitemaker *et al.* [165] reported that primary monocyte derived MAC treated for 5 days with 1,25(OH)$_2$D3 (10^{-8} M) were markedly protected from HIV replication. Finally, Pauza *et al.* [157] observed large variability and contradictory results in 1,25(OH)$_2$D3 effects between MAC from different blood donors; in some cases the treatment produced a 50% reduction in viral replication but in others it induced a slight increase in viral production.

Another experimental strategy to evaluate the effects of 1,25(OH)$_2$D3 signalling on HIV-1 replication parameters has been done by an evaluation of HIV-1 LTR promoter activity after 1,25(OH)$_2$D3 stimulation in transfected HeLa, Cos-1 and U937 cells. $1,25(OH)_2D3$ stimulated the LTR transcription in a dose-response manner, with 4-fold induction with 100 nM $1,25(OH)_2D3$ [17]. We have observed the same effect in primary monocyte- derived MAC from healthy blood donors and more interestingly, the intensity of the induction showed a relationship between *VDR BsmI* genotype polymorphism (unpublished data from AC laboratory).

Data regarding the significance of $1,25(OH)_2D3$ in the course of HIV-1 infection are scarce; Arpadi *et al.* [10] evaluated the effect of $1,25(OH)_2D3$ supplementation in children and adolescents at a dosage of 10^5 IU every 2 months and they have found no difference in progression of HIV-1 disease as measured by CD4$^+$ cell count, viral load, rate of disease progression or antiviral treatment failure.

In conclusion, the $1,25(OH)_2D3$ effects on viral replication depend on several parameters, such as the maturation stage of the cells, the timing of treatment and probably individual genotypes for *VDR* and the genes coding for enzymes regulating the metabolism of $1,25(OH)_2D3$. Additional efforts will be necessary to unveil the specific role of $1,25(OH)_2D3$ signaling in HIV-1 replication and receptors expression especially in primary cells of monocyte/MAC lineage. The upregulation of CXCR4 by $1,25(OH)_2D3$ in cells of myeloid lineage has been demonstrated by several studies [163], although in this context the evaluation of the influence of VDR genotypes on the *in vivo* selection of X4 or double tropic R5X4 strains is warranted. MAC are capable to perform both hydroxylation steps of the $1,25(OH)_2D3$ metabolism suggesting a possible role of local $1,25(OH)_2D3$ synthesis by myeloid cells, although we cannot exclude the possibility that $1,25(OH)_2D3$ is already present in these cells, especially after an initiation of differentiation process, pathogen encounter or cytokines stimulation. A promising experimental strategy could be to test the effects of antagonists of $1,25(OH)_2D3$ or siRNA against VDR during the course of HIV-1 infection of primary MAC as well as the use of steroids deprived of serum (charcoal-dextran treated) or ketoconazole (24 hydroxylase inhibitor).

Action of Vitamin D on Innate Immune Response has Contrasting Effects on HIV Infection

The most well characterised antimicrobial peptides in humans are defensins and cathelicidin (also named LL-37).

Defensins belong to the family of microbicide and cytotoxic peptides involved in innate defense. They are abundant in the granules of neutrophils (5% of total protein content) and are also found in epithelia of mucosal surfaces such as those of the intestine, respiratory tract, urinary tract, skin and vagina. Members of the defensin family are highly similar in protein sequence and distinguished by a conserved cysteine motif.

α-defensins and most of the β-defensins genes are clustered on chromosome 8p23.1 locus that exhibits copy number variation from 2 to 12 copies per diploid genome. β-defensins are widely expressed throughout human epithelia. More than 30 *loci* exist, but only 4 (HBD1 to HBD4) have been studied in detail. α-defensins 1-4 and β-defensins 2-3 show anti-HIV-1 activity *in vitro*. *In vivo* expression correlates with protection in mother-to-child transmission, as demonstrated by the strong association between high α-defensin concentrations and a decreased risk of partum and postnatal HIV transmission has been observed. On the contrary α-defensins 5 and 6 increase HIV-1 infectivity and may play a role in enhancing HIV-1 transmission through genital mucosa [166]. The relationships between vitamin D and defensin expression have not been studied in detail. One report described the upregulation of defensins expression in mouse skin after UV stimulation mediated by vitamin D production [167]; in humans the defensin-β2 promoter contains a VDRE, and the gene transcription can be slightly enhanced by 24 hours treatment with $1,25(OH)_2D3$ (1,5-2,0 fold) in epithelial cells but not in neutrophils or monocytes. On the contrary, $1,25(OH)_2D3$ partially blocks the defensin-β2 expression at 48 hours in head and neck squamous carcinoma cells and adult keratinocytes [49].

In humans there is only one cathelicidin gene that is expressed on all epithelial surfaces (mouth, tongue, esophagus, lungs, intestine, cervix and vagina, sweat glands, etc.) and circulating white cells, including neutrophils, monocytes, natural killer cells, and γδT cells. In general, the expression of cathelicidin in most epithelial sites is constitutive but can be increased by local injury or infection. The interaction between vitamin D signalling and cathelicidin expression has been described in detail; cathelicidin gene is a direct target of VDR, because its promoter contains a VDRE and vitamin D treatment induces a strong up-regulation of cathelicidin mRNA. Cathelicidin is able to block HIV-1 infection *in vitro* [168, 169] but the concentration required to reach 50% of inhibition of infection (30-50 mg/ml) is more than 2000- fold higher than the mean concentration observed in cervicovaginal secretion (13 ng/ml, range 2-191 ng/ml) [170]. The same study observed that the presence of sexually transmitted infections was associated with higher risk of HIV-1 acquisition (especially *N. gonorrhoeae*, *C. trachomatis* or both) and increased levels of several defensins and cathelicidin.

Cathelicidin is an agonist of the formyl peptide receptors and induces increased cell migration, phagocytosis and release of proinflammatory mediators [171], being the neutrophils, monocytes, and T cells the main target cells; this peptide has also been related to neovascularization and wound healing [172]. We hypothesise that although cathelicidin shows minor antiviral effect at physiological concentration [168-170], it might induce a more permissive environment for HIV-1 replication through attraction of neutrophils, monocytes and T cells to the tissues exposed to viral infection [170]. New data concerning the functional relationship between antimicrobial peptides levels, HIV-1 susceptibility and polymorphisms in VDR or the enzymes of vitamin D synthesis and degradation might provide a more accurate model of the complex interaction between this arm of innate immune response and HIV-1 infection. In addition to microbicide and cytotoxic peptides, host factors with specific antiviral properties have been described. Among them, the human apolipoprotein B mRNA-editing enzyme-catalytic polipeptide-like-3G (APOBEC3G) has raised special interest as an interfering agent of HIV dissemination. APOBEC3G belongs to a family of cytidine deaminases that, in absence of the viral protein *Vif*, is incorporated in the nascent viral particle. Virions carrying APOBEC3G express cytidine deaminase activity during reverse transcription that induces deamination of cytosines to uracil, resulting in G to A hypermutation on DNA positive strand. Hypermutated viral DNA leads to aberrant viral products aborting viral propagation [173]. Antiviral APOBEC3G activity can be abrogated by the interaction with viral protein *Vif* that induces proteasoma-dependent degradation of APOBEC3G. Studies on exposed uninfected individuals (EUI) indicate that variations on APOBEC3G levels might influence vulnerability to HIV infection. APOBEC3G expression is up-regulated by IFN-α and IFN-γ, induced in response to viral exposure [174]. Expression levels of IFN-γ vary among T-helper subtypes, being mainly expressed after Th1-polarization. Following this, it has been shown that CD4+ T-helper type 2 lymphocytes express lower levels of APOBEC3G than T-helper type 1 lymphocytes. As a result, differences on infectivity among Th1- and Th2-produced HIV particles have been correlated with changes in APOBEC3G expression levels [175]. It is tempting to speculate that the 1,25(OH)$_2$D3-mediated inhibition of IFN-γ production [63] contributes to inhibition of Th1 polarization and the subsequent displacement to a Th2 profile that could be reflected as a lower expression of APOBEC3G which favours the not restricted Th2-produced HIV particles. Evaluation of APOBEC3G response on CD4+ T cells to 1,25(OH)$_2$D3 treatment could be of interest to assess this hypothesis.

Vitamin D Action on Acquired Immune Response: Tolerogenic vs. Activation Strategies on Persistence of HIV Infection

Although immunopathogenesis of HIV infection has been largely studied, mechanisms underlying viral persistence and inability of host immune response to control infection remain obscure. T cell immune responses, that are capital for the control of many viral infections, are often unable to control HIV replication. The incapability to mount an efficient T cell response seems to be a common feature of chronic viral infections, such as HIV, hepatitis virus B (HVB) and C (HVC) infections. It has been found that viruses causing persistent viral infection develop a variety of strategies to evade or overcome the host immune response. Among mechanisms developed on such a way, avoiding T cell activation by the promotion of a tolerogenic status [176] and induction of T cell exhaustion by T cell overstimulation [177], there are two strategies used by HIV to evade an efficient T cell mediated immune response. We can expect contrasting effects of vitamin D immunomodulation on these two mechanisms.

HIV infection is characterised by several disturbances in the cytokine expression pattern. Among these, a general decrease in the expression of pro-inflammatory cytokines, as a consequence of a reduced Th1 polarization, seems to contribute to the host-inability for mounting a proper T cell mediated response [107]. It is remarkable that vitamin D and HIV infection exert similar action on Th1- Th2-polarization, both of them favouring Th2 polarization. As for vitamin D action on Th cell polarization, HIV infection is characterised by a down-regulation of IL-12 and IFN-γ as a result of the interaction of HIV-1-specific T cells with APC inducing CTL dysfunction [178-180]. IL-12 is a key cytokine required for the correct priming of CD4+ T cells to provide help to CD8+ T cells to respond to HIV infection [181]. In addition, as for vitamin D mediated induction of IL-10, HIV *Tat* protein, a key viral protein involved in viral replication, interferes the host cytokine production by the induction of IL-10 [182]. IL-10 is up- regulated during HIV infection, contributing to maintain a tolerogenic status that favours HIV mediated immunodeficiency. Finally, it has been proposed by several authors that the Th2-polarization that characterises HIV infection could resemble an allergic response to viral antigens [183,184] and that *gp120* envelope and *Tat* viral proteins could act as potent viral allergens [185-188]. Also, a high frequency of hypersensitivity reactions in HIV infected patients has been described to contribute to HIV disease progression [184]. As formerly mentioned, vitamin D promotes allergy [115] and predisposes to allergic syndromes [116]. Following this, vitamin D could contribute to reinforce the HIV-promoted allergy associated with disease progression.

Despite the presence of HIV induced immunodeficiency, almost all cellular components of the immune system, B cells, NK cells, T cells and MAC show evidence of immune activation. Early steps of HIV infection are characterised by an acute T cell response, mainly CD8+ T cells, which can be maintained during the chronic phase of infection, and with a lower magnitude CD4+ T cells, probably due by their preferential depletion by the virus [189]. In addition, microbial products, mainly derived from the gastrointestinal tract, contribute to HIV-related systemic immune activation [190]. In spite of this T cell response, HIV infection can be established and reach successful persistence. Paradoxically, T cell activation, that may be considered a positive response against viral pathogens, could be detrimental in the context of HIV infection, as new targets for viral replication, in particular CD4+ T cells, can contribute to promote HIV infection. This intuitive observation is supported by experimental data indicating that there is indeed a direct correlation between T cell activation levels and HIV disease progression [191,192]. This paradoxical effect of immune activation is exploited and promoted by HIV in a perverse strategy [193,194], inducing an altered homeostasis of T cells (i.e., T cell turnover and apoptosis). Continuous and persistent differentiation of *naïve* T lymphocytes to antigen experienced cells and subsequent apoptosis reach boundaries on the regenerative capacity of the immune system. As a consequence HIV infected individuals lose their capability to replenish *naïve* T cell pool, exhibiting characteristics of replicative senescence [195] that exhaust the capacity of the immune system to control HIV infection [177].

It has been proposed by several authors that suppression of the activated immune response in HIV infection can contribute to control infection. In fact, antiretroviral therapy (ART), which is until now the best strategy to combat HIV, inhibits virus replication by contributing to the deactivation of the immune responses in HIV infected individuals [196]. Treatment of HIV infection with immunosuppresent drugs as ART coadjuvants has been considered, assuming that a decreased immune activation associated with HIV infection may be beneficial [197]. However, concerns have been raised about this strategy; changing initial parameters may have effects on long-term infection, by establishing a new immunological set point that may affect the rate of disease progression [198].

It is intuitive to consider vitamin D treatment as an immunomodulatory adjuvant in HIV infection. As previously mentioned, vitamin D acts on T cell polarization promoting Treg cells while inhibiting T effectors cells, mainly Th1 cells. Thus, vitamin D may contribute to avoid the early exacerbating T cell response that HIV could have taken in advantage. Nevertheless, the contribution of Treg on HIV infection must be considered with caution, as beneficial and detrimental effects are expected [199]. In support for a beneficial effect of Treg on HIV infection is the negative association between Tregs and immune activation showed during HIV infection [200] that may contribute to the attenuation of HIV-specific T cell immune responses in the early stages of HIV disease [201]. On the other hand, in support for a detrimental effect is an association of Treg cells with more severe stages of infection and induction of Th2 polarization [202]. An increase in Treg function could impair cellular immunity that is able to block HIV spread. In the simian immunodeficiency virus (SIV) infection a premature induction of immunosuppressive regulatory cells has been shown to contribute to viral persistence by limiting early antiviral response [176].

Another concern about using vitamin D as an immunosuppressant agent on HIV infection comes from the expected promotion of T cell exhaustion and viral persistence induced by vitamin D, as consequent to an altered pattern of cytokines expression. As pointed before, vitamin D induces Th2 and Treg cells, with a IL-4/IL-5/IL-10 and TGF-β/IL-10 profiles. IL-10 is an immunomodulatory cytokine that attenuates inflammatory response by suppressing Th1 cytokine production and proliferation of CD4+ and CD8+ cells [203]. Recently, a key role of IL-10 cytokine on T cell exhaustion and viral persistence has been proposed [204]. Increased IL-10 production has been reported during persistent viral infection of lymphocytic choriomeningitis virus (LCMV), whereas anti-IL10 receptor antibodies unleash the viral persistence [205]. Thereafter, IL-10 receptor antagonists have been proposed for the treatment of chronic viral infections in humans [206]. Thus, vitamin D-induced IL-10 production could contribute to virus persistency and favouring viral persistence.

Lesson Learned from Vitamin D Receptor Polymorphisms and Association Studies

Several VDR polymorphisms have been described in the regulatory, coding and 3' UTR regions with functional effects (Fig. **8**). Two common polymorphisms, *Cdx* (rs1568820) and *A1012G* (rs4516035), have been located in the 5' regulatory region that influence binding of transcription factors. The *Cdx* polymorphism is a G to A transition located between exons 1f and 1e that alters the recognition site for the intestinal-specific transcription factor caudal-related homeodomain protein (Cdx)-2 affecting 1,25(OH)$_2$D3-VDR mediated intestinal calcium absorption [207]. The *A1012G* polymorphism is an A to G transition located between 1e and 1a exons that modify the GATA binding protein (GATA)-3 transcription factor recognition sequence, involved in the regulation of Th2 polarization. Cdx-2 and GATA promoter SNPs are included in single haplotype block of the VDR promoter region [208].

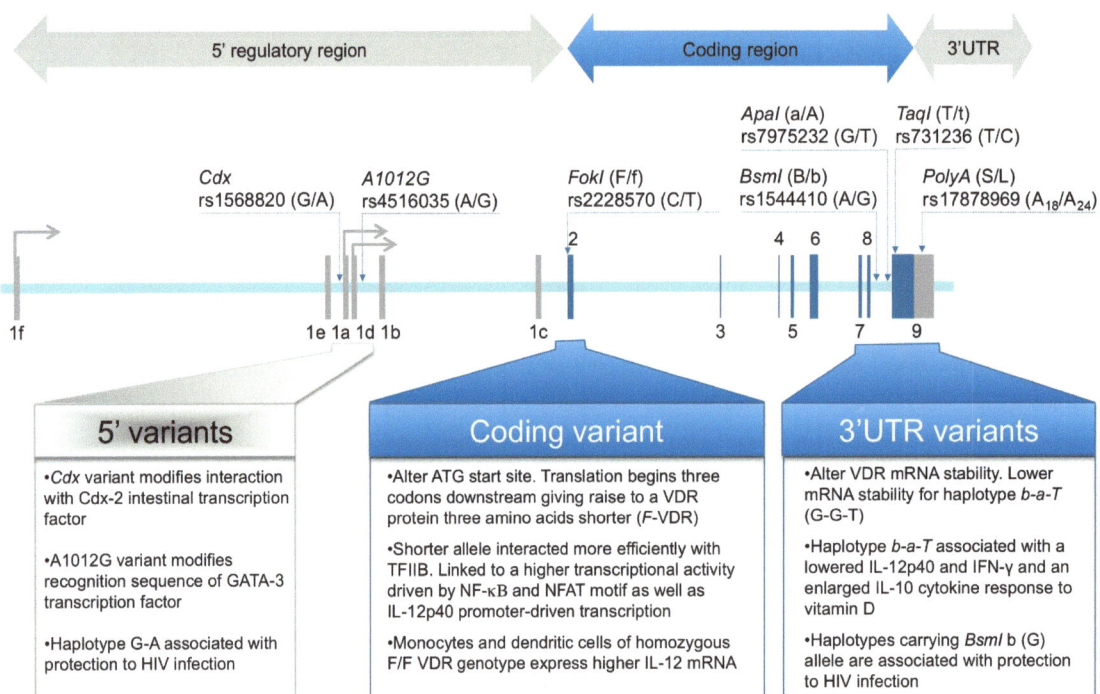

Figure 8. The most relevant VDR polymorphic markers are all along *VDR* gene structure. Two markers are located in the promoter-5'UTRs region, rs11568820 (*Cdx*) upstream exon 1e and rs4516035 (*A1012G*) between exons 1e and 1a. Marker rs2228570 (*FokI*) is located in exon 2. Finally, four additional markers are located in the 3'UTR region, rs1544410 (*BsmI*) and rs7975232 (*ApaI*), between exons 8 and 9 and rs731236 (*TaqI*) and rs17878969 (*PolyA*) in exon 9. SNP markers rs11568820, rs4516035, rs2228570, rs1544410, rs7975232 and rs731236 are biallelic. Marker rs17878969 is a mononucleotide repeats of adenines, showing a bimodal distribution of allele frequency [213] with short (S) allele expanding 18 A repeats and long (L) allele expanding 24 A repeats. Alleles have been coded according to coding *VDR* sequence. Restriction fragment length polymorphism (*FokI*, *BsmI*, *ApaI* and *TaqI*) alleles are also coded according to cutting (small letter) and un-cutting (capital letter) alleles. Functional effects of polymorphic variants on immune function are depicted at the bottom of the Figure.

In addition, a common *FokI* polymorphism (rs10735810) has been described in the VDR coding region that alters the first ATG start site to an alternate ACG sequence. By this polymorphism two potential starting sites for the VDR translation seems to appear [209]. Messenger RNA transcripts with the ACG sequence begin translation of three codons downstream, expressing a VDR protein that is three amino acids shorter (424 aa vs 427 aa). Functional differences among *FokI* genotypes show that VDR protein coded by the F-VDR (short, 424 aa) allele interacted more efficiently with Transcription Factor II B (TFIIB) and showed greater transcriptional activity than the full-length VDR protein coded by f-VDR allele [210]. The impact of *FokI* polymorphism on $1,25(OH)_2D3$-VDR mediated immune modulations has been recently evaluated [211]. The shorter F-VDR form was linked to a higher transcriptional activity driven by NF-Kβ and NFAT motif as well as IL-12p40 promoter-driven transcription.

Consequently, it was also shown that monocytes and DCs of homozygous subjects for short F/F VDR genotype express higher IL-12 mRNA and protein than cells with a long f/f VDR genotype, concluding that the short F-VDR allele is associated with a more active immune response.

Finally, three restriction fragment length polymorphisms (RFLP), designed as *BsmI* (rs1544410), *ApaI* (rs7975232) and *TaqI* (rs731236), and a *PolyA* (rs17878969) microsatellite polymorphism, have been described in the 3'-UTR region of the VDR gene, showing strong linkage disequilibrium in Caucasian population [212,213].

Functional effects of 3'-UTR variants have been related to alterations in VDR mRNA stability [208]. Functional effects of 3'UTR haplotypes on VDR mediated immune modulation have been evaluated. Haplotype b-a-T (for *BsmI* and *ApaI* RFLP, cut allele, and *TaqI* RFLP, uncut allele) was associated with decreased IL-12p40 and IFN-γ and increased IL-10 cytokine response of $1,25(OH)_2D3$ treated peripheral blood mononuclear cells [214].

This seems to indicate that $1,25(OH)_2D3$-VDR mediated Th1 polarization is haplotype dependent with the b-a-T haplotype producing lower Th1 polarization effect.

The 3' UTR polymorphisms have been associated with an increased susceptibility to infection by bacteria and viruses, including *Mycobacterium tuberculosis* [215,216], *Mycobacterium leprae* [217], Dengue Virus [218], HTLV-1 [219], HBV [220] and Respiratory Syncytial Virus [221].

$1,25(OH)_2D3$-mediated signals appear to have a protective role in tuberculosis, *in vitro* [15] as well as *in vivo* [216, 222]. However, *in vivo* $1,25(OH)_2D3$ treatment exhibits a negative influence on the clinical course of both toxoplasmosis [223,224] and leishmaniosis [16] in a mouse.

On the contrary, a clinical trial evaluating the effect of vitamin D as a supplementary treatment for tuberculosis showed no overall effect on human beings [225].

In the context of HIV-1 infection, two *VDR* polymorphisms (*BsmI* and *FokI*) have been associated with susceptibility to faster progression towards AIDS-defining illness on a Spanish cohort of HIV-1 positive intravenous drug users. *BsmI* B/B homozygotes [22] and *FokI* F/f heterozygotes [21] were over represented among those reaching AIDS outcome. Both genotypes are associated with functional effects, enhanced VDR activity (*FokI*-F allele) and increased mRNA stability (*BsmI*-B allele).

Apart from the association of *VDR* gene variants with progression to AIDS, these gene variants could also influence the susceptibility to HIV-1 infection. Studies comparing Spanish HIV-1 positive intravenous drug users *vs.* HIV-1 exposed uninfected controls [20] and Indians HIV-1 positive *vs.* healthy controls [19] have suggested that the promoter *Cdx-A1012G* (G-A) haplotype and the 3' UTR haplotypes containing the *BsmI*-b allele are associated with protection to HIV-1 infection. Since protective haplotypes confer a lower efficiency on the vitamin D pathway, it was inferred that hampering vitamin D signalling could confer protection to HIV-1 transmission.

CONCLUDING REMARKS: VITAMIN D, FRIEND OR FOE IN HIV INFECTION?

There is a general agreement that vitamin D sufficiency contributes to good health, being essential to regulate the absorption and metabolism of calcium and phosphorus resulting in health bones [226]. In addition, vitamin D protects from bacterial infections and controls cell proliferation that could give rise to cancer cells. A general concern is about vitamin D insufficiency that seems to affect a great proportion of the population in both developed and developing countries. However, we would have to be cautious about vitamin D contribution to a chronic and persistent infection such as HIV. We have found in the literature evidences supporting a protective role of vitamin D in HIV infection by inducing antimicrobial agents and modulating host to exacerbate immune responses. Nevertheless, we have also found solid data bearing for a deleterious role of the hormone by promoting HIV replication and helping virus to mount evading strategies. The major mistake we can do is to try to resolve this dilemma in terms of friend and foe. There is not a single and simple answer that allows us to understand the complexity of this phenomenon.

There is no data in the literature about the effect of HIV-1 infection in the expression of VDR and vitamin D-related enzymes. In the case of the chronic retroviral infection with MuLV, it has been observed an alteration on both the local vitamin D metabolism and the VDR expression by immune cells [227]. Over 30% of the myeloid cells from MuLV infected mice expressed VDR, whereas less than 1% of the uninfected cells did so. This suggests that retroviral infection induces the VDR expression in monocyte/MAC. There is a correlation between the increase in functional receptor protein and increased response to 1,25-(OH)2D3 in many cellular systems [5]. In this retroviral infection the vitamin D treatment leads to increased cytopathic effects and lower survival. Unfortunately a similar experimental approach has not been investigated in the case HIV-1 infection. Although the literature about vitamin D and HIV-1 is abundant, some critical questions remain to be answered. The relationship between vitamin D metabolism and HIV-1 infection might be elucidated using an approach that might include: investigation of epistatical interactions with vitamin D pathway (including sex) or gene-environment effects (diet, sun exposure); test for associations between genetic polymorphisms in the whole vitamin D pathway including the genes in charge for the synthesis and degradation of this hormone, especially in individuals at risk for sexual transmission of HIV-1; the functional validation of the genetic polymorphisms identified in the vitamin D pathway; the quantification of mRNA and protein of VDR and the enzymes of vitamin D metabolism in cellular subpopulations of HIV-1 infected individuals and healthy controls.

Recent studies demonstrated that inhibition of antigen-presentation attenuator drastically boosts memory HIV-specific T- and B-cell responses induced by DC- and DNA-based HIV vaccines [228]. Therefore, inhibition of antigen-presentation attenuators has been considered as an alternative strategy for enhancing the effectiveness of different prophylactic and therapeutic vaccine strategies against HIV [229]. Vitamin D inhibits APC maturation and antigen presentation acting as antigen-presentation attenuator. Subsequently, the use of VDR antagonists and/or inhibitors of the vitamin D pathway enzymes could be proposed as co-adjuvants in HIV therapeutic approaches. Further investigations are warranted to develop vitamin D related drugs that, avoiding non-desired side effects, could be used in such strategies.

ACKNOWLEDGMENTS

This work was supported by Grants "Fondo de Investigaciones Sanitarias" (FIS) to J.F. (ref.: PI021476 and PI051778) and A.C. (ref.: PI021205). "Fundació Marató TV3" to J.F. (ref.: 020730) and A.C. (ref.: 020732).

REFERENCES

[1]   Lin R, White JH. The pleiotropic actions of vitamin D. Bioessays. 2004;26(1):21-8.
[2]   Rigby WF. The immunobiology of vitamin D. Immunol Today. 1988;9(2):54-8.
[3]   Deluca HF, Cantorna MT. Vitamin D: its role and uses in immunology. *FASEB* J. 2001;15(14):2579-85.
[4]   Lips P. Vitamin D physiology. Prog Biophys Mol Biol. 2006;92(1):4-8.
[5]   Pike JW. Vitamin D3 receptors: structure and function in transcription. Annu Rev Nutr. 1991;11:189-216.
[6]   Hewison M. Vitamin D and the immune system. J Endocrinol. 1992;132(2):173-5.

[7]   White JH. Vitamin D signaling, infectious diseases, and regulation of innate immunity. Infect Immun; 2008;9:3837–43.

[8]   8. Hewison M. Vitamin D and innate immunity.   Curr Opin Investig Drugs. 2008;9(5):485-90.

[9]   Vincek V. Sunlight induced progression of AIDS. Med Hypotheses. 1995;44(2):119-23.

[10] Arpadi SM, McMahon D, Abrams EJ, Bamji M, Purswani M, Engelson ES, *et al.* Effect of bimonthly supplementation with oral cholecalciferol on serum 25-hydroxyvitamin D concentrations in HIV-infected children and adolescents. Pediatrics. 2009;123(1):e121-6.

[11] Ramayo E, González-Moreno MP, Macías J, Cruz-Ruíz M, Mira JA, Villar-Rueda AM, *et al.* Relationship between osteopenia, free testosterone, and vitamin D metabolite levels in HIV-infected patients with and without highly active antiretroviral therapy. AIDS Res Hum Retroviruses. 2005;21(11):915-21.

[12] Stephensen CB, Marquis GS, Kruzich LA, Douglas SD, Aldrovandi GM, Wilson CM. Vitamin D status in adolescents and young adults with HIV infection. Am J Clin Nutr. 2006;83(5):1135-41.

[13] Van Den Bout-Van Den Beukel CJ, Fievez L, Michels M, Sweep FC, Hermus AR, Bosch ME, *et al.* Vitamin D deficiency among HIV type 1-infected individuals in the Netherlands: effects of antiretroviral therapy. AIDS Res Hum Retroviruses. 2008;24(11):1375-82.

[14] Villamor E. A potential role for vitamin D on HIV infection? Nutr Rev. 2006;64(5):226-33.

[15] Liu PT, Stenger S, Li H, Wenzel L, Tan BH, Krutzik SR, *et al.* Toll-like receptor triggering of a vitamin D-mediated human antimicrobial response. Science. 2006;311(5768):1770-3.

[16] Ehrchen J, Helming L, Varga G, Pasche B, Loser K, Gunzer M, *et al.* Vitamin D receptor signaling contributes to susceptibility to infection with Leishmania major. *FASEB* J. 2007;21(12):3208-18.

[17] Nevado J, Tenbaum SP, Castillo AI, Sánchez-Pacheco A, Aranda A. Activation of the human immunodeficiency virus type I long terminal repeat by 1alpha,25-dihydroxyvitamin D3. J Mol Endocrinol. 2007;38(6):587-601.

[18] Locardi C, Petrini C, Boccoli G, Testa U, Dieffenbach C, Butto S, *et al.* Increased human immunodeficiency virus (HIV) expression in chronically infected U937 cells upon in vitro differentiation by hydroxyvitamin D3: roles of interferon and tumor necrosis factor in regulation of HIV production. J Virol. 1990;64(12):5874-82.

[19] Alagarasu K, Selvaraj P, Swaminathan S, Narendran G, Narayanan PR. 5' Regulatory and 3' Untranslated Region Polymorphisms of Vitamin D Receptor Gene in South Indian HIV and HIV-TB Patients. J Clin Immunol. 2008.

[20] de la Torre MS, Torres C, Nieto G, Vergara S, Carrero AJ, Macías J, *et al.* Vitamin D receptor gene haplotypes and susceptibility to HIV-1 infection in injection drug users. J Infect Dis. 2008;197(3):405-10.

[21] Nieto G, Barber Y, Rubio MC, Rubio M, Fibla J. Association between AIDS disease progression rates and the Fok-I polymorphism of the VDR gene in a cohort of HIV-1 seropositive patients. J Steroid Biochem Mol Biol. 2004; 89-90(1-5):199-207.

[22] Barber Y, Rubio C, Fernández E, Rubio M, Fibla J. Host genetic background at CCR5 chemokine receptor and vitamin D receptor loci and human immunodeficiency virus (HIV) type 1 disease progression among HIV-seropositive injection drug users. J Infect Dis. 2001;184(10):1279-88.

[23] DeLuca HF. The vitamin D system in the regulation of calcium and phosphorus metabolism. Nutr Rev. 1979;37(6):161-93.

[24] Zehnder D, Bland R, Walker EA, Bradwell AR, Howie AJ, Hewison M, *et al.* Expression of 25-hydroxyvitamin D3-1alpha-hydroxylase in the human kidney. J Am Soc Nephrol. 1999;10(12):2465-73.

[25] Adams JS, Sharma OP, Gacad MA, Singer FR. Metabolism of 25-hydroxyvitamin D3 by cultured pulmonary alveolar macrophages in sarcoidosis. J Clin Invest. 1983;72(5):1856-60.

[26] Zehnder D, Bland R, Williams MC, McNinch RW, Howie AJ, Stewart PM, *et al.* Extrarenal expression of 25-hydroxyvitamin d(3)-1 alpha-hydroxylase. J Clin Endocrinol Metab. 2001;86(2):888-94.

[27] Monkawa T, Yoshida T, Hayashi M, Saruta T. Identification of 25-hydroxyvitamin D3 1alpha-hydroxylase gene expression in macrophages. Kidney Int. 2000;58(2):559-68.

[28] Hewison M, Freeman L, Hughes SV, Evans KN, Bland R, Eliopoulos AG, *et al.* Differential regulation of vitamin D receptor and its ligand in human monocyte-derived dendritic cells. J Immunol. 2003;170(11):5382-90.

[29] Al-Ali H, Yabis AA, Issa E, Salem Z, Tawil A, Khoury N, *et al.* Hypercalcemia in Langerhans' cell granulomatosis with elevated 1,25 dihydroxyvitamin D (calcitriol) level. Bone. 2002;30(1):331-4.

[30] Cadranel J, Garabedian M, Milleron B, Guillozo H, Akoun G, Hance AJ. 1,25(OH)$_2$D3 production by T lymphocytes and alveolar macrophages recovered by lavage from normocalcemic patients with tuberculosis. J Clin Invest. 1990;85(5):1588-93.

[31] Fetchick DA, Bertolini DR, Sarin PS, Weintraub ST, Mundy GR, Dunn JF. Production of 1,25-dihydroxyvitamin D3 by human T cell lymphotrophic virus-I-transformed lymphocytes. J Clin Invest. 1986;78(2):592-6.

[32]   Schuessler M, Astecker N, Herzig G, Vorisek G, Schuster I. Skin is an autonomous organ in synthesis, two-step activation and degradation of vitamin D(3): CYP27 in epidermis completes the set of essential vitamin D(3)-hydroxylases. Steroids. 2001;66(3-5):399-408.

[33]   Vantieghem K, Overbergh L, Carmeliet G, De Haes P, Bouillon R, Segaert S. UVB-induced 1,25(OH)2D3 production and vitamin D activity in intestinal CaCo-2 cells and in THP-1 macrophages pretreated with a sterol Delta7-reductase inhibitor. J Cell Biochem. 2006;99(1):229-40.

[34]   Gottfried E, Rehli M, Hahn J, Holler E, Andreesen R, Kreutz M. Monocyte-derived cells express CYP27A1 and convert vitamin D3 into its active metabolite. Biochem Biophys Res Commun. 2006;349(1):209-13.

[35]   Matsumoto K, Azuma Y, Kiyoki M, Okumura H, Hashimoto K, Yoshikawa K. Involvement of endogenously produced 1,25-dihydroxyvitamin D-3 in the growth and differentiation of human keratinocytes. Biochim Biophys Acta. 1991;1092(3):311-8.

[36]   Norman AW, Henry HL, Bishop JE, Song XD, Bula C, Okamura WH. Different shapes of the steroid hormone 1alpha,25(OH)(2)-vitamin D(3) act as agonists for two different receptors in the vitamin D endocrine system to mediate genomic and rapid responses. Steroids. 2001;66(3-5):147-58.

[37]   Norman AW. Minireview: vitamin D receptor: new assignments for an already busy receptor. Endocrinology. 2006;147(12):5542-8.

[38]   Mizwicki MT, Keidel D, Bula CM, Bishop JE, Zanello LP, Wurtz JM, *et al*. Identification of an alternative ligand-binding pocket in the nuclear vitamin D receptor and its functional importance in 1alpha,25(OH)2-vitamin D3 signaling. Proc Natl Acad Sci USA. 2004;101(35):12876-81.

[39]   Nemere I, Dormanen MC, Hammond MW, Okamura WH, Norman AW. Identification of a specific binding protein for 1 alpha,25-dihydroxyvitamin D3 in basal-lateral membranes of chick intestinal epithelium and relationship to transcaltachia. J Biol Chem. 1994;269(38):23750-6.

[40]   Nemere I, Safford SE, Rohe B, DeSouza MM, Farach-Carson MC. Identification and characterization of 1,25D3-membrane-associated rapid response, steroid (1,25D3-MARRS) binding protein. J Steroid Biochem Mol Biol. 2004;89-90(1-5):281-5.

[41]   Rohe B, Safford SE, Nemere I, Farach-Carson MC. Identification and characterization of 1,25D3-membrane-associated rapid response, steroid (1,25D3-MARRS)-binding protein in rat IEC-6 cells. Steroids. 2005;70(5-7):458-63.

[42]   Garbi N, Hämmerling G, Tanaka S. Interaction of ERp57 and tapasin in the generation of MHC class I-peptide complexes. Curr Opin Immunol. 2007;19(1):99-105.

[43]   Lindquist JA, Jensen ON, Mann M, Hämmerling GJ. ER-60, a chaperone with thiol-dependent reductase activity involved in MHC class I assembly. EMBO J. 1998;17(8):2186-95.

[44]   Khanal R, Nemere I. Membrane receptors for vitamin D metabolites. Crit Rev Eukaryot Gene Expr. 2007;17(1):31-47.

[45]   Turano C, Coppari S, Altieri F, Ferraro A. Proteins of the PDI family: unpredicted non-ER locations and functions. J Cell Physiol. 2002;193(2):154-63.

[46]   Abell BA, Brown DT. Sindbis virus membrane fusion is mediated by reduction of glycoprotein disulfide bridges at the cell surface. J Virol. 1993;67(9):5496-501.

[47]   Ryser HJ, Levy EM, Mandel R, DiSciullo GJ. Inhibition of human immunodeficiency virus infection by agents that interfere with thiol-disulfide interchange upon virus-receptor interaction. Proc Natl Acad Sci USA. 1994;91(10):4559-63.

[48]   Whitfield GK, Hsieh JC, Jurutka PW, Selznick SH, Haussler CA, MacDonald PN, *et al*. Genomic actions of 1,25-dihydroxyvitamin D3. J Nutr. 1995;125(6 Suppl):1690S-4S.

[49]   Wang TT, Nestel FP, Bourdeau V, Nagai Y, Wang Q, Liao J, *et al*. Cutting edge: 1,25-dihydroxyvitamin D3 is a direct inducer of antimicrobial peptide gene expression. J Immunol. 2004;173(5):2909-12.

[50]   St-Arnaud R. The direct role of vitamin D on bone homeostasis. Arch Biochem Biophys. 2008;473(2):225-30.

[51]   Bouillon R, Eelen G, Verlinden L, Mathieu C, Carmeliet G, Verstuyf A. Vitamin D and cancer. J Steroid Biochem Mol Biol. 2006;102(1-5):156-62.

[52]   Garcion E, Wion-Barbot N, Montero-Menei CN, Berger F, Wion D. New clues about vitamin D functions in the nervous system. Trends Endocrinol Metab. 2002;13(3):100-5.

[53]   Etten E, Mathieu C. Immunoregulation by 1,25-dihydroxyvitamin D: Basic concepts. J Steroid Biochem Mol Biol. 2005;97(1-2):93-101.

[54]   Crofts LA, Hancock MS, Morrison NA, Eisman JA. Multiple promoters direct the tissue-specific expression of novel N-terminal variant human vitamin D receptor gene transcripts. Proc Natl Acad Sci USA. 1998;95(18):10529-34.

[55]   Kato S, Takeyama K, Kitanaka S, Murayama A, Sekine K, Yoshizawa T. In vivo function of VDR in gene expression-VDR knock-out mice. J Steroid Biochem Mol Biol. 1999;69(1-6):247-51.

[56]   Bouillon R, Carmeliet G, Verlinden L, van Etten E, Verstuyf A, Luderer HF, *et al.* Vitamin D and human health: lessons from vitamin D receptor null mice. Endocr Rev. 2008;29(6):726-76.

[57]   Hakim I, Bar-Shavit Z. Modulation of TNF-alpha expression in bone marrow macrophages: involvement of vitamin D response element. J Cell Biochem. 2003;88(5):986-98.

[58]   Panichi V, De Pietro S, Andreini B, Bianchi AM, Migliori M, Taccola D, *et al.* Calcitriol modulates in vivo and in vitro cytokine production: a role for intracellular calcium. Kidney Int. 1998;54(5):1463-9.

[59]   Cohen-Lahav M, Shany S, Tobvin D, Chaimovitz C, Douvdevani A. Vitamin D decreases NF{kappa}B activity by increasing I{kappa}B{alpha} levels. Nephrol Dial Transplant. 2006;21(4):889.

[60]   Cohen ML, Cohen ML, Douvdevani A, Douvdevani A, Chaimovitz C, Chaimovitz C, *et al.* Regulation of TNF-alpha by 1-alpha-25-dihydroxyvitamin D3 in human macrophages from CAPD patients. Kidney Int. 2001;59(1):69.

[61]   Sadeghi K, Wessner B, Laggner U, Ploder M, Tamandl D, Friedl J, *et al.* Vitamin D3 down-regulates monocyte TLR expression and triggers hyporesponsiveness to pathogen-associated molecular patterns. Eur J Immunol. 2006;36(2):361-70.

[62]   Schauber J, Gallo R. Antimicrobial peptides and the skin immune defense system. J Allergy Clin Immunol. 2008;122(2):261-6.

[63]   Cippitelli M, Santoni A. Vitamin D3: a transcriptional modulator of the interferon-gamma gene. Eur J Immunol. 1998;28(10):3017-30.

[64]   Towers TL, Freedman LP. Granulocyte-macrophage colony-stimulating factor gene transcription is directly repressed by the vitamin D3 receptor. Implications for allosteric influences on nuclear receptor structure and function by a DNA element. J Biol Chem. 1998;273(17):10338-48.

[65]   Dong X, Lutz W, Schroeder TM, Bachman LA, Westendorf JJ, Kumar R, *et al.* Regulation of relB in dendritic cells by means of modulated association of vitamin D receptor and histone deacetylase 3 with the promoter. Proc Natl Acad Sci USA. 2005;102(44):16007-12.

[66]   D'Ambrosio D, Cippitelli M, Cocciolo MG, Mazzeo D, Di Lucia P, Lang R, *et al.* Inhibition of IL-12 production by 1,25-dihydroxyvitamin D3. Involvement of NF-kappaB downregulation in transcriptional repression of the p40 gene. J Clin Invest. 1998;101(1):252-62.

[67]   Harant H, Andrew PJ, Reddy GS, Foglar E, Lindley IJ. 1alpha,25-dihydroxyvitamin D3 and a variety of its natural metabolites transcriptionally repress nuclear-factor-kappaB-mediated interleukin-8 gene expression. Eur J Biochem. 1997;250(1):63-71.

[68]   Alroy I, Towers TL, Freedman LP. Transcriptional repression of the interleukin-2 gene by vitamin D3: direct inhibition of NFATp/AP-1 complex formation by a nuclear hormone receptor. Mol Cell Biol. 1995;15(10):5789-99.

[69]   Cippitelli M, Fionda C, Di Bona D, Di Rosa F, Lupo A, Piccoli M, *et al.* Negative regulation of CD95 ligand gene expression by vitamin D3 in T lymphocytes. J Immunol. 2002;168(3):1154-66.

[70]   Moeenrezakhanlou A, Nandan D, Reiner NE. Identification of a Calcitriol-Regulated Sp-1 Site in the Promoter of Human CD14 using a Combined Western Blotting Electrophoresis Mobility Shift Assay (WEMSA).   Biol Proced Online. 2008;10:29-35.

[71]   Provvedini DM, Tsoukas CD, Deftos LJ, Manolagas SC. 1,25-dihydroxyvitamin D3 receptors in human leukocytes. Science. 1983;221(4616):1181-3.

[72]   Veldman CM, Cantorna MT, DeLuca HF. Expression of 1,25-dihydroxyvitamin D(3) receptor in the immune system. Arch Biochem Biophys. 2000;374(2):334-8.

[73]   Brennan A, Katz DR, Nunn JD, Barker S, Hewison M, Fraher LJ, *et al.* Dendritic cells from human tissues express receptors for the immunoregulatory vitamin D3 metabolite, dihydroxycholecalciferol. Immunology. 1987;61(4):457-61.

[74]   Milde P, Hauser U, Simon T, Mall G, Ernst V, Haussler MR, *et al.* Expression of 1,25-dihydroxyvitamin D3 receptors in normal and psoriatic skin. J Invest Dermatol. 1991;97(2):230-9.

[75]   Dam TN, Møller B, Hindkjaer J, Kragballe K. The vitamin D3 analog calcipotriol suppresses the number and antigen-presenting function of Langerhans cells in normal human skin. J Investig Dermatol Symp Proc. 1996;1(1):72-7.

[76]   Hewison M, Burke F, Evans KN, Lammas DA, Sansom DM, Liu P, *et al.* Extra-renal 25-hydroxyvitamin D3-1alpha-hydroxylase in human health and disease. J Steroid Biochem Mol Biol. 2007;103(3-5):316-21.

[77]   Adams JS, Hewison M. Unexpected actions of vitamin D: new perspectives on the regulation of innate and adaptive immunity. Nat Clin Pract Endocrinol Metab. 2008;4(2):80-90.

[78]   Dasari P, Nicholson IC, Zola H. Toll-like receptors. J Biol Regul Homeost Agents. 2008;22(1):17-26.

[79] Adams JS. Vitamin D as a defensin. J Musculoskelet Neuronal Interact. 2006;6(4):344-6.

[80] Bhalla AK, Amento EP, Serog B, Glimcher LH. 1,25-Dihydroxyvitamin D3 inhibits antigen-induced T cell activation. J Immunol. 1984;133(4):1748-54.

[81] Penna G, Adorini L. 1 Alpha,25-dihydroxyvitamin D3 inhibits differentiation, maturation, activation, and survival of dendritic cells leading to impaired alloreactive T cell activation. J Immunol. 2000;164(5):2405-11.

[82] Griffin MD, Lutz W, Phan VA, Bachman LA, McKean DJ, Kumar R. Dendritic cell modulation by 1alpha,25 dihydroxyvitamin D3 and its analogs: a vitamin D receptor-dependent pathway that promotes a persistent state of immaturity in vitro and in vivo. Proc Natl Acad Sci USA. 2001;98(12):6800-5.

[83] Boonstra A, Barrat FJ, Crain C, Heath VL, Savelkoul HF, O'Garra A. 1alpha,25-Dihydroxyvitamin d3 has a direct effect on naive CD4(+) T cells to enhance the development of Th2 cells. J Immunol. 2001;167(9):4974-80.

[84] Lemire JM, Archer DC, Beck L, Spiegelberg HL. Immunosuppressive actions of 1,25-dihydroxyvitamin D3: preferential inhibition of Th1 functions. J Nutr. 1995;125(6 Suppl):1704S-8S.

[85] Yu XP, Bellido T, Manolagas SC. Down-regulation of NF-kappa B protein levels in activated human lymphocytes by 1,25-dihydroxyvitamin D3. Proc Natl Acad Sci USA. 1995;92(24):10990-4.

[86] Gregori S, Giarratana N, Smiroldo S, Uskokovic M, Adorini L. A 1alpha,25-dihydroxyvitamin D(3) analog enhances regulatory T-cells and arrests autoimmune diabetes in NOD mice. Diabetes. 2002;51(5):1367-74.

[87] Tobler A, Gasson J, Reichel H, Norman AW, Koeffler HP. Granulocyte-macrophage colony-stimulating factor. Sensitive and receptor-mediated regulation by 1,25-dihydroxyvitamin D3 in normal human peripheral blood lymphocytes. J Clin Invest. 1987;79(6):1700-5.

[88] Mahon BD, Wittke A, Weaver V, Cantorna MT. The targets of vitamin D depend on the differentiation and activation status of CD4 positive T cells. J Cell Biochem. 2003;89(5):922-32.

[89] Piemonti L, Monti P, Sironi M, Fraticelli P, Leone BE, Dal Cin E, et al. Vitamin D3 affects differentiation, maturation, and function of human monocyte-derived dendritic cells. J Immunol. 2000;164(9):4443-51.

[90] Xu H, Soruri A, Gieseler RK, Peters JH. 1,25-Dihydroxyvitamin D3 exerts opposing effects to IL-4 on MHC class-II antigen expression, accessory activity, and phagocytosis of human monocytes. Scand J Immunol. 1993;38(6):535-40.

[91] Matsuzaki J, Tsuji T, Zhang Y, Wakita D, Imazeki I, Sakai T, et al. 1alpha,25-Dihydroxyvitamin D3 downmodulates the functional differentiation of Th1 cytokine-conditioned bone marrow-derived dendritic cells beneficial for cytotoxic T lymphocyte generation. Cancer Sci. 2006;97(2):139-47.

[92] Adorini L, Giarratana N, Penna G. Pharmacological induction of tolerogenic dendritic cells and regulatory T cells. Semin Immunol. 2004;16(2):127-34.

[93] Penna G, Amuchastegui S, Giarratana N, Daniel KC, Vulcano M, Sozzani S, et al. 1,25-Dihydroxyvitamin D3 selectively modulates tolerogenic properties in myeloid but not plasmacytoid dendritic cells. J Immunol. 2007;178(1):145-53.

[94] Gauzzi MC, Purificato C, Donato K, Jin Y, Wang L, Daniel KC, et al. Suppressive effect of 1alpha,25-dihydroxyvitamin D3 on type I IFN-mediated monocyte differentiation into dendritic cells: impairment of functional activities and chemotaxis. J Immunol. 2005;174(1):270-6.

[95] Spittler A, Willheim M, Leutmezer F, Ohler R, Krugluger W, Reissner C, et al. Effects of 1 alpha,25-dihydroxyvitamin D3 and cytokines on the expression of MHC antigens, complement receptors and other antigens on human blood monocytes and U937 cells: role in cell differentiation, activation and phagocytosis. Immunology. 1997;90(2):286-93.

[96] Helming L, Böse J, Ehrchen J, Schiebe S, Frahm T, Geffers R, et al. 1alpha,25-Dihydroxyvitamin D3 is a potent suppressor of interferon gamma-mediated macrophage activation. Blood. 2005;106(13):4351-8.

[97] Canning MO, Grotenhuis K, de Wit H, Ruwhof C, Drexhage HA. 1-alpha,25-Dihydroxyvitamin D3 (1,25(OH)$_2$D3) hampers the maturation of fully active immature dendritic cells from monocytes. Eur J Endocrinol. 2001;145(3):351-7.

[98] Giovannini L, Panichi V, Migliori M, De Pietro S, Bertelli AA, Fulgenzi A, et al. 1,25-dihydroxyvitamin D(3) dose-dependently inhibits LPS-induced cytokines production in PBMC modulating intracellular calcium. Transplant Proc. 2001;33(3):2366-8.

[99] Chen S, Sims GP, Chen XX, Gu YY, Chen S, Lipsky PE. Modulatory effects of 1,25-dihydroxyvitamin D3 on human B cell differentiation. J Immunol. 2007;179(3):1634-47.

[100] Gombart AF, Borregaard N, Koeffler HP. Human cathelicidin antimicrobial peptide (CAMP) gene is a direct target of the vitamin D receptor and is strongly up-regulated in myeloid cells by 1,25-dihydroxyvitamin D3. *FASEB* J. 2005;19(9):1067-77.

[101] Ren S, Nguyen L, Wu S, Encinas C, Adams JS, Hewison M. Alternative splicing of vitamin D-24-hydroxylase: a novel mechanism for the regulation of extrarenal 1,25-dihydroxyvitamin D synthesis. J Biol Chem. 2005;280(21):20604-11.

[102] Akira S, Takeda K, Kaisho T. Toll-like receptors: critical proteins linking innate and acquired immunity. Nat Immunol. 2001;2(8):675-80.

[103] Kidd P. Th1/Th2 balance: the hypothesis, its limitations, and implications for health and disease. Altern Med Rev. 2003;8(3):223-46.

[104] Penna G, Giarratana N, Amuchastegui S, Mariani R, Daniel KC, Adorini L. Manipulating dendritic cells to induce regulatory T cells. Microbes Infect. 2005;7(7-8):1033-9.

[105] Muthian G, Raikwar HP, Rajasingh J, Bright JJ. 1,25 Dihydroxyvitamin-D3 modulates JAK-STAT pathway in IL-12/IFNgamma axis leading to Th1 response in experimental allergic encephalomyelitis. J Neurosci Res. 2006;83(7):1299-309.

[106] Pavlovitch JH RM, Garabedian M Enhancing effect of 1,25-dihydroxy-vitamin D3 on murine retroviral immunodeficiency syndrome. Immunol Infect Dis 1996;6:93-7.

[107] Norris PJ, Rosenberg ES. Cellular immune response to human immunodeficiency virus. AIDS. 2001;15 (Suppl 2):S16-21.

[108] Harrer T, Harrer E, Kalams SA, Barbosa P, Trocha A, Johnson RP, *et al*. Cytotoxic T lymphocytes in asymptomatic long-term nonprogressing HIV-1 infection. Breadth and specificity of the response and relation to in vivo viral quasispecies in a person with prolonged infection and low viral load. J Immunol. 1996;156(7):2616-23.

[109] Clerici M, Shearer GM. A TH1-->TH2 switch is a critical step in the etiology of HIV infection. Immunol Today. 1993;14(3):107-11.

[110] Klein SA, Dobmeyer JM, Dobmeyer TS, Pape M, Ottmann OG, Helm EB, *et al*. Demonstration of the Th1 to Th2 cytokine shift during the course of HIV-1 infection using cytoplasmic cytokine detection on single cell level by flow cytometry. AIDS. 1997;11(9):1111-8.

[111] Majumder B, Janket ML, Schafer EA, Schaubert K, Huang XL, Kan-Mitchell J, *et al*. Human immunodeficiency virus type 1 Vpr impairs dendritic cell maturation and T-cell activation: implications for viral immune escape. J Virol. 2005;79(13):7990-8003.

[112] Romagnani S, Del Prete G, Manetti R, Ravina A, Annunziato F, De Carli M, *et al*. Role of TH1/TH2 cytokines in HIV infection. Immunol Rev. 1994;140:73-92.

[113] Galli G, Annunziato F, Cosmi L, Manetti R, Maggi E, Romagnani S. Th1 and th2 responses, HIV-1 coreceptors, and HIV-1 infection. J Biol Regul Homeost Agents. 2001;15(3):308-13.

[114] Adorini L. Immunomodulatory effects of vitamin D receptor ligands in autoimmune diseases. Int Immunopharmacol. 2002;2(7):1017-28.

[115] Hyppönen E, Sovio U, Wjst M, Patel S, Pekkanen J, Hartikainen AL, *et al*. Infant vitamin d supplementation and allergic conditions in adulthood: northern Finland birth cohort 1966. Ann N Y Acad Sci. 2004;1037:84-95.

[116] Wjst M. The vitamin D slant on allergy. Pediatr Allergy Immunol. 2006;17(7):477-83.

[117] Nnoaham KE, Clarke A. Low serum vitamin D levels and tuberculosis: a systematic review and meta-analysis. Int J Epidemiol. 2008;37(1):113-9.

[118] Falkenbach, A, Sedlmeyer, A. Travel to sunny countries is associated with changes in immunological parameters. Photodermatol Photoimmunol Photomed. 1997;13(4):139-42.

[119] Chan TY. Vitamin D deficiency and susceptibility to tuberculosis. Calcif Tissue Int. 2000;66(6):476-8.

[120] Cannell JJ, Vieth R, Umhau JC, Holick MF, Grant WB, Madronich S, *et al*. Epidemic influenza and vitamin D. Epidemiol Infect. 2006;134(6):1129-40.

[121] Fleming DM, Elliot AJ. Epidemic influenza and vitamin D. Epidemiol Infect. 2007;135(7):1091-2; author reply 2-5.

[122] Yusuf S, Piedimonte G, Auais A, Demmler G, Krishnan S, Van Caeseele P, *et al*. The relationship of meteorological conditions to the epidemic activity of respiratory syncytial virus. Epidemiol Infect. 2007;135(7):1077-90.

[123] Li-Ng M, Aloia JF, Pollack S, Cunha BA, Mikhail M, Yeh J, *et al*. A randomized controlled trial of vitamin D3 supplementation for the prevention of symptomatic upper respiratory tract infections. Epidemiol Infect. 2009:1-9.

[124] Rietveld WJ, Boon ME, Meulman JJ. Seasonal fluctuations in the cervical smear detection rates for (pre)malignant changes and for infections. Diagn Cytopathol. 1997;17(6):452-5.

[125] Vogel J, Cepeda M, Tschachler E, Napolitano LA, Jay G. UV activation of human immunodeficiency virus gene expression in transgenic mice. J Virol. 1992;66(1):1-5.

[126] Meola T, Soter NA, Ostreicher R, Sanchez M, Moy JA. The safety of UVB phototherapy in patients with HIV infection. J Am Acad Dermatol. 1993;29(1):216-20.

[127] Akaraphanth R, Lim HW. HIV, UV and immunosuppression. Photodermatol Photoimmunol Photomed. 1999;15(1):28-31.

[128] Saah AJ, Horn TD, Hoover DR, Chen C, Whitmore SE, Flynn C, *et al*. Solar ultraviolet radiation exposure does not appear to exacerbate HIV infection in homosexual men. The Multicenter AIDS Cohort Study. AIDS. 1997;11(14):1773-8.

[129] Maas J, Termorshuizen F, Geskus RB, Goettsch W, Coutinho RA, Miedema F, *et al*. Amsterdam Cohort Study on HIV and AIDS: impact of exposure to UVR as estimated by means of a 2-year retrospective questionnaire on immune parameters in HIV positive males. Int J Hyg Environ Health. 2002;205(5):373-7.

[130] Termorshuizen F, Geskus RB, Roos MT, Coutinho RA, Van Loveren H. Seasonal influences on immunological parameters in HIV-infected homosexual men: searching for the immunomodulating effects of sunlight. Int J Hyg Environ Health. 2002;205(5):379-84.

[131] EuroHIV. The HIV epidemic associated with injecting drug use in Europe. HIV/AIDS surveillance in Europe: 1996. 1996;50:34-42.

[132] Hamers FF, Batter V, Downs AM, Alix J, Cazein F, Brunet JB. The HIV epidemic associated with injecting drug use in Europe: geographic and time trends. AIDS. 1997;11(11):1365-74.

[133] Jablonski N. The evolution of human skin coloration. J Hum Evol. 2000;39(1):57-106.

[134] Holick M. Environmental factors that influence the cutaneous production of vitamin D. Am J Clin Nutr. 1995;61(3):638S.

[135] Webb AR, Engelsen O. Calculated ultraviolet exposure levels for a healthy vitamin D status. Photochem Photobiol. 2006;82(6):1697-703.

[136] EuroHIV. HIV/AIDS Surveillance in Europe: Mid-year report 2007. Saint-Maurice: Institut de Veille Sanitaire. 2007(76).

[137] Bautista CT, Sateren WB, Sanchez JL, Singer DE, Scott P. Geographic mapping of HIV infection among civilian applicants for United States military service. Health Place. 2008;14(3):608-15.

[138] Dawson-Hughes B, Heaney RP, Holick MF, Lips P, Meunier PJ, Vieth R. Estimates of optimal vitamin D status. Osteoporos Int. 2005;16(7):713-6.

[139] Holick MF. Sunlight, UV-radiation, vitamin D and skin cancer: how much sunlight do we need? Adv Exp Med Biol. 2008;624:1-15.

[140] Coodley GO, Coodley MK, Nelson HD, Loveless MO. Micronutrient concentrations in the HIV wasting syndrome. AIDS. 1993;7(12):1595-600.

[141] Haug C, Müller F, Aukrust P, Frøland SS. Subnormal serum concentration of 1,25-vitamin D in human immunodeficiency virus infection: correlation with degree of immune deficiency and survival. J Infect Dis. 1994;169(4):889-93.

[142] Haug CJ, Aukrust P, Haug E, Mørkrid L, Müller F, Frøland SS. Severe deficiency of 1,25-dihydroxyvitamin D3 in human immunodeficiency virus infection: association with immunological hyperactivity and only minor changes in calcium homeostasis. J Clin Endocrinol Metab. 1998;83(11):3832-8.

[143] Mayur N, Lewis S, Catherwood BD, Nanes MS. Tumor necrosis factor alpha decreases 1,25-dihydroxyvitamin D3 receptors in osteoblastic ROS 17/2.8 cells. J Bone Miner Res. 1993;8(8):997-1003.

[144] Aukrust P, Haug CJ, Ueland T, Lien E, Müller F, Espevik T, *et al*. Decreased bone formative and enhanced resorptive markers in human immunodeficiency virus infection: indication of normalization of the bone-remodeling process during highly active antiretroviral therapy. J Clin Endocrinol Metab. 1999;84(1):145-50.

[145] Dusso AS. Protease inhibitors inhibit in vitro conversion on 25(OH)-vitamin D to 1,25 (OH)2-vitamin D. 2nd International Workshop on Adverse Drug Interactions and Lipodystrophy Toronto. 2000;abstract 030.

[146] Cozzolino M, Vidal M, Arcidiacono MV, Tebas P, Yarasheski KE, Dusso AS. HIV-protease inhibitors impair vitamin D bioactivation to 1,25-dihydroxyvitamin D. AIDS. 2003;17(4):513-20.

[147] Urso R, Visco-Comandini U, Antonucci G. Bone dysmetabolism in HIV infection: a melting pot of opinions. AIDS. 2003;17(9):1416-7.

[148] Madeddu G, Spanu A, Solinas P, Calia GM, Lovigu C, Chessa F, *et al*. Bone mass loss and vitamin D metabolism impairment in HIV patients receiving highly active antiretroviral therapy. Q J Nucl Med Mol Imaging.2004;48(1):39-48.

[149] McComsey GA, Kendall MA, Tebas P, Swindells S, Hogg E, Alston-Smith B, *et al*. Alendronate with calcium and vitamin D supplementation is safe and effective for the treatment of decreased bone mineral density in HIV. AIDS. 2007;21(18):2473-82.

[150] Kitano K, Baldwin GC, Raines MA, Golde DW. Differentiating agents facilitate infection of myeloid leukemia cell lines by monocytotropic HIV-1 strains. Blood. 1990;76(10):1980-8.

[151] Makuta Y, Sonoda Y, Yamamoto D, Funakoshi-Tago M, Aizu-Yokota E, Takebe Y, *et al*. Interleukin-10-induced CCR5 expression in macrophage like HL-60 cells: involvement of Erk1/2 and STAT-3. Biol Pharm Bull. 2003;26(8):1076-81.

[152] Loetscher M, Geiser T, O'Reilly T, Zwahlen R, Baggiolini M, Moser B. Cloning of a human seven-transmembrane domain receptor, LESTR, that is highly expressed in leukocytes. J Biol Chem. 1994;269(1):232-7.

[153] Savli H, Aalto Y, Nagy B, Knuutila S, Pakkala S. Gene expression analysis of 1,25(OH)$_2$D3-dependent differentiation of HL-60 cells: a cDNA array study. Br J Haematol. 2002;118(4):1065-70.

[154] Gupta SK, Pillarisetti K, Aiyar N. CXCR4 undergoes complex lineage and inducing agent-dependent dissociation of expression and functional responsiveness to SDF-1alpha during myeloid differentiation. J Leukoc Biol. 2001;70(3):431-8.

[155] Sundstrom C, Nilsson K. Establishment and characterization of a human histiocytic lymphoma cell line (U-937). Int J Cancer. 1976;17(5):565-77.

[156] Cassol E, Alfano M, Biswas P, Poli G. Monocyte-derived macrophages and myeloid cell lines as targets of HIV-1 replication and persistence. J Leukoc Biol. 2006;80(5):1018-30.

[157] Pauza CD, Kornbluth R, Emau P, Richman DD, Deftos LJ. Vitamin D3 compounds regulate human immunodeficiency virus type 1 replication in U937 monoblastoid cells and in monocyte-derived macrophages. J Leukoc Biol. 1993;53(2):157-64.

[158] Skolnik PR, Jahn B, Wang MZ, Rota TR, Hirsch MS, Krane SM. Enhancement of human immunodeficiency virus 1 replication in monocytes by 1,25-dihydroxycholecalciferol. Proc Natl Acad Sci USA. 1991;88(15):6632-6.

[159] Goletti D, Kinter AL, Biswas P, Bende SM, Poli G, Fauci AS. Effect of cellular differentiation on cytokine-induced expression of human immunodeficiency virus in chronically infected promonocytic cells: dissociation of cellular differentiation and viral expression. J Virol. 1995;69(4):2540-6.

[160] Boulerice F, Geleziunas R, Bour S, Li HL, D'Addario M, Roulston A, *et al*. Differential susceptibilities of U-937 cell clones to infection by human immunodeficiency virus type 1. J Virol. 1992;66(2):1183-7.

[161] Kameoka M, Kimura T, Okada Y, Nakaya T, Kishi M, Ikuta K. High susceptibility of U937-derived subclones to infection with human immunodeficiency virus type 1 is correlated with virus-induced cell differentiation and superoxide generation. Immunopharmacology. 1995;30(1):89-101.

[162] Moriuchi H, Moriuchi M, Arthos J, Hoxie J, Fauci AS. Promonocytic U937 subclones expressing CD4 and CXCR4 are resistant to infection with and cell-to-cell fusion by T-cell-tropic human immunodeficiency virus type 1. J Virol. 1997;71(12):9664-71.

[163] Biswas P, Mengozzi M, Mantelli B, Delfanti F, Brambilla A, Vicenzi E, *et al*. 1,25-Dihydroxyvitamin D3 upregulates functional CXCR4 human immunodeficiency virus type 1 coreceptors in U937 minus clones: NF-kappaB-independent enhancement of viral replication. J Virol. 1998;72(10):8380-3.

[164] Honda Y, Rogers L, Nakata K, Zhao BY, Pine R, Nakai Y, *et al*. Type I interferon induces inhibitory 16-kD CCAAT/ enhancer binding protein (C/EBP)beta, repressing the HIV-1 long terminal repeat in macrophages: pulmonary tuberculosis alters C/EBP expression, enhancing HIV-1 replication. J Exp Med. 1998;188(7):1255-65.

[165] Schuitemaker H, Kootstra NA, Koppelman MH, Bruisten SM, Huisman HG, Tersmette M, *et al*. Proliferation-dependent HIV-1 infection of monocytes occurs during differentiation into macrophages. J Clin Invest. 1992;89(4):1154-60.

[166] Klotman ME, Rapista A, Teleshova N, Micsenyi A, Jarvis GA, Lu W, *et al*. Neisseria gonorrhoeae-induced human defensins 5 and 6 increase HIV infectivity: role in enhanced transmission. J Immunol. 2008;180(9):6176-85.

[167] Hong SP, Kim MJ, Jung MY, Jeon H, Goo J, Ahn SK, *et al*. Biopositive effects of low-dose UVB on epidermis: coordinate upregulation of antimicrobial peptides and permeability barrier reinforcement. J Invest Dermatol. 2008;128(12):2880-7.

[168] Bergman P, Walter-Jallow L, Broliden K, Agerberth B, Söderlund J. The antimicrobial peptide LL-37 inhibits HIV-1 replication. Curr HIV Res. 2007;5(4):410-5.

[169] Wang G, Watson KM, Buckheit RW. Anti-human immunodeficiency virus type 1 activities of antimicrobial peptides derived from human and bovine cathelicidins. Antimicrob Agents Chemother. 2008;52(9):3438-40.

[170] Levinson P, Kaul R, Kimani J, Ngugi E, Moses S, MacDonald KS, *et al*. Levels of innate immune factors in genital fluids: association of alpha defensins and LL-37 with genital infections and increased HIV acquisition. AIDS. 2009;23(3):309-17.

[171] Nagaoka I, Tamura H, Hirata M. An antimicrobial cathelicidin peptide, human CAP18/LL-37, suppresses neutrophil apoptosis via the activation of formyl-peptide receptor-like 1 and P2X7. J Immunol. 2006;176(5):3044-52.

[172] Carretero M, Escámez MJ, García M, Duarte B, Holguín A, Retamosa L, *et al*. In vitro and in vivo wound healing-promoting activities of human cathelicidin LL-37. J Invest Dermatol. 2008;128(1):223-36.

[173] Mangeat B, Turelli P, Caron G, Friedli M, Perrin L, Trono D. Broad antiretroviral defence by human APOBEC3G through lethal editing of nascent reverse transcripts. Nature. 2003;424(6944):99-103.

[174] Peng G, Lei KJ, Jin W, Greenwell-Wild T, Wahl SM. Induction of APOBEC3 family proteins, a defensive maneuver underlying interferon-induced anti-HIV-1 activity. J Exp Med. 2006;203(1):41-6.

[175] Vetter ML, Johnson ME, Antons AK, Unutmaz D, D'Aquila RT. Differences in APOBEC3G expression in CD4+ T helper lymphocyte subtypes modulate HIV-1 infectivity. PLoS Pathog. 2009;5(2):e1000292.

[176] Estes JD, Li Q, Reynolds MR, Wietgrefe S, Duan L, Schacker T, *et al*. Premature induction of an immunosuppressive regulatory T cell response during acute simian immunodeficiency virus infection. J Infect Dis. 2006;193(5):703-12.

[177] El-Far M, Halwani R, Said E, Trautmann L, Doroudchi M, Janbazian L, *et al*. T-cell exhaustion in HIV infection. Curr HIV/AIDS Rep. 2008;5(1):13-9.

[178] Chehimi J, Starr SE, Frank I, D'Andrea A, Ma X, MacGregor RR, *et al*. Impaired interleukin 12 production in human immunodeficiency virus-infected patients. J Exp Med. 1994;179(4):1361-6.

[179] Nagy-Agren SE, Cooney EL. Interleukin-12 enhancement of antigen-specific lymphocyte proliferation correlates with stage of human immunodeficiency virus infection. J Infect Dis. 1999;179(2):493-6.

[180] Ma X, Montaner LJ. Proinflammatory response and IL-12 expression in HIV-1 infection. J Leukoc Biol. 2000;68(3):383-90.

[181] Gupta S, Boppana R, Mishra GC, Saha B, Mitra D. Interleukin-12 is necessary for the priming of CD4+ T cells required during the elicitation of HIV-1 gp120-specific cytotoxic T-lymphocyte function. Immunology. 2008;124(4):553-61.

[182] Leghmari K, Bennasser Y, Bahraoui E. HIV-1 Tat protein induces IL-10 production in monocytes by classical and alternative NF-kappaB pathways. Eur J Cell Biol. 2008;87(12):947-62.

[183] Paganelli R, Scala E, Ansotegui IJ, Mezzaroma I, Pinter E, Ferrara R, *et al*. Hyper IgE syndrome induced by HIV infection. Immunodeficiency. 1993;4(1-4):149-52.

[184] Dikeacou T, Katsambas A, Lowenstein W, Romana C, Balamotis A, Tsianakas P, *et al*. Clinical manifestations of allergy and their relation to HIV infection. Int Arch Allergy Immunol. 1993;102(4):408-13.

[185] Becker Y. HIV-1 induced AIDS is an allergy and the allergen is the Shed gp120--a review, hypothesis, and implications. Virus Genes. 2004;28(3):319-31.

[186] Marone G, Florio G, Petraroli A, de Paulis A. Dysregulation of the IgE/Fc epsilon RI network in HIV-1 infection. J Allergy Clin Immunol. 2001;107(1):22-30.

[187] Dugas N, Dereuddre-Bosquet N, Goujard C, Dormont D, Tardieu M, Delfraissy JF. Role of nitric oxide in the promoting effect of HIV type 1 infection and of gp120 envelope glycoprotein on interleukin 4-induced IgE production by normal human mononuclear cells. AIDS Res Hum Retroviruses. 2000;16(3):251-8.

[188] Patella V, Florio G, Petraroli A, Marone G. HIV-1 gp120 induces IL-4 and IL-13 release from human Fc epsilon RI+ cells through interaction with the VH3 region of IgE. J Immunol. 2000;164(2):589-95.

[189] Betts MR, Ambrozak DR, Douek DC, Bonhoeffer S, Brenchley JM, Casazza JP, *et al*. Analysis of total human immunodeficiency virus (HIV)-specific CD4(+) and CD8(+) T-cell responses: relationship to viral load in untreated HIV infection. J Virol. 2001;75(24):11983-91.

[190] Brenchley JM, Price DA, Schacker TW, Asher TE, Silvestri G, Rao S, *et al*. Microbial translocation is a cause of systemic immune activation in chronic HIV infection. Nat Med. 2006;12(12):1365-71.

[191] Hazenberg MD, Otto SA, van Benthem BH, Roos MT, Coutinho RA, Lange JM, *et al*. Persistent immune activation in HIV-1 infection is associated with progression to AIDS. AIDS. 2003;17(13):1881-8.

[192] Giorgi JV, Liu Z, Hultin LE, Cumberland WG, Hennessey K, Detels R. Elevated levels of CD38+ CD8+ T cells in HIV infection add to the prognostic value of low CD4+ T cell levels: results of 6 years of follow-up. The Los Angeles Center, Multicenter AIDS Cohort Study. J Acquir Immune Defic Syndr. 1993;6(8):904-12.

[193] Shan M, Klasse P, Banerjee K, Dey A, Iyer S, Dionisio R, *et al*. HIV-1 gp120 mannoses induce immunosuppressive responses from dendritic cells. PLoS Pathog. 2007;3(11):e169.

[194] Stevceva L, Yoon V, Anastasiades D, Poznansky MC. Immune responses to HIV Gp120 that facilitate viral escape. Curr HIV Res. 2007;5(1):47-54.

[195] Papagno L, Spina CA, Marchant A, Salio M, Rufer N, Little S, *et al*. Immune activation and CD8+ T-cell differentiation towards senescence in HIV-1 infection. Plos Biol. 2004;2(2):E20.

[196] Autran B, Carcelain G, Li TS, Blanc C, Mathez D, Tubiana R, *et al*. Positive effects of combined antiretroviral therapy on CD4+ T cell homeostasis and function in advanced HIV disease. Science. 1997;277(5322):112-6.

[197] Rizzardi GP, Lazzarin A, Pantaleo G. Potential role of immune modulation in the effective long-term control of HIV-1 infection. J Biol Regul Homeost Agents. 2002;16(1):83-90.

[198] Fumero E, García F, Gatell JM. Immunosuppressive drugs as an adjuvant to HIV treatment. J Antimicrob Chemother. 2004;53(3):415-7.

[199] Seddiki N, Kelleher AD. Regulatory T cells in HIV infection: who's suppressing what? Curr HIV/AIDS Rep. 2008;5(1):20-6.

[200] Eggena MP, Barugahare B, Jones N, Okello M, Mutalya S, Kityo C, *et al*. Depletion of regulatory T cells in HIV infection is associated with immune activation. J Immunol. 2005;174(7):4407-14.

[201] Kinter AL, Hennessey M, Bell A, Kern S, Lin Y, Daucher M, *et al*. CD25(+)CD4(+) regulatory T cells from the peripheral blood of asymptomatic HIV-infected individuals regulate CD4(+) and CD8(+) HIV-specific T cell immune responses in vitro and are associated with favorable clinical markers of disease status. J Exp Med. 2004;200(3):331-43.

[202] Tsunemi S, Iwasaki T, Imado T, Higasa S, Kakishita E, Shirasaka T, *et al*. Relationship of CD4+CD25+ regulatory T cells to immune status in HIV-infected patients. AIDS. 2005;19(9):879-86.

[203] Moore KW, de Waal Malefyt R, Coffman RL, O'Garra A. Interleukin-10 and the interleukin-10 receptor. Annu Rev Immunol. 2001;19:683-765.

[204] Blackburn SD, Wherry EJ. IL-10, T cell exhaustion and viral persistence. Trends Microbiol. 2007;15(4):143-6.

[205] Brooks DG, Trifilo MJ, Edelmann KH, Teyton L, McGavern DB, Oldstone MB. Interleukin-10 determines viral clearance or persistence in vivo. Nat Med. 2006;12(11):1301-9.

[206] Ejrnaes M, Filippi CM, Martinic MM, Ling EM, Togher LM, Crotty S, *et al*. Resolution of a chronic viral infection after interleukin-10 receptor blockade. J Exp Med. 2006;203(11):2461-72.

[207] Arai H, Miyamoto KI, Yoshida M, Yamamoto H, Taketani Y, Morita K, *et al*. The polymorphism in the caudal-related homeodomain protein Cdx-2 binding element in the human vitamin D receptor gene. J Bone Miner Res. 2001;16(7):1256-64.

[208] Fang Y, van Meurs JB, d'Alesio A, Jhamai M, Zhao H, Rivadeneira F, *et al*. Promoter and 3'-untranslated-region haplotypes in the vitamin d receptor gene predispose to osteoporotic fracture: the rotterdam study. Am J Hum Genet. 2005;77(5):807-23.

[209] Gross C, Eccleshall TR, Malloy PJ, Villa ML, Marcus R, Feldman D. The presence of a polymorphism at the translation initiation site of the vitamin D receptor gene is associated with low bone mineral density in postmenopausal Mexican-American women. J Bone Miner Res. 1996;11(12):1850-5.

[210] Jurutka PW, Remus LS, Whitfield GK, Thompson PD, Hsieh JC, Zitzer H, *et al*. The polymorphic N terminus in human vitamin D receptor isoforms influences transcriptional activity by modulating interaction with transcription factor IIB. Mol Endocrinol. 2000;14(3):401-20.

[211] van Etten E, Verlinden L, Giulietti A, Ramos-Lopez E, Branisteanu DD, Ferreira GB, *et al*. The vitamin D receptor gene FokI polymorphism: functional impact on the immune system. Eur J Immunol. 2007;37(2):395-405.

[212] Morrison NA, Qi JC, Tokita A, Kelly PJ, Crofts L, Nguyen TV, *et al*. Prediction of bone density from vitamin D receptor alleles. Nature. 1994;367(6460):284-7.

[213] Ingles SA, Ross RK, Yu MC, Irvine RA, La Pera G, Haile RW, *et al*. Association of prostate cancer risk with genetic polymorphisms in vitamin D receptor and androgen receptor. J Natl Cancer Inst. 1997;89(2):166-70.

[214] Selvaraj P, Vidyarani M, Alagarasu K, Prabhu Anand S, Narayanan PR. Regulatory role of promoter and 3' UTR variants of vitamin D receptor gene on cytokine response in pulmonary tuberculosis. J Clin Immunol. 2008;28(4):306-13.

[215] Bellamy R, Ruwende C, Corrah T, McAdam KP, Thursz M, Whittle HC, *et al*. Tuberculosis and chronic hepatitis B virus infection in Africans and variation in the vitamin D receptor gene. J Infect Dis. 1999;179(3):721-4.

[216] Wilkinson RJ, Llewelyn M, Toossi Z, Patel P, Pasvol G, Lalvani A, *et al*. Influence of vitamin D deficiency and vitamin D receptor polymorphisms on tuberculosis among Gujarati Asians in west London: a case-control study. Lancet. 2000;355(9204):618-21.

[217] Roy S, Frodsham A, Saha B, Hazra SK, Mascie-Taylor CG, Hill AV. Association of vitamin D receptor genotype with leprosy type. J Infect Dis. 1999;179(1):187-91.

[218] Loke H, Bethell D, Phuong CX, Day N, White N, Farrar J, *et al*. Susceptibility to dengue hemorrhagic fever in vietnam: evidence of an association with variation in the vitamin d receptor and Fc gamma receptor IIa genes. Am J Trop Med Hyg. 2002;67(1):102-6.

[219] Saito M, Eiraku N, Usuku K, Nobuhara Y, Matsumoto W, Kodama D, *et al*. ApaI polymorphism of vitamin D receptor gene is associated with susceptibility to HTLV-1-associated myelopathy/tropical spastic paraparesis in HTLV-1 infected individuals. J Neurol Sci 2005;232(1-2):29-35.

[220] Suneetha PV, Sarin SK, Goyal A, Kumar GT, Shukla DK, Hissar S. Association between vitamin D receptor, CCR5, TNF-alpha and TNF-beta gene polymorphisms and HBV infection and severity of liver disease. J Hepatol. 2006;44(5):856-63.

[221] Janssen R, Bont L, Siezen CL, Hodemaekers HM, Ermers MJ, Doornbos G, *et al.* Genetic susceptibility to respiratory syncytial virus bronchiolitis is predominantly associated with innate immune genes. J Infect Dis. 2007;196(6):826-34.

[222] Gibney KB, MacGregor L, Leder K, Torresi J, Marshall C, Ebeling PR, *et al.* Vitamin D deficiency is associated with tuberculosis and latent tuberculosis infection in immigrants from sub-Saharan Africa. Clin Infect Dis. 2008;46(3):443-6.

[223] Rajapakse R, Uring-Lambert B, Andarawewa KL, Rajapakse RP, Abou-Bacar A, Marcellin L, *et al.* 1,25(OH)$_2$D3 inhibits in vitro and in vivo intracellular growth of apicomplexan parasite Toxoplasma gondii. J Steroid Biochem Mol Biol. 2007;103(3-5):811-4.

[224] Rajapakse R, Mousli M, Pfaff AW, Uring-Lambert B, Marcellin L, Bronner C, *et al.* 1,25-Dihydroxyvitamin D3 induces splenocyte apoptosis and enhances BALB/c mice sensitivity to toxoplasmosis. J Steroid Biochem Mol Biol. 2005;96(2):179-85.

[225] Wejse C, Gomes VF, Rabna P, Gustafson P, Aaby P, Lisse IM, *et al.* Vitamin D as Supplementary Treatment for Tuberculosis - A Double-blind Randomized Placebo-controlled Trial. Am J Respir Crit Care Med. 2009; 179: 843-50.

[226] Norman AW. From vitamin D to hormone D: fundamentals of the vitamin D endocrine system essential for good health. Am J Clin Nutr. 2008;88(2):491S-9S.

[227] Nguyen TM, Pavlovitch J, Papiernik M, Guillozo H, Walrant-Debray O, Pontoux C, *et al.* Changes in 1,25-(OH)2D3 synthesis and its receptor expression in spleen cell subpopulations of mice infected with LPBM5 retrovirus. Endocrinology. 1997;138(12):5505-10.

[228] Evel-Kabler K, Chen SY. Inhibition of antigen-presentation attenuators to augment vaccines. Curr Opin Mol Ther. 2006;8(1):24-30.

[229] Song XT, Evel-Kabler K, Rollins L, Aldrich M, Gao F, Huang XF, *et al.* An alternative and effective HIV vaccination approach based on inhibition of antigen presentation attenuators in dendritic cells. PLoS Med. 2006;3(1):e11.

CHAPTER 8

The Complement System and HIV-1 Infection

Heribert Stoiber, Zoltan Banki and Doris Wilflingseder*

Department of Hygiene and Medical Microbiology, Innsbruck Medical University, Innsbruck, Austria.

Abstract: Already at the endothelial barrier of the host, HIV triggers responses of the innate immune system. A prominent component of the innate immunity is the complement system, which is immediately activated upon viral entry. Although the complement contributes to the control of viral replication by various strategies, HIV has evolved mechanisms to escape from complement-meditated neutralization and turns this part of the immune system to its advantage. Here we discuss the complex interactions of complement and complement receptors with HIV and review the escape mechanisms, which protect HIV from complement-mediated destruction.

THE COMPLEMENT ACTIVATION PATHWAYS

The complement system has evolved early during evolution. Already invertebrates such as ascidians (subphylum *Urochordata*), Amphioxus (subphylum *Cephalochordata*) or *Nematostella vectensis* exhibit an almost complete set of complement gene family members [1-3]. In vertebrates the complement system consists of more than 30 proteins present in an inactive state [4]. Activation of the classical, the lectin or the alternative pathway triggers a cascade multiplier by generating an intrinsic amplification loop. The classical pathway is initiated by binding of C1q, a subcomponent of the C1-complex, to IgM or IgG molecules in complex with antigens. Activation of the C1-complex leads to formation of C3-convertase by activation and association of C2 and C4 components. The lectin and alternative pathways can be activated independently of the presence of immunoglobulins. The lectin pathway is induced by recognition of carbohydrate patterns on the surface of pathogens by mannose binding lectin (MBL). Beside its permanent background activation by the spontaneous decay of C3 into $C3(H_2O)$, the alternative pathway is activated by molecules embedded in the surface membranes of invading microorganisms. All three pathways converge in the activation of C3. Cleavage of C3 to C3b induces the formation of C5-convertases and the sequential activation of complement components C5, C6, C7, C8 and the assembly of C9 within the membrane attack complex (MAC). The arrangement of the MAC on the cell surface results in death of the target by osmotic lysis. To prevent damage from the host cell, several regulatory proteins, referred to as regulators of complement activation (RCAs) disrupt the complement activation process [4]. Key elements of the complement cascade (C4, C3, C5 and formation of MAC) are controlled by different plasma and membrane-localized RCAs. Soluble factors such as factor H (fH) act in concert with membrane-anchored structures such as membrane cofactor protein (MCP, CD46), decay accelerating factor (DAF, CD55) and CD59, to protect the host-cell against possible self-destruction by the complement system. A further important mechanism in controlling the complement cascade is degradation of C3b to inactive iC3b and C3d. The key protein in this process is factor I (fI), a soluble serine protease, which requires co-factors such as fH, complement receptor 1 (CR1) or DAF for efficient cleavage of C3b. Although iC3b and C3d do not further participate in the complement cascade, they are important opsonins mediating several complement receptor-dependent actions, such as phagocytosis [4].

COMPLEMENT RECEPTORS

Complement Receptor Type 1 (CR1)

Human CR1 is a large and multifunctional member of the RCA protein family [5]. A common feature of these proteins are repeats of sequentially arranged modules of about 60 amino acids, referred to as short consensus repeats (SCRs). Seven or more SCRs are further grouped to form larger structural elements called long homologous repeats (LHRs), each encoding approximately 45 kDa of protein and designated LHR-A, -B, -C,

---

*Address Correspondence to this Author Doris Wilflingseder, Ph.D. at:** Department of Hygiene and Medical Microbiology, Innsbruck Medical University, A-6020 Innsbruck, Austria.

and -D. In total four polymorphic forms of human CR1 are known, which differ in the number of SCRs (up to 34) or LHRs. The distribution of the respective allele frequencies varies between 0.83 for *CR1*1* and 0.01 for *CR1*4* [6]. The ligand binding sites for C3b and C4b are mapped in LHR B (SCR 8-10) and LHR C (SCR 15-17). LHR A harbours an additional C4b binding region. These modular arrangements provide the basis for multivalent CR1-C3b/C4b interactions [5]. A further important feature of CR1 is its decay accelerating activity for classical and alternative C3 and C5 convertases, which is also located in LHR A [5]. The tissue distribution of CR1 covers a broad spectrum of peripheral blood cells. Only platelets, NK cells and T cell subsets are CR1 negative. In germinal centres (GC) of the lymphoid follicles, follicular dendritic cells (FDCs) express CR1, which may be of importance in the induction of immunological memory. Due to the numerical predominance of erythrocytes about 90% of the total CR1 in the body is expressed on this cell type. A main function of CR1 on erythrocytes is the transport of C3b/C4b-opsonized immune complexes (IC) to the liver and spleen. In these organs, IC are transferred to phagocytic cells and are finally removed [5].

Complement Receptor Type 2 (CR2)

CR2 (CD21) belongs to the family of complement regulatory proteins and consists of 15 or 16 SCRs. The two isoforms are differentially expressed; CD21L, the long isoform, is found on FDCS, while the shorter isoform CD21S is expressed on B lymphocytes, endothelial cells and some activated T cells [4]. Although the main ligand is the terminal degradation product of C3 cleavage, C3d, CR2 also interacts with C3dg and iC3b. On B lymphocytes, CR2 is non-covalently associated in a receptor complex with CD19 and CD81 within lipid rafts [7,8]. The CR2/CD19/CD81 complex bridges innate and adaptive immunity by decreasing the threshold level for B cell activation through the cross-linking opsonized antigens with the surface immunoglobulin receptor and the CR2 [9]. In GC reactions, CR2 is involved in antibody maturation and B cell memory [7].

Complement Receptor Type 3 and 4 (CR3 and CR4)

In contrast to CR1 and CR2, which are single chain receptors and belong to the RCA family, CR3 is a representative of the family of β_2 integrins, a superfamily of heterodimeric adhesion molecules [10]. These receptors consist of non-covalently associated α and β chains. The α chain is a 165 kD molecule (CD11b), whereas the independently anchored β chain has a molecular weight of 95 kD (CD18). In addition to CR3, LFA-1 (CD11a/CD18) and CR4 (CD11c/CD18) belong to the β_2 integrin family [10].The α chain of CR3 is a transmembrane protein with 7 tandem repeats of approximately 65 amino acids at its amino terminus. It contains the I-domain harbouring the binding sites for most ligands and binds C3-fragments in a Ca^{++} dependent manner [11]. Among all C3 fragments interacting with CR3, iC3b exhibits the highest affinity for this receptor. Additionally other molecules ligate CR3 including ICAM-1 (CD54) and ICAM-2, proteins of the clotting system like fibrinogen, kininogen and factor X or molecules of microbial origin [10]. CR3 is present on a number of different cell types including monocytes, macrophages, T lymphocytes, dendritic cells, follicular dendritic cells, granulocytes, natural killer cells, microglia, synovial cells, osteoclasts as well as histocytes [20].

A further member of the β_2 integrin family is CR4, consisting of CD11c and CD18 [4]. Due to these structural similarities the ligand specificities of CR3 and CR4 resemble each other. Tissue distribution of CD11c/CD18 is comparable to CR3, although CR4 seems to be more prominent on distinct dendritic cell subsets.

Anaphylatoxin Receptors C3a and C5a (C3aR and C5aR)

Activation of the complement system by pathogens leads to the N-terminal cleavage of components C3, C4 and C5, thereby generating complement fragments C3a, C4a and C5a [12,13]. These anaphylatoxins have been shown to mediate many biological effects: chemotactic migration, cellular adhesion, stimulation of oxidative metabolism, and release of lysosomal enzymes and numerous mediators of inflammation, such as histamine and cytokines [13].

The functional responses mediated by C3a and C5a are due to high-affinity binding of these fragments to the cell surface receptors C3aR and C5aR. C3aR and C5aR (CD88) belong to the rhodopsin subfamily of G protein-coupled receptors with seven transmembrane segments [14,15]. C3aR and C5aR share 37% nucleotide identity with the highest homology in the transmembrane regions and in the second intracellular loop. C3aR is unique among this family since it has an unusually large extracellular domain between the fourth and fifth transmembrane region [14,15].

The expression of the genes for C3aR and C5aR was, until recently, thought to be largely restricted to cells of the myeloid lineage, such as neutrophils, macrophages, eosinophils, basophils and mast cells. However, in recent years, many studies have demonstrated widespread localization of these receptors throughout many tissues and cell types outside the immune system, including epithelial, endothelial and smooth muscle cells, the human liver and lung, human keratinocytes of the inflamed skin, as well as astrocytes, microglia and neurons [16,17].

INTERACTIONS OF COMPLEMENT WITH HIV.

Complement Activation by HIV

Similarly to other pathogens, HIV infection results in activation of the complement system. HIV triggers the classical pathway, even in the absence of HIV-specific antibodies. Direct binding of the viral envelope protein gp41 to C1q causes this activation mediating the deposition of C3 fragments on the viral surface [18,19]. By epitope mapping three C1q-binding sites on gp41 were identified, which depend on hydrophobic interactions [20]. After seroconversion, HIV-specific antibodies further enhance complement activation [21]. In addition, MBL, the triggering molecule of the lectin pathway, was also described to bind HIV [22]. MBL interacts with the virus via high mannose carbohydrates on gp120 and the interaction of MBL with HIV depends on sialysation [22].

Inactivation of HIV Through Complement-Mediated Lysis

Several antibodies that induce complement-mediated lysis (CoML) of HIV have been described [23,24]. In vivo, such CoML-inducing antibodies are supposed to contribute to the control of the viral spread during the acute phase of infection. Mainly non-neutralizing antibodies seem to dominate this process [25,26]. The responses are thought to be found in the chronic phase of infection, too [25-29] (Fig. **1A**). However, substantial amounts of the virus seem to be resistant against the lytic attacks by the complement system [20,30,31].

Responsible for this intrinsic resistance of HIV against human complement are membrane proteins derived from the human cells, which are acquired by the virus during the budding process [32]. Among them are RCAs such as CD46 (MCP), CD55 (DAF) or CD59, which down-regulate complement activation at several stages of the cascade [33-35]. In addition, HIV can bind fH, an RCA in fluid phase, which further favours the protection of the virus against lysis by the complement system [36-39]. The crucial role of fH for protection of the virus is evident, since incubation of HIV with fH-depleted sera results in up to 80% of complement-dependent virolysis in the presence of HIV-specific antibodies [40].

Similar to fH-depleted sera, which promote CoML, fH-derived peptide is able to enhance C3 deposition on HIV-infected cells by inhibition of fH deposition on HIV and thus to induce virolysis [41].

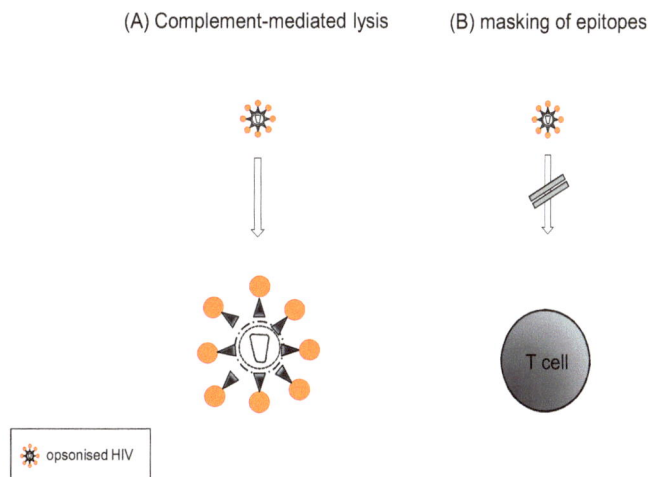

Figure 1: Inactivation of HIV by complement: (A) The complement system contributes to the control of the viral burden in infected individuals. In addition (B), opsonisation of the viral surface with C3-fragments may mask viral epitopes crucial for the adherence to target cells and/or the fusion process.

Inactivation Through Opsonization

Non-neutralizing Abs produced at early stages of infection is correlated with reduced infectivity, which seems to depend on complement [26]. Although some lysis was observed (see above), the covering of HIV with C3-fragments, i.e. opsonization, may also play an important role in controlling viral replication. *In vitro* data indicate that the masking of viral epitopes by deposition of C3-fragments on the viral envelope reduces the infectivity of complement-receptor-negative T cells [42,43]. This neutralization mechanism has been described for other viruses, too, [44] and may contribute, at least in part, to lower viral loads during the acute HIV infection (Fig. **1B**).

Inactivation Through Phagocytosis

The coating with antibodies and complement tags HIV for uptake and destruction by phagocytes, such as dendritic cells (DCs), monocytes/macrophages or polymorphonuclear granulocytes [45]. Phagocytic cells internalize immune complexed viruses via their Fc and complement receptors (CRs), which upon engagement trigger uptake and subsequent degradation. In CR-mediated phagocytosis, all cell-bound C3-fragments act as opsonins and favor binding to the phagocyte via CRs [46]. In as much phagocytosis contributes to the reduction in viral loads of HIV-infected individuals is not completely elucidated yet. Defects in both complement and Fc receptor-dependent phagocytosis of macrophages and neutrophils are reported during disease progression [47-51].

Complement-Mediated Enhancement of HIV Infection

Without intervention HIV remains resistant to human serum. Due to the protection mechanisms, described above, opsonized HIV accumulates in several compartments of the host, such as blood, lymphatic tissue (LT), brain, mother's milk, seminal fluid or mucosal surfaces and can interact with CR expressing cells. The infectivity of opsonized virions may be rescued, or even enhanced, through exploitation of CRs on target and bystander cells (Fig. **2**). By these mechanisms, the infection, dissemination and establishment of viral reservoirs is facilitated, as outlined below.

Complement-Mediated Enhancement of HIV Infection in CIS

Complement-mediated enhancement of infection is the topic of various reviews [20,52-56]. Such an enhancement in *cis* is reported after cross-linking of the CR1 on T cells with antibodies against this CR [57] (Fig. **2A**). Similarly, aggregated C3b enhances transcription of viral genes in HIV-infected cells *in vitro* and in T lymphocytes isolated from HIV-infected individuals [57]. However, only a small subset of CD4$^+$ T cells express CR1. Thus, the *in vivo* role of the CR1 for an infection of T cells in *cis* remains to be elucidated. Enhancement of infection has further been observed in CR2$^+$ cell lines of T [58-61] or B cell origin [62,63] as well as in primary cultures of B lymphocytes [64,65] and syncytio-trophoblasts [66]. In most of these *in vitro* studies, simultaneous expression of CD4 is required for productive infection, although some studies demonstrated CD4-independent infection of CR2$^+$ cells [67,68] (Fig. **2A**).

Not only CR2, but also CR3 mediates enhancement HIV infection in *cis*, since on the one hand viral particles acquire ICAM-1 and CR3 during the budding process from monocytic cells [32], on the other hand complement-coated HIV interacts with CR3$^+$ cells [69]. The host-derived ICAM-1 glycoprotein on the viral surface was shown to be biologically active and enhance viral infectivity in a CD4 independent manner [70], probably due to interaction with its counter-receptors LFA-1 and CR3 on the surface of the target cell. Incorporation of the intercellular adhesion molecule ICAM-1 into viral particles increased virus infectivity on peripheral blood mononuclear cells (PBMCs) by two- to sevenfold [71]. Treatment of target PBMCs with an antibody against LFA-1, a main ICAM-1 receptor, was able to block the ICAM-1-mediated enhancement. Adhesion between ICAM-1 on the target cell and CR3 on the virions could also mediate enhancement of viral infectivity, even without opsonising complement fragments on the viral surface due to C3-homolgy regions in gp41 [37]. Experiments with monocytic cells have shown that viral replication is increased, when monocytic cells were infected with iC3b-opsonized viral particles [72]. Simultaneous binding of iC3b to CR3 and of gp120 to CD4 and CCR5 has been suggested. Latently infected monocytes may be activated during a secondary infection by binding of opsonized particles or immune complexes to CR3, thereby inducing NFκB translocation and viral transcription.

(A) Enhancement of infection in cis   (B) Enhancement of infection in trans

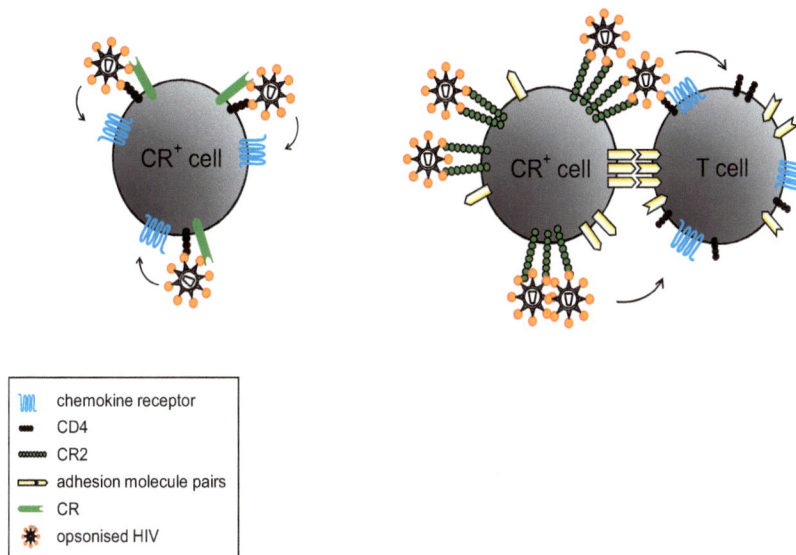

Legend:
- chemokine receptor
- CD4
- CR2
- adhesion molecule pairs
- CR
- opsonised HIV

Figure 2: Complement-mediated enhancement of infection: (A) Binding of opsonized virus to CRs expressed on the target cells favours the infection of CD4- and chemokine receptor-positive cells. (B) Trapping of HIV on CD4- and chemokine receptor-negative cells via CRs promotes the transfer of HIV to T cells.

Such activated monocytes release high amounts of viral particles and secrete inflammatory cytokines [73]. As mentioned above CR3 is present on a large variety of cell types. Many aspects of the interaction between HIV and CR3 still remain to be elucidated. One example is the presence of CR3 on epithelial cells, which has been suggested to be involved in HIV transmission through rectal and cervicovaginal mucosa [74]. Another open question touches the FcR- and CR-mediated internalization of opsonized HIV which may profoundly affects intracellular sorting and antigen presentation [75].

Complement-Mediated Enhancement of HIV Infection in Trans

CR1 seems to play a role for the pathogenesis of complement-opsonized HIV by contributing to the infection in *trans*. Immune-complexed HIV adhere to erythrocytes of infected individuals through CR1-C3b interactions [76,77] and transfer the virus - at least in vitro- to T cells (Fig. **2A**). Additionally, CR1 on erythrocytes might be important for processing of complement fragments on the surface of HIV to generate C3dg [78]. This in turn can mediate the trapping of viral particles to CR2$^+$ cells, thus enhancing the infection in *trans* [12] (Fig. **2B**). In line with this observation, trapping of complement-coated virions to CR2$^+$ cells has been shown with peripheral B lymphocytes isolated from HIV-infected patients [79] and in *ex vivo* studies for follicular dendritic cells (FDCs) [80-82]. The FDCs in the LT represents by far the largest viral reservoir in the body; up to 90 % of viral particles are extracellularly bound to FDCs [83,84]. Since FDCs express substantial amounts of CR1 and CR2 as well as lesser quantities of CR3 [85], they interact with all major C3 degradation products. *In vitro*, FDC-trapping of HIV is dependent on complement and on HIV-specific antibodies [81,86], although, accumulation of retroviruses in LT reservoirs is already observable in the acute phase of infection [87-90], when Abs are absent and HIV is covered with complement-fragments only [91]. Trapped virions were shown to remain infectious for T cells migrating through GC even in the presence of neutralising antibodies [92]. Although HAART reduces the pool of FDCS-associated HIV by over 2500-fold, viral RNA can still be detected in some GC [93].

In an *ex vivo* study with tonsilar specimen of a presymptomatic HIV-positive patients, CR2 was identified as the main ligand for *in vivo* complement-coated virus [80,81]. Monoclonal antibodies blocking C3d-CR2 interaction but not antibodies against CR1 or CR3 could detach the main part of trapped virions from the FDC network. Since the same antibodies could detach virus from tonsillar cell suspensions of patients receiving

HAART, trapping mechanisms do not seem to change in individuals during treatment [80]. Beside CR, other molecules such as Fcγ receptors or adhesion molecules like ICAM-1 and LFA-1 have been suggested to contribute to FDC-mediated trapping of HIV [94].

In addition to FDCs, B lymphocytes have been implicated in virus trapping and dissemination. Expression of CR1 and CR2 allows binding of immune-complexed HIV on peripheral and lymphoid B cells, which subsequently transmit the virus to T lymphocytes and promote infection [95-98]. B cells isolated from peripheral blood and LT of chronically infected individuals were shown to carry immune-complexed HIV on their surface [79]. Since B cells circulate, they potentially disseminate infectious virus throughout the body. In the LT, they pass through T cell zones containing CD4⁺ T lymphocytes and vice versa. In these areas, but alos in GCs, the promotion of B cell-T cell contacts sets the stage for direct transmission of trapped HIV from B to T cells (Fig. **2B**). Indeed, in autologous tonsillar B cell-T cell co-cultures opsonized virus was found to preferentially bind to CR2 on B lymphocytes [98]. In this system, T cell infection occured independently of pre-stimulation of primary T lymphocytes [98]. The mechanism responsible for infection of un-stimulated primary T cells seems to involve direct interaction between B and T cells, in which B cells act as continuous supply of infectious virus. Additionally, the stabilization of B cell-T cell contacts through adhesion molecules facilitates membrane fusion between HIV and T cells [98].

It has been reported that CR3⁺/CR4⁺ dendritic cells pulsed with HIV-1 transmit the virus to freshly isolated blood monocytes and also to monocyte-derived macrophages with high efficiency [73]. Inhibition experiments using mAb against β₂ integrins have demonstrated that anti-CD18 mAb significantly inhibited transmission of HIV-1 from dendritic cells to monocytes. In addition, weak inhibition of HIV-1 transmission was observed with anti-CD11b mAb, suggesting an involvement of CR3 in this process. Efficient transfer of complement-opsonized HIV was also observed from DCs to T cells in short- and long-term transmission experiments [75].

CR3 has also been detected on microglia, a functional analogue of monocytes in the brain, which play an important role in HIV neuropathology. Using an anti-CR3 monoclonal antibody, microglia can be activated and induced to proliferate via their CR3 molecules [99]. Such activated microglia cells secrete proinflammatory cytokines such as IL-1, TNF-α, IL-6 and GM-CSF. These cytokines regulate the activity of interacting cell types, induce expression of complement proteins and propagate HIV infection in the CNS [100,101].

Enhancement of HIV Infection by Anaphylatoxins

Monocytic cells of healthy subjects express high amounts of C5aR and C3aR on their surface [102,103] In contrast, studies on peripheral blood monocytes and neutrophils from AIDS patients demonstrated significantly impaired migratory activity to complement anaphylatoxins and lower expression of C5aR. As a consequence, it has been supposed that this defective migratory function may contribute to the depressed inflammatory response frequently observed in patients with AIDS [104,105].

Recently, C5a has been shown to prime monocyte-derived macrophages for HIV infection. Treatment of monocyte-derived macrophages with C5a enhanced infectivity of R5 strains up to 40-times and a similar effect was observed with a C5a derivative, C5a$_{desArg}$. Kinetic analyses demonstrated that exposure to C5a accelerates productive infection in these cells. C5aR-blocking mAb reversed the susceptibility of macrophages [106] and also DCs for HIV infection [107].

Thus, increased secretion of proinflammatory cytokines correlated with higher susceptibility of macrophages to HIV infection upon cultivation in the presence of C5a and C5a$_{desArg}$ [106]. These observations provide a possible explanation for higher likelihood of HIV infection at the mucosal sites in individuals with sexually transmissible infections [108].

OUTLOOK

Although complement and even non-neutralizing Abs may contribute to control viral replication at several stages of the disease, HIV has developed mechanisms to turn complement-activation and opsonization to its advantage while avoiding CoML. Further elucidating the fine-tuned interplay between the humoral (complement) and cell-associated (complement receptors) sites with HIV will provide further insights in the complex interaction between HIV and the immune system.

CONFLICT OF INTEREST STATEMENT

The authors declare that they have no conflict of interest.

ACKNOWLEDGMENT

The authors are supported by the 6th frame work of the EU (DEC-VAC 2005-018685), grants of the Austrian Research Fund FWF (P18960 to DW and P17914 to HS) and the Federal Government of Tyrol (Tiroler Wissenschaftsfonds TWF-2008-1-562). The secretarial support of L. Hahn and Mag. B. Mullauer is gratefully acknowledged.

REFERENCES

[1]   Azumi K, De Santis R, De Tomaso A, Rigoutsos I, Yoshizaki F, Pinto MR, *et al*. Genomic analysis of immunity in a Urochordate and the emergence of the vertebrate immune system: "waiting for Godot". Immunogenetics 2003; 55:570-81.

[2]   He Y, Tang B, Zhang S, Liu Z, Zhao B, Chen L. Molecular and immunochemical demonstration of a novel member of Bf/C2 homolog in amphioxus Branchiostoma belcheri: implications for involvement of hepatic cecum in acute phase response. Fish Shellfish Immunol 2008; 24:768-78.

[3]   Kimura A, Sakaguchi E, Nonaka M. Multi-component complement system of Cnidaria: C3, Bf, and MASP genes expressed in the endodermal tissues of a sea anemone, Nematostella vectensis. Immunobiology 2009; 214:165-78.

[4]   Speth C, Prodinger WM, Würzner R, Stoiber H, Dierich MP. In: Fundamental Immunology, Paul W E, Ed. Complement. Lippincott-Raven Publishers, PA. 2007; pp.1048-1078.

[5]   Krych M, Molina H, Atkinson JP. CD35: complement receptor type 1. J Biol Regul Homeost Agents 1999; 13:229-33.

[6]   Cohen JH, Atkinson JP, Klickstein LB, Oudin S, Subramanian VB, Moulds JM. The C3b/C4b receptor (CR1, CD35) on erythrocytes: methods for study of the polymorphisms. Mol Immunol 1999; 36:819-25.

[7]   Fearon DT, Carroll MC. Regulation of B lymphocyte responses to foreign and self-antigens by the CD19/CD21 complex. Annu Rev Immunol 2000; 18:393-422.

[8]   Cherukuri A, Cheng PC, Sohn HW, Pierce SK. The CD19/CD21 complex functions to prolong B cell antigen receptor signaling from lipid rafts. Immunity 2001; 14:169-79.

[9]   Dempsey PW, Allison ME, Akkaraju S, Goodnow CC, Fearon DT. C3d of complement as a molecular adjuvant: bridging innate and acquired immunity. Science 1996; 271:348-350.

[10]   Ehlers MR. Microbes Infect. 2000; 2:289-94.

[11]   Diamond MS, Garcia-Aguilar J, Bickford JK, Corbi AL, Springer TA. The I domain is a major recognition site on the leukocyte integrin Mac-1 (CD11b/CD18) for four distinct adhesion ligands. Cell Biol. 1993; 120:1031-43.

[12]   Stoiber H, Banki Z, Wilflingseder D, Dierich MP. Complement-HIV interactions during all steps of viral pathogenesis. Vaccine 2008; 26:3046-54.

[13]   Gerard C, Gerard NP. C5A anaphylatoxin and its seven transmembrane-segment receptor. Annu Rev Immunol. 1994; 12:775-808.

[14]   Gerard C, Gerard NP. The chemotactic receptor for human C5a anaphylatoxin. Nature. 1991; 349:614-7.

[15]   Crass T, Raffetseder U, Martin U, Grove M, Klos A, Köhl J, *et al*. Expression cloning of the human C3a anaphylatoxin receptor (C3aR) from differentiated U-937 cells. Eur J Immunol. 1996; 26:1944-50.

[16]   Nataf S, Stahel PF, Davoust N, Barnum SR. Complement anaphylatoxin receptors on neurons: new tricks for old receptors? Trends Neurosci. 1999; 22:397-402.

[17]   Zwirner J, Fayyazi A, Götze O. Expression of the anaphylatoxin C5a receptor in non-myeloid cells. Mol Immunol. 1999; 36:877-84.

[18]   Ebenbichler CF, Thielens NM, Vornhagen R, Marschang P, Arlaud GJ, Dierich MP. Human immunodeficiency virus type 1 activates the classical pathway of complement by direct C1 binding through specific sites in the transmembrane glycoprotein gp41. J Exp Med 1991;174:1417-1424.

[19]   Spear GT, Jiang HX, Sullivan BL, Gewurz H, Landay AL, Lint TF. Direct binding of complement component C1q to human immunodeficiency virus (HIV) and human T lymphotrophic virus-I (HTLV-I) coinfected cells. AIDS Res Hum Retroviruses 1991; 7:579-585.

[20]   Stoiber H, Clivio A, Dierich MP. Role of complement in HIV infection. Annu Rev Immunol 1997; 15:649-674.

[21]   Prohaszka Z, Hidvegi T, Ujhelyi E, Stoiber H, Dierich MP, Süsal C, et al. Interaction of complement and specific antibodies with the external glycoprotein (gp120) of human immunodeficiency virus type 1 (HIV-1). Immunology 1995; 85:184-189.

[22]   Ji X, Gewurz H, Spear GT. Mannose binding lectin (MBL) and HIV. Mol Immunol. 2005; 42:145-52.

[23]   Spear GT, Takefman DM, Sullivan BL, Landay AL, Zolla-Pazner S. Complement activation by human monoclonal antibodies to human immunodeficiency virus. J Virol 1993; 67: 53–9.

[24]   Gregersen JP, Mehdi S, Baur A, Hilfenhaus J. Antibody- and complement-mediated lysis of HIV-infected cells and inhibition of viral replication. J Med Virol 1990; 30: 287–93.

[25]   Aasa-Chapman MM, Holuigue S, Aubin K, Wong M, Jones NA, Cornforth D, et al. Detection of antibody-dependent complement-mediated inactivation of both autologous and heterologous virus in primary human immunodeficiency virus type 1 infection. J Virol 2005; 79: 2823–30.

[26]   Huber M, Fischer M, Misselwitz B, Manrique A, Kuster H, Niederöst B, et al. Complement lysis activity in autologous plasma is associated with lower viral loads during the acute phase of HIV-1 infection. PLoS Med 2006; 3: 441.

[27]   Spear GT, Olinger GG, Saifuddin M, Gebel HM. Human antibodies to major histocompatibility complex alloantigens mediate lysis and neutralization of HIV-1 primary isolate virions in the presence of complement. J Acquir Immune Defic Syndr 2001; 26:103–10.

[28]   Spear GT, Sullivan BL, Landay AL, Lint TF. Neutralization of human immunodeficiency virus type 1 by complement occurs by viral lysis. J Virol 1990; 64: 5869–73.

[29]   Sullivan BL, Knopoff EJ, Saifuddin M, Takefman DM, Saarloos MN, Sha BE, et al. Susceptibility of HIV-1 plasma virus to complement-mediated lysis. Evidence for a role in clearance of virus in vivo. J Immunol 1996; 157: 1791–8.

[30]   Dierich MP, Stoiber H, Clivio A. A "Complementary" AIDS vaccine. Nature Med. 1996; 2:153-155.

[31]   Banki Z, Soederholm A, Mullauer B, Dierich MP, Stoiber H. Tracing complement-retroviral interactions from mucosal surfaces to the lymphatic tissue. Front Biosci. 2007; 12:2096-2106.

[32]   Frank I, Stoiber H, Godar S, Möst J, Stockinger H, Dierich MP. Acquisition of host cell-surface-derived molecules by HIV-1. AIDS 1996; 10:1611-1620.

[33]   Saifuddin M, Hedayati T, Atkinson JP, Holguin MH, Parker CJ, Spear GT. Human immunodeficiency virus type 1 incorporates both glycosyl phosphatidylinositol-anchored CD55 and CD59 and integral membrane CD46 at levels that protect from complement-mediated destruction. J Gen Virol 1997; 78: 1907–11.

[34]   Marschang P, Sodroski J, Wurzner R, Dierich MP. Decay-accelerating factor (CD55) protects human immunodeficiency virus type 1 from inactivation by human complement. Eur J Immunol 1995; 25: 285–90.

[35]   Montefiori DC, Cornell RJ, Zhou JY, Zhou JT, Hirsch VM, Johnson PR. Complement control proteins, CD46, CD55, and CD59, as common surface constituents of human and simian immunodeficiency viruses and possible targets for vaccine protection. Virology 1994; 205: 82–92.

[36]   Stoiber H, Schneider R, Janatova J, Dierich MP. Human complement proteins C3b, C4b, factor H and properdin react with specific sites in gp120 and gp41, the envelope proteins of HIV-1. Immunobiology 1995; 193: 98–113.

[37]   Stoiber H, Ebenbichler CF, Schneider R, Janatova J, Dierich MP. Interaction of several complement proteins with gp120 and gp41, the two envelope glycoproteins of HIV-1. AIDS 1995; 9:19-26.

[38]   Pinter C, Siccardi AG, Longhi R, Clivio A. Direct interaction of complement factor H with the C1 domain of HIV type 1 glycoprotein 120. AIDS Res Hum Retroviruses 1995; 11: 577–88.

[39]   Pinter C, Siccardi AG, Lopalco L, Longhi R, Clivio A. HIV glycoprotein 41 and complement factor H interact with each other and share functional as well as antigenic homology. AIDS Res Hum Retroviruses 1995; 11: 971–80.

[40]   Stoiber H, Pinter C, Siccardi AG, Clivio A, Dierich MP. Efficient destruction of human immunodeficiency virus in human serum by inhibiting the protective action of complement factor H and decay accelerating factor (DAF, CD55). J Exp Med 1996; 183: 307–10.

[41]   Stoiber H, Ammann C, Spruth M, Müllauer B, Eberhart A, Harris CL, et al. Enhancement of complement-mediated lysis by a peptide derived from SCR13 of complement factor H. Immunobiology 2001; 203:670-686.

[42]   Sullivan BL, Takefman DM, Spear GT. Complement can neutralize HIV-1 plasma virus by a C5-independent mechanism. Virology 1998; 248, 173-81.

[43]   Scherl M, Posch U, Obermoser G, Ammann C, Sepp N, Ulmer H, et al. Targeting human immunodeficiency virus type 1 with antibodies derived from patients with connective tissue disease. Lupus 2006; 15, 865-72.

[44]   Nemerow GR, Cooper NR. Isolation of Epstein Barr-virus and studies of its neutralization by human IgG and complement. J Immunol 1981; 127, 272-278.

[45]   Rabinovitch M. Professional and non-professional phagocytes: an introduction. Trends Cell Biol 1995; 5: 85–7.

[46]   Brown EJ. Complement receptors and phagocytosis. Curr Opin Immunol 1991; 3: 76–82.

[47]   Kedzierska K, Azzam R, Ellery P, Mak J, Jaworowski A, Crowe SM. Defective phagocytosis by human monocyte/macrophages following HIV-1 infection: underlying mechanisms and modulation by adjunctive cytokine therapy. J Clin Virol 2003; 26: 247.

[48]   Bender BS, Davidson BL, Kline R, Brown C, Quinn TC. Role of the mononuclear phagocyte system in the immunopathogenesis of human immunodeficiency virus infection and the acquired immunodeficiency syndrome. Rev Infect Dis 1988; 10: 1142–54.

[49]   Monari C, Casadevall A, Pietrella D, Bistoni F, Vecchiarelli A. Neutrophils from patients with advanced human immunodeficiency virus infection have impaired complement receptor function and preserved Fcgamma receptor function. J Infect Dis 1999; 180: 1542–9.

[50]   Thomas CA, Weinberger OK, Ziegler BL, Greenberg S, Schieren I, Silverstein SC, et al. Human immunodeficiency virus-1 env impairs Fc receptor-mediated phagocytosis via a cyclic adenosine monophosphate-dependent mechanism. Blood 1997; 90:3760-5.

[51]   Azzam R, Kedzierska K, Leeansyah E, Chan H, Doischer D, Gorry PR, et al. Impaired complement-mediated phagocytosis by HIV type-1-infected human monocyte-derived macrophages involves a cAMP-dependent mechanism. AIDS Res Hum Retroviruses 2006; 22:619-29.

[52]   Beck Z, Prohászka Z, Füst G. Traitors of the immune system-enhancing antibodies in HIV infection: their possible implication in HIV vaccine development. Vaccine 2008 ; 26:3078-85.

[53]   Freissmuth D, Dierich MP, Stoiber H. Role of complement in the pathogenesis of SIV infection. Front Biosci. 2003; 8:733-9.

[54]   Bánki Z, Stoiber H, Dierich MP. HIV and human complement: inefficient virolysis and effective adherence. Immunol Lett., 2005; 97:209-214.

[55]   Willey S, Aasa-Chapman MM. Humoral immunity to HIV-1: neutralisation and antibody effector functions. Trends Microbiol. 2008; 16:596-604.

[56]   Huber M, Trkola A. Humoral immunity to HIV-1: neutralization and beyond. J Intern Med. 2007; 262:5-25.

[57]   Mouhoub A, Delibrias CC, Fischer E, Boyer V, Kazatchkine MD. Ligation of CR1 (C3b receptor, CD35) on CD4+ T lymphocytes enhances viral replication in HIV-infected cells. Clin Exp Immunol. 1996; 106:297-303.

[58]   June RA, Schade SZ, Bankowski MJ, Kuhns M, McNamara A, Lint TF, et al. Complement and antibody mediate enhancement of HIV infection by increasing virus binding and provirus formation. AIDS 1991; 5:269-74.

[59]   Zhou J, Montefiori DC. Complement-activating antibodies in sera from infected individuals and vaccinated volunteers that target human immunodeficiency virus type 1 to complement receptor type 1 (CR1, CD35). Virology 1996; 226:13-21.

[60]   Robinson WE Jr, Montefiori DC, Mitchell WM. Complement-mediated antibody-dependent enhancement of HIV-1 infection requires CD4 and complement receptors. Virology 1990; 175:600-4.

[61]   Robinson WE Jr, Montefiori DC, Mitchell WM. Antibody-dependent enhancement of human immunodeficiency virus type 1 infection. Lancet 1988; 1: 790–4.

[62]   Gras GS, Dormont D. Antibody-dependent and antibody-independent complement-mediated enhancement of human immunodeficiency virus type 1 infection in a human, Epstein-Barr virus-transformed B-lymphocytic cell line. J Virol. 1991; 65:541-5.

[63]   Tremblay M, Meloche S, Sekaly RP, Wainberg MA. Complement receptor 2 mediates enhancement of human immunodeficiency virus 1 infection in Epstein-Barr virus-carrying B cells. J Exp Med. 1990; 171:1791-6.

[64]   Gras G, Richard Y, Roques P, Olivier R, Dormont D. Complement and virus-specific antibody-dependent infection of normal B lymphocytes by human immunodeficiency virus type 1. Blood 1993; 81:1808-18.

[65]   Delibrias CC, Mouhoub A, Fischer E, Kazatchkine MD. CR1(CD35) and CR2(CD21) complement C3 receptors are expressed on normal human thymocytes and mediate infection of thymocytes with opsonized human immunodeficiency virus. Eur J Immunol. 1994; 24:2784-8.

[66]   Toth FD, Mosborg-Petersen P, Kiss J, Aboagye-Mathiesen G, Zdravkovic M, Hager H, et al. Antibody-dependent enhancement of HIV-1 infection in human term syncytiotrophoblast cells cultured in vitro. Clin Exp Immunol. 1994; 96:389-94.

[67]   Boyer V, Delibrias C, Noraz N, Fischer E, Kazatchkine MD, Desgranges C. Complement receptor type 2 mediates infection of the human CD4-negative Raji B-cell line with opsonized HIV. Scand J Immunol. 1992 ; 36:879-83.

[68] Boyer V, Desgranges C, Trabaud MA, Fischer E, Kazatchkine MD. Complement mediates human immunodeficiency virus type 1 infection of a human T cell line in a CD4- and antibody-independent fashion. J Exp Med. 1991; 173:1151-8.

[69] Pruenster M, Wilflingseder D, Bánki Z, Ammann CG, Muellauer B, Meyer M, *et al.* C-type lectin-independent interaction of complement opsonized HIV with monocyte-derived dendritic cells. Eur J Immunol. 2005; 35:2691-8.

[70] Rizzuto CD, Sodroski JG. Contribution of virion ICAM-1 to human immunodeficiency virus infectivity and sensitivity to neutralization. J Virol. 1997; 71:4847-51.

[71] Stoiber H, Frank I, Spruth M, Schwendinger M, Mullauer B, Windisch JM, *et al.* Inhibition of HIV-1 infection in vitro by monoclonal antibodies to the complement receptor type 3 (CR3): an accessory role for CR3 during virus entry? Mol Immunol. 1997; 34:855-63.

[72] Thieblemont N, Haeffner-Cavaillon N, Haeffner A, Cholley B, Weiss L, Kazatchkine MD. Triggering of complement receptors CR1 (CD35) and CR3 (CD11b/CD18) induces nuclear translocation of NF-kappa B (p50/p65) in human monocytes and enhances viral replication in HIV-infected monocytic cells. J Immunol. 1995; 155:4861-7.

[73] Kacani L, Frank I, Spruth M, Schwendinger MG, Müllauer B, Sprinzl GM, *et al.* Dendritic cells transmit human immunodeficiency virus type 1 to monocytes and monocyte-derived macrophages. J Virol. 1998; 72:6671-7.

[74] Hussain LA, Kelly CG, Rodin A, Jourdan M, Lehner T. Investigation of the complement receptor 3 (CD11b/CD18) in human rectal epithelium. Clin Exp Immunol. 1995; 102:384-8.

[75] Wilflingseder D, Banki Z, Garcia E, Pruenster M, Pfister G, Muellauer B, *et al.* gG opsonization of HIV impedes provirus formation in and infection of dendritic cells and subsequent long-term transfer to T cells. J Immunol. 2007; 178:7840-8.

[76] Hess C, Klimkait T, Schlapbach L, Del Zenero V, Sadallah S, Horakova E, *et al.* Association of a pool of HIV-1 with erythrocytes in vivo: a cohort study. Lancet 2002; 359: 2230-2234.

[77] Horakova E, Gasser O, Sadallah S, Inal JM, Bourgeois G, Ziekau I, *et al.* Complement mediates the binding of HIV to erythrocytes. J. Immunol. 2004; 173: 4236-4241.

[78] Bánki Z, Wilflingseder D, Ammann CG, Pruenster M, Müllauer B, Holländer K, *et al.* Factor I-mediated processing of complement-fragments on HIV immune-complexes targets HIV to CR2-expressing B cells and facilitates B cell-mediated transmission of opsonized HIV to T cells. J Immunol. 2006; 177:3469-76.

[79] Moir S, Malaspina A, Li Y, Chun TW, Lowe T, Adelsberger J, *et al.* B cells of HIV-1-infected patients bind virions through CD21-complement interactions and transmit infectious virus to activated T cells. J Exp Med. 2000; 192:637-46.

[80] Joling P, Bakker LJ, Van Strijp JA, Meerloo T, de Graaf L, Dekker ME, *et al.* Binding of human immunodeficiency virus type-1 to follicular dendritic cells in vitro is complement dependent. J. Immunol. 1993; 150: 1065-1073.

[81] Kacani L, Prodinger WM, Sprinzl GM, Schwendinger MG, M. Spruth, H. Stoiber, *et al.* Detachment of human immunodeficiency virus type 1 from germinal centers by blocking complement receptor type 2. J Virol. 2000; 74: 7997-8002.

[82] Banki Z, Kacani L, Rusert P, Pruenster M, Wilflingseder D, Falkensammer B, *et al.* Complement dependent trapping of infectious HIV in human lymphoid tissues. AIDS 2005; 19: 481-486.

[83] Pantaleo G, Fauci AS. Immunopathogenesis of HIV infection. Annu. Rev. Microbiol. 1996; 50: 825-854.

[84] Haase AT, Henry K, Zupancic M, Sedgewick G, Faust RA, Melroe H, *et al.* Quantitative image analysis of HIV-1 infection in lymphoid tissue. Science 1996; 274: 985-989.

[85] Stingl G, Wolff-Schreiner EC, Pichler WJ, Gschnait F, Knapp W, Wolff K. Epidermal Langerhans cells bear Fc and C3 receptors. Nature 1977; 268: 245-246.

[86] Smith-Franklin BA, Keele BF, Tew JG, Gartner S, Szakal AK, Estes JD, *et al.* Follicular dendritic cells and the persistence of HIV infectivity: the role of antibodies and Fcgamma receptors. J. Immunol. 2002; 168: 2408-2414.

[87] Chakrabarti L, Cumont MC, Montagnier L, Hurtrel B. Kinetics of primary SIV infection in lymph nodes. J. Med. Primatol. 1994; 23: 117-1124.

[88] Hurtrel B, Chakrabarti L, Hurtrel M, Bach JM, Ganiere JP, Montagnier L. Early events in lymph nodes during infection with SIV and FIV. Res. Virol. 1994 ; 145 : 221-227.

[89] Stahl-Hennig C, Steinman RM, Tenner-Racz K, Pope M, Stolte N, Matz-Rensing K, *et al.* Rapid infection of oral mucosal-associated lymphoid tissue with simian immunodeficiency virus. Science 1999; 285: 1261-1265.

[90] Milush JM, Kosub D, Marthas M, Schmidt K, Scott F, Wozniakowski A, *et al.* Rapid dissemination of SIV following oral inoculation. AIDS 2004; 18: 2371-2380.

[91]   Stoiber H, Prünster M, Ammann CG, Dierich MP. Complement- opsonized HIV: the free rider on its way to infection. Mol. Immunol. 2005; 42:153-160.

[92]   Heath SL, Tew JG, Szakal AK Burton GF. Follicular dendritic cells and human immunodeficiency virus infectivity. *Nature* 1995; 377: 740-744.

[93]   Cavert W, Notermans DW, Staskus K, Wietgrefe SW, Zupancic M, Gebhard K, *et al.* Kinetics of response in lymphoid tissues to antiretroviral therapy of HIV-1 infection. *Science* 1997; 276: 960-964.

[94]   Fujiwara M, Tsunoda R, Shigeta S, Yokota T, Baba M. Human follicular dendritic cells remain uninfected and capture human immunodeficiency virus type 1 through CD54-CD11a interaction. J. Virol. 1999; 73: 3603-3607.

[95]   Jakubik JJ, Saifuddin M, Takefman DM, Spear GT. B lymphocytes in lymph nodes and peripheral blood are important for binding immune complexes containing HIV-1. Immunology 1999; 96: 612-619.

[96]   Doepper S, Stoiber H, Kacani L, Sprinzl G, Steindl F, Prodinger WM, *et al.* B cell-mediated infection of stimulated and unstimulated autologous T lymphocytes with HIV-1: role of complement. Immunobiology 2000; 202; 293-305.

[97]   Jakubik JJ, Saifuddin M, Takefman DM, Spear GT. Immune complexes containing human immunodeficiency virus type 1 primary isolates bind to lymphoid tissue B lymphocytes and are infectious for T lymphocytes. J. Virol. 2000; 74: 552-555.

[98]   Dopper S, Wilflingseder D, Prodinger WM, Stiegler G, Speth C, Dierich MP, *et al.* Mechanism(s) promoting HIV-1 infection of primary unstimulated T lymphocytes in autologous B cell/T cell co-cultures. Eur J Immunol. 2003; 33: 2098-2107.

[99]   Reid DM, Perry VH, Andersson PB, Gordon S. Mitosis and apoptosis of microglia in vivo induced by an anti-CR3 antibody which crosses the blood-brain barrier. Neuroscience. 1993; 56:529-33.

[100]   Bruder C, Hagleitner M, Darlington G, Mohsenipour I, Würzner R, Höllmüller I, *et al.* HIV-1 induces complement factor C3 synthesis in astrocytes and neurons by modulation of promoter activity. Mol Immunol. 2004; 40:949-61.

[101]   Speth C, Schabetsberger T, Mohsenipour I, Stöckl G, Würzner R, Stoiber H, *et al.* Mechanism of human immunodeficiency virus-induced complement expression in astrocytes and neurons. J Virol. 2002; 76:3179-88.

[102]   Fearon DT. Identification of the membrane glycoprotein that is the C3b receptor of the human erythrocyte, polymorphonuclear leukocyte, B lymphocyte, and monocyte. J. Exp. Med. 1980; 152: 20-30.

[103]   Paccaud JP, Carpentier JL, Schifferli JA. Direct evidence for the clustered nature of complement receptors type 1 on the erythrocyte membrane. J. Immunol. 1988; 141: 3889-3894.

[104]   Monari C, Casadevall A, Pietrella D, Bistoni F, Vecchiarelli A. Neutrophils from patients with advanced human immunodeficiency virus infection have impaired complement receptor function and preserved Fcgamma receptor function. J Infect Dis. 1999; 180:1542-9.

[105]   Wahl SM, Allen JB, Gartner S, Orenstein JM, Popovic M, Chenoweth DE, *et al.* HIV-1 and its envelope glycoprotein down-regulate chemotactic ligand receptors and chemotactic function of peripheral blood monocytes. J Immunol. 1989; 142:3553-9.

[106]   Kacani L, Bánki Z, Zwirner J, Schennach H, Bajtay Z, Erdei A, *et al.* C5a and C5a(desArg) enhance the susceptibility of monocyte-derived macrophages to HIV infection. J Immunol. 2001; 166:3410-5.

[107]   Soederholm A, Bánki Z, Wilflingseder D, Gassner C, Zwirner J, López-Trascasa M, *et al.* HIV-1 induced generation of C5a attracts immature dendriticcells and promotes infection of autologous T cells. Eur J Immunol. 2007; 37:2156-63.

[108]   Wasserheit JN. HIV infection and other STDs: so close and yet so far. Sex Transm Dis. 1999; 26:549-50.

INDEX

Integrin; 84-88, 93, 102, 146, 150.

L
Lectin; 54, 55, 71, 145, 147.
LFA-1; 146, 148, 150.
Lymphoid; 3, 7, 11, 17, 21, 28-30, 32, 56, 71, 92, 93, 109, 113, 146.
LPS; 24, 25, 27, 65, 66, 69-71, 91, 117.
LTNP; 5, 11, 23, 56.
LTR; 5, 6, 19, 25, 26, 28, 72, 74, 123, 128, 129.

M
Macrophage; 1, 7, 9, 11, 18-22, 24-27, 29, 32, 52-55, 64, 65, 68, 69, 71, 74, 76, 82, 83, 85, 87-91, 111-113, 146-148, 150.
Mannose; 145, 147.
M-CSF; 24, 25, 27, 29, 32.
Memory; 3, 4, 8, 9, 20, 22, 24, 28-32, 53, 92, 93, 107-108, 119, 134, 146.

N
Naïve; 2, 3, 5, 7, 9-11, 20-24, 26, 30, 32, 71, 83, 92, 93, 107, 108, 120, 128, 131.
Nef; 17, 18, 32.
Neutralization; 9, 145, 148.
Neutrophil; 6, 7, 18, 22, 23, 51-55, 68, 69, 83-86, 93, 129, 130.
NK; 18-24, 27, 30-32, 69, 71, 83, 91, 106, 107, 131, 146.
NF-Kb; 19, 21, 25-28, 67, 70, 71, 74, 115-120.

P
PAMPs; 52, 67, 117.
PBMC; 2, 11, 18-32, 53, 55, 56, 73, 89, 91, 93, 104, 148.
PMA; 23, 25, 52, 89, 90.
Polymorphism; 112, 129, 130, 132-134.

R
Raft; 85, 87, 88, 114, 146.
RAGE; 64, 65, 67-72, 74.

S
SCID; 2, 27, 30.
Sexual; 28, 56, 71, 123, 130, 134, 150.
SIV; 4, 5, 10, 11, 19-22, 25-29, 31, 92, 102, 131.
STAT; 6.

T
TAT; 3, 4, 17, 18, 21, 23, 27.
Th; 7, 18, 21-26, 68, 71, 107, 118, 120-122, 127, 130-133.
TLR; 24, 26, 51, 53, 67-71, 116, 118-120.

U
uPA; 1, 6, 81-94.

ABBREVIATIONS

AIDS	:	Acquired ImmunoDeficiency Syndrome
AMPs	:	AntiMicrobial Peptides
APOBEC	:	Apolipoprotein B m-RNA-editing enzyme-catalytic polypeptide-like
CAF	:	CD8 antiviral factor
CCR5	:	C-C chemokine receptor type 5
CTL	:	Cytotoxic CD8+ T cell
DAMPs	:	Damage-Associated Molecule Patterns
DC	:	Dendritic Cell
Env	:	Envelope
ESN	:	HIV-exposed SeroNegative
FDC	:	Follicular Dendritic Cell
G-CSF	:	Granulocyte-colony stimulating factor
GM-CSF	:	Granulocyte-macrophage colony stimulating factor
HAART	:	Highly Active Anti Retroviral Therapy
HNP	:	Human Neutrophil Defensin
ICAM	:	Inter-Cellular Adhesion Molecule 1
IRIS	:	Immune Reconstitution Inflammatory Syndrome
IFN	:	Interferon
Ig	:	Immunoglobulin
IL	:	Interleukin
LFA-1	:	Lymphocyte function-associated antigen 1
LPS	:	Lypopolysaccharide
LTNP	:	Long Term Non Progressor
LTR	:	Long Terminal Repeat
M-CSF	:	Macrophage colony-stimulating factor
Nef	:	Negative Factor

NK   :   Natural Killer

NF-Kb   :   Nuclear Factor-Kb

PAMPs   :   Pathogen-associated molecular patterns

PBMC   :   Peripheral Blood Mononuclear Cell

PMA   :   Phorbol-Myristate-Acetate

RAGE   :   Receptor for Advanced Glycation End-products

SCID   :   Severe Combined Immunodeficiency Syndrome

SIV   :   Simian Immunodeficiency Virus

STAT   :   Signal Transducer and Activator of Transcription

Tat   :   Trans-Activator of Transcription

Th   :   T helper lymphocyte

TLR   :   Toll-Like Receptor

uPA   :   urokinase Plasminogen Activator